Therapy of Inflammatory Bowel Disease

INFLAMMATORY DISEASE AND THERAPY

Series Editor

Daniel E. Furst
University of Medicine and Dentistry of New Jersey
Robert Wood Johnson Medical School
New Brunswick, New Jersey
and Pharmaceuticals Division
CIBA-GEIGY Corporation
Summit, New Jersey

1. Methotrexate Therapy in Rheumatic Disease, *edited by William S. Wilke*
2. Therapy of Inflammatory Bowel Disease: New Medical and Surgical Approaches, *edited by Mark A. Peppercorn*

Additonal Volumes in Preparation

Platelet Activating Factor in Endotoxin and Immune Diseases, *edited by Dean A. Handley, Robert N. Saunders, William J. Houlihan, and John C. Tomesch*

Therapy of Inflammatory Bowel Disease

New Medical and Surgical Approaches

edited by

MARK A. PEPPERCORN

Beth Israel Hospital
Harvard Medical School
Boston, Massachusetts

MARCEL DEKKER, INC. New York and Basel

Library of Congress Cataloging-in-Publication Data

Therapy of inflammatory bowel disease : new medical and surgical approaches / edited by Mark A. Peppercorn.
p. cm. -- (Inflammatory disease and therapy ; 2)
ISBN 0-8247-8169-4 (alk. paper)
1. Enteritis, Regional--Treatment. 2. Enteritis, Regional--Surgery. 3. Ulcerative colitis--Treatment. 4. Ulcerative colitis--Surgery. I. Peppercorn, Mark A. II. Series.
[DNLM: 1. Inflammatory Bowel Diseases--diet therapy. 2. Inflammatory Bowel Diseases--drug therapy. 3. Intestines--surgery. WI 522 T398]
RC862.E52T48 1990
616.3'4406--dc20
DNLM/DLC
for Library of Congress 89-17123
CIP

This book is printed on acid-free paper.

MARCEL DEKKER, INC.
270 Madison Avenue, New York, New York 10016

Current printing (last digit):
10 9 8 7 6 5 4 3 2 1

PRINTED IN THE UNITED STATES OF AMERICA

To my wife, Margie, for her love and understanding;
to my sons, Jeffrey and Danny, for their inspiration;
and to my parents, Adelle and David Peppercorn, for their
lifelong encouragement

Series Introduction

As knowledge of inflammation has flourished over the last decade, understanding of the pathogenesis and therapy of inflammatory diseases has also improved. This has been particularly true in the rheumatic diseases, including infectious rheumatic diseases, those rheumatic diseases associated with gastrointestinal inflammation, immunologically mediated illnesses, various forms of vasculitis, and so forth.

Marcel Dekker, Inc., which specializes in high-quality monographs in a variety of focused medical disciplines, has supplied up-to-date, detailed, and practical information for the practicing physician and research scientist. The Inflammatory Disease and Therapy series will address a number of carefully chosen topics of interest to practicing physicians, rheumatologists, and research scientists.

Daniel E. Furst

Preface

Inflammatory bowel disease (IBD) affects nearly two million Americans, and almost 10,000 new cases each of ulcerative colitis and Crohn's disease are diagnosed annually in the United States alone. Although more common in "developed" areas of the world, IBD knows no geographical, ethnic, or racial boundaries. For some persons, these disorders are devastating, with continual symptoms resulting in much time lost from family, school, and work and often culminating in surgery which can have profound physical and psychic implications. Fortunately, the majority of patients with IBD can be treated successfully with one or more therapeutic agents during acute flares and be kept in remission for prolonged periods between exacerbations.

As a clinician caring for such patients, it has been gratifying to see the recent advances in the area of drug therapy of IBD. For many years that drug therapy was limited to sulfasalazine and either a topical or systemic corticoid. In the past few years metronidazole and the immunosuppressives 6-mercaptopurine and azathioprine have assumed accepted roles in the treatment of Crohn's disease. Now topical and oral aminosalicylates have been introduced and promise to be of major benefit. Preliminary studies have raised hopes that one day topical cromolyn, cyclosporin, chloroquine, methotrexate, and antituberculous agents may prove useful.

Paralleling the exciting developments in drug therapy have been advances in the nutritional aspects of IBD and in alternatives to colectomy and conventional ileostomy. Indeed, if the early successes of the ileal pouch–anal anastomosis procedure are sustained, then patients with ulcerative colitis will not have to face colectomy with the horror that so many now do.

With this proliferation of new drugs, new nutritional considerations, and ileostomy alternatives, those who care for patients with IBD need a resource that comprehensively but concisely reviews and updates the latest in IBD therapy. In *Therapy of Inflammatory Bowel Disease: New Medical and Surgical Approaches*, we have tried to provide the students of ulcerative colitis and Crohn's disease, house officers, fellows, investigators, and practitioners with just such a comprehensive resource. Part I details the pharmacology, clinical utility, modes of action, and toxicity of the various therapeutic agents, with specific recommendations for usage. Part I concludes with chapters on nutrition and ileostomy alternatives designed to complement the sections on the individual drugs.

As anyone who cares for patients with IBD knows, a variety of clinical situations are encountered over and over again and require specialized knowledge. Moreover, no two patients with IBD are alike, each presenting a different therapeutic challenge. Part II provides information dealing with certain general conditions, including extraintestinal and malignant complications, the pediatric patient, pregnancy and nursing, and psychosocial issues. The last chapter deals with specific patient presentations commonly faced by the clinician and enables the reader to learn how experienced clinicians apply the tools described in earlier chapters to the office and bedside practice of IBD.

I am grateful to my fellow contributors for their cooperation and thoroughness. I am indebted to Wendy-Sue Porter for her diligence in preparing the manuscripts and to Peggy Prahl and Donna Abbott for their additional secretarial assistance. Finally, I want to thank my colleague, Raj K. Goyal, for his unswerving and total support.

Mark A. Peppercorn

Contributors

Lawrence J. Brandt Division of Gastroenterology, Department of Medicine, Montefiore Medical Center/Albert Einstein College of Medicine, Bronx, New York

Francis A. Farraye* Division of Gastroenterology, Beth Israel Hospital, Harvard Medical School, Boston, Massachusetts

C. Richard Fleming Division of Gastroenterology, Department of Medicine, Mayo Clinic, Jacksonville, Florida, and Mayo Medical School, Rochester, Minnesota

Gerald Friedman Division of Gastroenterology, Department of Medicine, Mount Sinai School of Medicine of the City University of New York, New York, New York

Richard J. Grand Division of Pediatric Gastroenterology and Nutrition, Department of Pediatrics, Boston Floating Hospital, New England Medical Center, Tufts University School of Medicine, Boston, Massachusetts

---

**Present affiliation*: Harvard Community Health Plan, Brigham and Women's Hospital, Beth Israel Hospital, Harvard Medical School, Boston, Massachusetts.

Stephen B. Hanauer Section of Gastroenterology, Department of Medicine, University of Chicago Medical Center, Chicago, Illinois

Keith A. Kelly Department of Surgery, Mayo Clinic and Mayo Medical School, Rochester, Minnesota

Burton I. Korelitz Section of Gastroenterology, Department of Medicine, Lenox Hill Hospital, New York, New York

Karen A. Kurlander Charlesbridge Counseling and Resource Center for People with Chronic Gastro-intestinal Illnesses, Watertown, Massachusetts

Samuel Meyers Division of Gastroenterology, Department of Medicine, Mount Sinai School of Medicine of the City University of New York, New York, New York

Kathleen J. Motil Department of Pediatrics, USDA/ARS Children's Nutrition Research Center, Baylor College of Medicine, Houston, Texas

Mary F. O'Brien Charlesbridge Counseling and Resource Center for People with Chronic Gastro-intestinal Illnesses, Watertown, Massachusetts

John H. Pemberton Section of Colon and Rectal Surgery, Department of Surgery, Mayo Clinic and Mayo Medical School, Rochester, Minnesota

Mark A. Peppercorn Division of Gastroenterology, Department of Medicine, Beth Israel Hospital, Harvard Medical School, Boston, Massachusetts

Contents

Therapy of Inflammatory Bowel Disease

I

DRUG, NUTRITIONAL, AND SURGICAL THERAPIES

1

Oral and Parenteral Corticoids

Samuel Meyers

Mount Sinai School of Medicine of the City University of New York, New York, New York

Both oral and parenteral corticosteroids are used widely for the therapy of inflammatory bowel disease (IBD) and their efficacy is well known. Their use in treating ulcerative colitis has been supported by several placebo-controlled studies (1-6) and in Crohn's disease by two recent multicentered controlled trials (7,8), all comparing oral therapy to placebo in an outpatient setting. Corticotropin (ACTH) is also frequently used in IBD, despite the paucity of rigorous supportive data (9-13).

I. PHARMACOKINETICS

A. Prednisone and Prednisolone

There are several considerations to be weighed in the choice of corticosteroid agents and doses used to treat IBD. Dose ratios of some of the most frequently used agents are reported as hydrocortisone, 20: prednisolone, 5: prednisone, 5: methylprednisolone, 4: dexamethasone, 0.75. Prednisone and prednisolone are the most commonly used agents and are interconvertible (14). Prednisone is the inactive form and is activated by 11-beta-hydroxy-dehydrogenase to the active prednisolone. Equilibrium strongly favors this reaction which is rapid and is achieved largely by first-pass metabolism through the liver (15,16).

The rate of appearance of prednisolone from different brands of prednisone is somewhat variable (time to peak, 1.3-3 hr), which correlates with the in vitro rates of tablet dissolution (17,18). However, the extent of availability is relatively uniform and almost total, with a concentration-time profile very similar to that after prednisolone is taken by mouth (15,17,20-23). Food does not alter the extent of prednisolone availability after ingestion of prednisolone (21,22).

Even though plasma drug levels of these and natural corticosteroids can be measured, the results are difficult to interpret in clinical terms because the biological effects of the drugs on endogenous cortisol secretion, or on experimentally induced inflammation persist longer than would be predicted from the plasma level. This is not surprising since the site of action of corticosteroids is intracellular and mediated by way of altered protein synthesis (24). Thus, the plasma half-life of prednisolone after intravenous administration is 3–4 hr, but the biological half-life is 18-36 hr (25-27). Furthermore. although anti-inflammatory activity appears to be qualitatively related to the concentration of active steroid in the tissue (25), no clear relation has been observed between the plasma level achieved and the therapeutic response in inflammatory bowel disease (28-30). The situation is further complicated by the fact that both therapeutic activity and liability to side effects are related, not to total drug levels, but to drug levels unbound to protein.

The protein binding of prednisolone is complex. It is bound reversibly to albumin and to a specific alpha-1-glycoprotein, corticosteroid-binding globulin. The specific globulin has a high affinity but a low capacity, and because of its low concentration in plasma, becomes saturated at therapeutic concentrations (31). Albumin has a lower affinity but a higher capacity for binding and does not appear to become saturated (32). Thus, at low concentrations of prednisolone, protein binding is high (80-90%), but declines at higher concentrations (60-70%), as the corticosteroid-binding globulin becomes saturated. Hypoalbuminemia, from any cause, results in a further decrease in binding (24, 33). At low concentrations there is a circadian variation related to changes in endogenous cortisol (34). The volume of distribution of prednisolone is closely related to the protein binding. It increases with the dose and is consistent with a saturable protein binding. In spite of these potential changes there is not likely to be any clinical effect of alterations in the parameters (16,34-36).

In Crohn's disease, absorption of orally administered prednisolone has been found to be reduced in some patients (37). These observations differ from an earlier report (38) which demonstrated normal mean peak plasma level and timing of absorption after oral prednisolone. An important difference in the studies was the greater proportion of patients with predominantly colonic disease in the earlier report. There is evidence that absorption of corticosteroids may be altered in ulcerative colitis. In severe acute colitis, the absorption of prednisolone after a 40 mg oral dose resulted in a lower peak level and a slower rate of fall, compared with normal volunteers (39). This was probably due to delayed gastrointestinal absorption. However, the total absorption was normal, since the area under the plasma drug curve was similar in patients with colitis and normal subjects. When prednisolone was given intravenously, thus bypassing the gastrointestinal tract, the serum levels achieved were similar to those obtained in normals (40).

Concentrations of prednisone in breast milk are minimal and do not appear to exceed 10% of the plasma concentration. The milk-to-plasma ratio increases with larger doses of prednisolone, as a result of the dose-dependent plasma protein binding. The increased free fraction allows a greater amount of drug to diffuse into breast milk (41).

Elimination of prednisone and prednisolone is largely metabolic by hydroxylation and conjugation (42). Only 2.5% of dose of prednisone and 11–14% of a dose of prednisolone appear in the urine unmetabolized after oral or intravenous administration (39). A major feature of prednisolone clearance is the increase seen with increasing doses (39). Dose-dependent clearance is accompanied by a similar change in the volume of distribution. Therefore, it is likely that the changes in the clearance and the volume of distribution both result from concentration-dependent changes in protein binding. As would be expected, no change in the plasma half-life has been noted (40,43). By contrast, others have noted a slight dose-dependent increase in the half-life of prednisolone (30,44). This may be explained by an increase in the volume of distribution or a decrease in the clearance over and above the changes that result from decreased protein binding. A saturable elimination pathway seems most likely, but the effect is minor. Several other factors may influence the elimination rate. Women appear to have a slightly higher clearance rate of prednisolone than men (45). Enzyme-inducing agents, including barbiturates, phenytoin, and rifampicin significantly increase the metabolic clearance of corticosteroid agents. The clearance almost doubles and the half-life of prednisolone decreases consequently to almost half the normal value (46,47). Oral contraceptive agents may increase the plasma half-life as much as 2.5-fold by raising the corticosteroid-binding globulin levels which causes a marked decrease in both the clearance and the volume of distribution of total prednisolone (48,49).

Circadian variation in the clearance of unbound prednisolone at low doses may be important (50). Normally higher morning cortisol concentrations result in a competitive decrease in the metabolism of prednisolone, which decreases the rate of clearance of the unbound fraction. These circadian effects may have clinical importance, since the area under the free prednisolone versus time curve would be greater with morning than with evening doses. Therefore, a greater effect per dose would be expected in the morning.

In summary, the complex pharmacokinetics of prednisone and prednisolone are more interesting in theory than important in practice. The rate of their availability certainly can vary, but is probably of little consequence as the action of these agents is not immediately related to their plasma concentrations. The extent of the availability of prednisolone is more important, but is very consistent, even when taken by mouth. The effects of altered protein binding are relatively predictable and result from the saturation of corticosteroid-binding globulin at low concentrations of prednisolone, and the nonsaturable nature of the albumin binding. The net effect is a dose-dependent increase in the measured volume of distribution and clearance with little change in the half-life. However, because the kinetics of free concentrations vary little with dose, the complex protein-binding effects are of little practical importance. The circadian effects favor the choice of morning rather than evening doses. The altered elimination of prednisolone that results from the coadministration of other drug agents certainly is important and doses should be adjusted accordingly.

The rate and method of drug administration may be clinically important. After a bolus of 20 mg intravenously, the maximum serum level was nearly five times greater than after 40 mg oral dose and the levels achieved remained significantly greater for 4 hr. When 20 mg prednisolone was given as an 8-hr infusion, the peak serum level was one third the maximum bolus level, but was also significantly greater than the maximum oral level achieved with an equivalent dose. It is unknown whether repeated high peaks after bolus infusions are of greater clinical benefit than more constant but lower concentrations of continuous infusion. One clinical trial, however, has shown that prednisolone given in one oral dose of 40 mg was therapeutically equivalent to four doses of 10 mg taken at intervals throughout the day (51). Although there is little correlation between plasma levels and clinical outcome, there must be a critical dose level below which corticosteroids are less effective. Oral prednisolone 20 mg daily has been shown to be less effective than 40 mg daily, though no further benefit was achieved using a 60-mg dose (52). The clinical implications of delayed oral absorption and the optimal oral and intravenous dose levels and timing remain to be determined in larger trials of patients with various degrees of disease severity.

B. Cortisone and Hydrocortisone

Cortisone is inactive and is converted to the active hydrocortisone by 11-beta-hydroxy-dehydrogenase (15). Compared with intravenous hydrocortisone, the availability of oral hydrocortisone is 54% and of cortisone 44% (measured as hydrocortisone) (53). A dose-dependent decrease in the bioavailability of oral hydrocortisone has been observed (71% from a 5 mg dose and 56% from a 20 mg dose) (54). Possible explanations include a saturable absorption or saturable binding to globulin in the protal system causing an increase in presystemc elimination (55). Based upon this information the availability after an oral dose should be greater if the same total daily dose were given in a divided regimen, rather than a single daily dose.

Hydrocortisone in physiological concentrations is 70% bound to plasma binding globulin, 20% to albumin, and 10% is free. At higher concentrations, similar to prednisolone, the plasma binding globulin becomes saturated and total binding of hydrocortisone is reduced to approximately 56% (56). Pregnancy and estrogen therapy increase the concentration of binding globulin and thus raise the total concentration of hydrocortisone, but free concentrations change little (31). The volume of distribution increases with dosage (55). As with prednisolone, this is predictable from the dose-dependent decrease in protein binding.

Elimination of hydrocortisone is predominantly via metabolism to tetrahydrocortisone. Clearance of hydrocortisone increases with dosage (57). As with the volume of distribution, this effect is explained largely by the saturation of plasma binding globulin. However, this does not explain a dose-dependent increase in the half-life from 1.2 to 1.8 hr since the saturation of protein binding would be expected to increase the volume of distribution and the clearance. This suggests there may be some saturation in the metabolism of hydrocortisone. The complex changes in protein binding and the resultant effects on the volume of distribution and clearance would have little clinical significance since unbound concentrations would not alter. However, the possibility of a saturable clearance might be important in long-term therapy and emphasizes the need to use as low a dose as possible in all circumstances.

Liver disease does not affect the conversion to active hydrocortisone, but it does prolong this half-life (58). Thyrotoxicosis increases the conversion of cortisone to hydrocortisone and shortens the half-life to approximately 1 hr (58,59). Phenytoin increases the clearance by about 20% with a concomitant decrease in the half-life (60).

C. Other Corticoid Agents

Several other agents have been used occasionally in the oral and parenteral therapy of IBD. The pharmacokinetics of these drugs have not been studied extensively. However, some information is available. Methylprednisolone availablity after an oral dose has been variably reported from 40 to 80% (61,62). Other pharmacokinetic parameters are similar to those of prednisolone, although elmination does not appear to be dose dependent (61). Betamethasone is also similar to prednisolone but has a half-life of 5 hr (63). The common factor of marked enzyme inducibility by drugs such as phenytoin is probably the most significant feature of clinical importance. Corticotropin (ACTH) is also used in therapy. ACTH is readily absorbed from parenteral sites, and is usually administered by intramuscular or intravenous routes. The hormone rapidly disappears from the circulation after intravenous use with a plasma half-life of 15 minutes.

II. CLINICAL INVESTIGATIONS

A. Ulcerative Colitis

Truelove and Witts in 1955 reported the earliest controlled trial of corticosteroids in the therapy of ulcerative colitis (1). They treated 109 subjects with oral cortisone (100 mg daily) and 101 with placebo for 6 weeks. Cortisone was superior, especially for those with their first attack of disease. Lennard-Jones et al. in 1960 then confirmed the superiority of oral prednisone over placebo (2). Thus, steroid therapy became an acceptably useful therapy in active ulcerative colitis, despite the small number of randomized double-blind clinical trials and their clear limitations.

Even less is known about the patient with severe ulcerative colitis. Lennard-Jones et al. (2) studied only mild or moderate patients. Truelove and Witts (1) did include some severely ill patients and reported oral cortisone to have a less favorable effect on this group, especially among those in relapse of established disease. Investigators from Oxford, England, have reported their uncontrolled experience with a 5-day intensive intravenous program for the therapy of severely ill patients with ulcerative colitis (64,65). The intensive regimen included bowel rest, intravenous nutrition, antibiotics, rectal corticosteroids, and intravenous prednisolone 60 mg/day. They gave 100 courses of therapy to 87 patients and noted 60% of the attacks responded. In an additional 15%, there was improvement, but the patients were not entirely symptom free. Remission was sustained with oral therapy in 33 patients (38%) over a mean follow-up period of 25 months. The absence of decisive improvement by the end of 5 days of this intensive therapy was considered an absolute indication for emergency colectomy. In Sweden, a similar intensive intravenous program for the therapy of 79 patients with severe colitis was used (66). Their regimen included bowel rest, parenteral nutrition, intravenous betamethasone (6 mg daily), corticosteroid enemas, and antibiotics in the majority of patients. The therapy was planned for a 5-day period but continued up to 21 days in patients who showed clinical or sigmoidoscopic improvement. Patients were referred to surgery if they showed no improvement within 5 days, or earlier if their condition deteriorated. Remission was achieved among 46.8% of those with total colitis and 88.2% with less extensive involvement. Remission was maintained by oral therapy in approximately 50% of the total group for one year, 35% for two years, and 20% for three years.

Despite significant methodological problems these studies add to our experience concerning the efficacy of corticosteroids for severe colitis (67). Since further placebo trials are unlikely, it is reassuring to see such high remission rates. These are clearly superior to the 2.9% response rate for the placebo group noted in an earlier study (1) and similar to the rates reported in more recent studies of corticoid therapy of severe acute colitis (29,30).

Finally, we must consider the role of corticosteroids in fulminant cases with toxic megacolon. Their use in these patients has been a matter of great debate but little study. Collective experiences must be drawn upon. Because most of these patients seen in the hospital developed their toxic dilatation while receiving steroid therapy, corticosteroid therapy must be maintained. Patients not promptly responding or those with colonic perforation or even suspected perforation require prompt surgical attention. In a small number of patients who develop toxic dilatation of the colon without prior corticosteroid therapy, it may be a rational move to add steroids to the present-day vigorous supportive medical program, provided failure to respond promptly does not lead to a progressive delay in performing colectomy and ileostomy when required (68,69).

Corticosteroids are worthy of a trial in all patients suffering from ulcerative colitis, regardless of the severity of the illness. The ideal patient for corticosteroid therapy is one undergoing a first attack, while the disease is still mild. In the more severely ill patients, corticosteroid therapy is usually administered parenterally. Corticotropin (ACTH) and hydrocortisone are both commonly used as parenteral therapy for severe ulcerative colitis. It has been suggested that ACTH is the superior of the two, but the issue remains controversial. Kirsner et al. reported the largest clinical experience: 240 patients treated over seven years (10). They concluded that intravenous or intramuscular aqueous ACTH was the most effective corticoid therapy. Other small clinical series, however, did not confirm the superiority of ACTH (9). In a randomized controlled study of 169 subjects, Truelove and Witts compared intramuscular ACTH gel (80 units daily) to oral cortisone (200 mg daily) (11). Both agents seemed to have similar efficacy overall and for a first attack, but ACTH appeared somewhat more effective for those with a relapse of established colitis. The apparent benefit of ACTH was offset by a higher relapse rate during the subsequent years. Powell-Tuck et al. compared intravenous hydrocortisone (400 mg daily) to intramuscular ACTH gel (80 units daily) among 16 patients (29). Both agents had similar overall efficacy but hydrocortisone was said to be the superior agent for those previously receiving corticosteroids. The first direct comparison of intravenous ACTH with intravenous hydrocortisone was performed by Kaplan et al. (28). They studied 22 patients in a prospective, double-blind manner, administering intravenous hydrocortisone (300 mg daily) or ACTH (40 units daily). The authors concluded that both agents were equally effective. Hydrocortisone, however, tended to be superior for patients who had been receiving corticosteroids prior to the study.

At the Mount Sinai Hospital in New York, patients with severe ulcerative colitis were studied in a prospective randomized clinical trial (30). They received either 120 U/day of intravenous ACTH or 300 mg/day of intravenous hydrocortisone for 10-days. Patients were separately stratified depending upon whether they had received previous oral corticosteroids (Group A, 35 patients) or had received no such recent prior treatment (Group B, 31 patients). Overall 24 of the

34 patients (41%) achieved remission with hydrocortisone therapy, compared to 14 of 32 (44%) receiving ACTH. In Group B however, the proportion of patients entering remission was greater with ACTH than with hydrocortisone (63% vs. 27%, $p > 0.05$). The opposite trend was observed in Group A, in which hydrocortisone appeared more effective (53% vs. 25%, $p = 0.06$). Because the 120 U/day dose of ACTH was higher than those usually recommended, these results cannot be extrapolated to lower doses of ACTH (9,10,28,29). But since 20 U/day is generally considered to elicit maximal adrenal responsiveness, it is unlikely that the use of any higher doses would alter the results (70,71). Not observed was the tendency reported by Truelove and Witts for ACTH-induced remissions to be shorter lived than hydrocortisone-induced remissions (11). Instead, 71% of the patients whose acute therapy was successful were still in remission one year after the study period, 86% of the ACTH-induced remission and 57% of the hydrocortisone-induced remissions were sustained.

This study is the second direct controlled comparison of intravenous ACTH with intravenous hydrocortisone in the treatment of ulcerative colitis. As in the Kaplan et al. study (28), patients were prospectively stratified and separately randomized to those receiving or not receiving prior steroids. In addition, four new features were introduced to the experimental design. First the study was restricted to patients with ulcerative colitis, to achieve more uniformity of the patient population. Second, for the same purpose, in advance specific clinical criteria of disease severity were established, that would determine eligibility for entry into the study. Third, to ensure that any benefits of therapy would not be obscured by intermittent doses, medications were given continuously over 24 hours during each day of the study. Finally, in an effort to achieve more statistically significant results, larger series of patients were studied.

The results indicate that the presence or absence of prior steroid therapy appears to be a determining factor in the preferential response to either ACTH or hydrocortisone. This is the same conclusion reached by the New Haven (28) and the London (29) studies. Unknown is the explanation for the opposite trends of the therapeutic superiority of ACTH or hydrocortisone in the two patient groups. There were no significant differences between the ACTH- and hydrocortisone-treated patients, either in Group A or Group B, that could account for the differences in the therapeutic response. Also, there was no evidence that the relatively poorer effectiveness of ACTH compared with hydrocortisone in Group A might be attributable to impaired adrenal responsiveness among those patients who received prior steroids. Mean serum cortisol levels were similar with either ACTH or hydrocortisone therapy, whether or not the patients received prior corticosteroid treatment. The dehydroepiandosterone-sulfate levels do not suggest that other adrenal factors besides cortisol are deficient in previously treated patients. Mean serum levels were substantially higher among ACTH-treated patients regardless of prior steroid exposure. Perhaps there were certain clinical differences between previously treated and previously untreated patient groups that determined the outcome. However, the trends for the superiority of ACTH or hydrocortisone in Groups A and B were maintained even when subgroups were separately analyzed according to a variety of clinical features beside recent corticosteroid therapy. Perhaps some other more subtle, unrecognized clinical characteristics may be contributing to the opposite trends in therapeutic response between the two groups. In any event, whatever the underlying pathophysiologic mechanism may be, on the basis of the data, it may be suggested that patients hospitalized with severe attacks of ulcerative colitis may respond better to intravenous hydrocortisone if they have been receiving prior corticosteroid therapy, and to intravenous ACTH if they have not received such prior therapy.

In this study group the median time in which clinical remission was achieved was 7.5 days (72). Although patients with more severe colitis achieved remission less often, those who did tended to do so earlier. In other similar studies of severe colitis, the time to clinical improvement was 4.4-5.3 days or to remission 8-10 days (28,110).

Prolonging therapy beyond 10 days by switching to the alternate corticoid drug did not improve the remission rate (72). Prolonged medical therapy of severe colitis is associated with an impressive rate of mortality and morbidity. Therefore, colectomy in those patients who do not respond promptly to optimal medical therapy should be considered (69). However, the failure of a patient to show decisive improvement after only 5 days of intravenous therapy should not be taken as a firm indication for colectomy (64,65). Such an early decision may inflict needless urgent operation on some patients. Yet, prolongation of therapy beyond 10 days did not induce a therapeutic response in any patient. Similar results were reported in two other patients who initially failed therapy with hydrocortisone and subsequently ACTH (28). Since minimal adverse effects and no mortality (30) were experienced, a 10-day period seems to safely allow an optimal opportunity for improvement with medical therapy for most patients with severe colitis.

Maintenance therapy for preventing relapses after successful treatment of an acute attack using 50-mg doses of cortisone has been ineffective (11). Because larger doses were useful to treat acute attacks is was postulated that larger doses would be useful for maintenance. Prednisone 15 mg daily was given in a placebo-controlled trial for 6 months to 32 patients whose acute colitis was successfully treated with corticosteroid therapy. The proceaure did not prevent relapses and resulted in side effects in 7 of the 32 patients. Even higher doses may be necessary to achieve therapeutic results, but this would result in a greater rate of adverse effects (73). Prednisolone 40 mg administered on alternatue days was tested in a placebo-controlled double-blind, crossover fashion for a 3-month period. The aim was to use the higher dose thought to be required in a way that would result in fewer side effects (74). Of 24 patients completing both trials, prednisone was significantly superior to placebo. Side effects attributable to the prednisolone were seen, although with the exception of the two patients who developed hyperglycemia, they were mild. Little is known about the effect of long-term alternate-day therapy on other serious side effects. There may be a role for alternate-day corticosteroids for a small group of patients whose disease causes considerable disability because of frequent relapses despite sulfasalazine or other therapy, and where surgery cannot be performed.

An acute episode of ulcerative colitis carries with it the risk of significant morbidity, and even death. It would be helpful to be able to predict the outcome of therapy in a given patient, and particularly to know what factors are most important to that prediction. One potent factor in predicting clinical remission was recent exposure to corticosteroids. Patients respond more often if they have been treated with intravenous hydrocortisone and had recent, continuously administered oral corticosteroids, or if they received intravenous ACTH and had no such prior oral therapy. Other variables, however, may have some predictive value. Certain clinical and laboratory factors indicative of relatively lesser degrees of colitis favored remission. These factors included limited disease anatomic location, fewer bowel movements, short duration of the present attack, a higher hemoglobin level, and a lower sedimentation rate. Although patients with disease characteristics compatible with more severe colitis activity achieved remission less often, those who did tended to do so earlier. An early response to initial therapy was the most important factor predicting the clinical outcome one year later. Prolonging therapy beyond 10 days did not improve the 1 year remission rate. In fact, a higher proportion of patients in this group required colectomy than did those who received a single 10-day course of therapy.

B. Crohn's Disease

Corticosteroids are widely used for the treatment of active, symptomatic Crohn's disease. Early uncontrolled clinical studies showed an initial symptomatic response was obtained in 75–90% of patients treated with 30 mg/day of prednisone or its equivalent (12,13,75). Fever, pain, and diarrhea subsided, appetite and well being improved, and, in the majority, hematocrit, sedimentation rate, or serum seromucoid levels returned toward normal. These favorable clinical responses were not necessarily associated with radiologic improvement. It appeared that steroid therapy produced satisfactory short-term benefit, but it was suspected that such therapy would not alter the long-term course of the disease.

A U.S. cooperative study (NCCDS) was the first controlled, prospective, double-blind study of corticosteroid therapy for Crohn's disease (7). Eighty-five patients received prednisone in doses determined by their disease activity (¼ to

¾ mg/kg). At the completion of the 17-week study, prednisone was found to be significantly more effective than placebo for Crohn's disease involving the small bowel. The cumulative percentage of patients achieving remission was 60% with prednisone therapy but less than 30% with placebo. Such superiority was not demonstrated when the disease was confined to the colon. However, the number of such patients was small. The extraintestinal and perianal complications of Crohn's disease were not responsive to prednisone therapy. Sulfasalazine therapy at entry to the study seemed to blunt the response to prednisone.

The European Cooperative Crohn's Disease Study confirmed the American results (8). In this study, 113 patients received 6-methylprednisolone for the therapy of active disease. The dosage was adjusted according to the disease activity, as measured by the Crohn's Disease Activity Index (CDAI) originally devised for the NCCDS. Therapy was initiated with 48 mg/day and reduced over 6 weeks to 12 mg daily. The initial dosage was higher than that used by the NCCDS (7), but the dosage reduction schedule was faster and automatic. This cycle of therapy continued for 6 weeks, but could be repeated two times if the patient's CDAI was > 150 (active disease) and none of the criteria of treatment failure were present. 6-Methylprednisolone was significantly more effective than placebo in previously treated or untreated patients, as well as among those with localization of disease in the small bowel, colon, or in both. Patients who achieved a CDAI of < 150 (inactive disease) after therapy could be continued on 6-methylprednisolone (8 mg daily) for up to 2 years. Such continued therapy was valuable in maintaining the remission of patients. The NCCDS also found some long-term benefit from continued prednisone therapy for periods up to 2 years (7). According to the ECCDS life-table analysis method, almost 80% of patients with active disease were in remission after 100 days and about 35% at 700 days compared with 15% and 8%, respectively, for the placebo group (8).

In clinical practice, when chronic corticosteroid therapy must be maintained, the dosage often cannot be reduced to less than 15 mg of prednisone daily. Indeed, in a substantial number of patients doses must be kept higher. Alternate-day therapy has been attempted in these circumstances and may be successful. The dose on alternate days should be between 50% and 100% hgiher than prior daily doses (76,77).

Beclomethasone 17, 21-dipropionate (BDP) is a topical corticosteroid, which in low doses has been shown to be free of any of the deleterious side effects associated with systematically absorbed corticosteroids. This is related to surface-active, anti-inflammatory properties of BDP which have been reported to be 5000 and 500 times more potent than hydrocortisone and dexamethasone, respectively (78,79). It would be appealing to treat patients with a locally acting drug that could be effective in such low doses that insufficient drug would be absorbed to produce systemic toxicity. BDP retention enemas have been used successfully to treat patients with distal ulcerative colitis or rectal Crohn's disease without producing clinical evidence of Cushing's syndrome or measurable suppression of hypothalamic-pituitary-adrenal axis (80–83). An oral form of BDP has been developed that allows controlled release of the active drug to the terminal ileum and right colon (84). Clinical trials of oral BDP in Crohn's disease and in conjunction with BDP enemas for the topical treatment of ulcerative colitis are awaited.

The effect of the combination of sulfasalazine and prednisone has been evaluated by the NCCDS (7). This combination was compared to that of prednisone and placebo among patients with active disease for 8 weeks. The combination was less effective than prednisone alone. Patients who were in remission at the end of the 8 weeks were rerandomized to receive either the two drugs together or prednisone plus placebo, while repeated attempts to withdraw the prednisone were made over the next 6 months. Sulfasalazine showed no prednisone-sparing effect. The addition of sulfasalazine to 6-methylprednisolone in the ECCDS also offered no advantage in the therapy of active or quiescent disease (8). The combination of sulfasalazine (3 g/day for 16 weeks and then 1.5 g/day for 17 weeks) and presdnisone (15 mg/day for 2 weeks, then 10 mg daily for 14 weeks, and for the last 17 weeks 5 mg daily) also conferred no advantage over placebo in the prevention of postoperative recurrence of Crohn's disease (85).

Intensive intravenous regimens using hdyrocortisone, prednisolone, betamethasone, or ACTH have been reported in the treatment of severely active ulcerative colitis (28–30,86,87). A similar approach has been retrospectively reviewed among a group of 49 patients with Crohn's disease (88). The therapy consisted of 5-day period of nothing by mouth, intravenous prednisolone (64 mg daily), intravenous fluids or parenteral nutrition, and an antibiotic (tetracycline or metronidazole). Hydrocortisone was infused rectally into those with colonic involvement. Remission was achieved in 38 (77%) patients with no significant difference between those with established disease and those seen for the first time. Patients with small bowel or colonic disease had similar good responses, but those with ileocolonic disease had the poorest outcome in both the long and short term. Ileocolonic disease has been previously noted to be the most refractory to therapy (89). Despite the good immediate results, there was no apparent change in the natural history of Crohn's disease after this intravenous therapy and remissions were not prolonged.

The role of corticosteroid therapy in both quiescent disease and after surgical disease resection has been examined in several trials. The long-term effect of prednisone 7.5 mg/day for up to three years after bowel resection with or without residual disease (90, or a decreasing dose from 15 mg to 5 mg of prednisone with a three-year subsequent follow-up (85), has been examined. In each study, prednisone-treated subjects fared no better than those receiving placebo. Neither the NCCDS (7) nor the ECCDS (9) showed benefit of corticosteroid therapy for those patients with inactive disease. Prophylactic steroid therapy is not beneficial for Crohn's disease.

C. Use in Pregnancy and Nursing

Corticosteroids can cross the placenta; fetal cortisol levels are low since cortisol is rapidly converted to the more inactive cortisone (91). Moreover, prednisone, prednisolone, and betamethasone levels in the fetal circulation are low (92), likely explaining the rarity of fetal hypothalmic-pituitary-adrenal suppression when corticosteroids are given to the mother during gestation (92-95). There have been occasional reports of neonatal death associated with high maternal corticosteroid doses in which adrenal atrophy has been noted at postmortem: such dosages should therefore be kept as low as possible (96).

Corticosteroids are well-known to cause fetal abnormalities in animals (94). Much of the data available on the outcome of human pregnancies where the mother received corticosteroids concern conditions other than inflammatory bowel disease. Some reports in humans suggest an increase in stillbirths or a reduction in birth weight (98,99). However, the majority of information is reassuring, especially in those studies of IBD where the results have been specifically analyzed in relation to the drug treatment the mother had received in these studies. The use of steroids does not appear to adversely affect the course and outcome of pregnanacy (100-106). The fetus, moreover, does not appear to be harmed by suppression of fetal ACTH (107). With regard to nursing, only small doses of adminstered steroid reach breast milk, and no restriction to breast feeding is considered necessary in mothers with IBD.

D. Recommendations for Therapy

Oral or parenteral administration of corticoids is indicated for moderate or severely active ulcerative colitis, as well as small or large bowel Crohn's disease. However, such therapy should not be initiated in the presence of major suppurative complications such as intra-abdominal or perineal abscess, although the physiologic stress imposed in some patients recently on corticosteroids may mandate therapy. In this stiuation, initial therapy with antibiotics or even surgery is safer and more useful. Corticoid agents may be introduced later, once the infection is controlled.

Initial therapy should be 45-60 mg/day of prednisone or its equivalent, given in divided doses, continued for approximately 10-14 days, and then tapered 5 mg every 7-10 days. The reduction should be made from the last dose of the day. Thus, as lower doses are achieved more will be administered in the morning, which helps minimize the side effects. If there is a relapse of disease activity, the dosage will need to be raised again. Once disease control is achieved the tapering process in resumed.

Corticosteroids are not used to maintain a remission for patients with ulcerative colitis. There may, however, be a role for prednisone, 40 mg every other day, for the patient who has frequent flareups with no other maintenance therapy alternatives and where surgery is not possible. For the patient with Crohn's disease whose symptoms improve but who continues to have low-grade clinical activity, I have found 5-10 mg of prednisone daily to keep the patient relatively asymptomatic. If possible, surgical removal of all diseased bowel should be considered rather than prolonged corticosteroid therapy, which even at low doses, is not desirable for more than one year. Immunosuppressive agents may have a role as "corticosteroid-sparing" agents. Their routine use in either Crohn's disease or ulcerative colitis, remains somewhat controversial and is discussed in detail in Chapter 6. For the patient with truly quiescent disease in remission, withdrawal of corticosteroids is usually successful, at least in the short term. There is no role for chronic maintenance corticosteroid therapy. Similarly, corticosteroids are not used for preventing postoperative recurrence of Crohn's disease.

Parenteral therapy is utilized in very ill patients who are not responding or not tolerating oral therapy. The choice of agents inlcudes prednisolone, betamethasone, hydrocortisone, or ACTH. No studies adequately establish the superiority of one of these agents, the proper dosage, or the best method of administration. Hydrocortisone or ACTH are, however, most often chosen. Studies performed in severe ulcerative colitis offer some guidance in choosing and administering the appropriate agent for the patient being considered. For example, I prefer hydrocortisone (300 mg daily) for patients who have received corticosteroids continuously for more than 30 days prior to hospitalization and ACTH (120 units daily) for patients not receiving such prior corticosteroid therapy. These agents are given as a continuous intravenous infusion mixed with 5% dextrose and water for 10 days. At that time the maximal benefit is achieved and oral prednisone is substituted, as previously described.

In both ulcerative colitis and Crohn's disease, sulfasalazine and oral prednisone can be combined in the hope of achieving synergy. If the patient is sick enough to be hospitalized, however, sulfasalazine is usually discontinued since it contributes little therapeutic benefit in this situation, and may add to a patient's discomfort because of side effects. I use antibiotics only for proven or strongly suspected infection or for suppurative manifestations of Crohn's disease. Metronidazole, however, may have a specific role for Crohn's disease, especially when it involves the large bowel or the perineal area (see Chapter 5). Metronidazole can be combined with corticosteroids instead of sulfasalazine, when there is extensive perineal involvement, when the sulfasalazine appears ineffective, or if the patient is intolerant or allergic to the drug.

III. MECHANISM OF ACTION

The mechanism by which corticoids exert their clinical usefulness is unknown. There are many abnormalities that have been postulated to occur in IBD. However, it is not known which of these are important in the initiation and/or maintenance of IBD. Therefore, an unequivocal statement as to where corticoid agents may operate is not possible. They most likely effect inflammation by inhibiting one or more mediators including cellular activities, prostaglandins, and the leukotriene system. An effect on bowel water and electrolyte transfer may also be important.

A. Cellular Activities

1. Subcellular Mechanisms

All steroid hormones enter the cell cytosol passively and bind to specific intracytoplasmic receptors. Then the steroid receptor complex translocates to the nucleus where it induces changes in the expression of specific genes and subsequent transcription and translation of the messenger RNA (mRNA) into proteins, which then exert their effect on target tissues. Steroid hormones may also indirectly increase protein synthesis by increasing the stability of mRNA (109). Intracytoplasmic corticosteroid receptors have been identified in human lymphocytes, monocytes, neutrophils, and eosinophils. Some effects of corticosteroids occur within minutes after exposure to sensitive cells. This suggests that protein synthesis is not always required for corticosteroid action. This direct action may be related to an effect on calcium influx or to interference with the phosphorylation of proteins (110).

2. Effect on Leukocyte Traffic

Corticosteroid-induced lymphopenia is mainly a consequence of the selective reversible depletion and redistribution of lymphocytes from the intravascular pool into lymphoid tissues (111). The bone marrow appears to be the major site of the corticosteroid-induced redistribution of lymphocytes in humans (112, 113). The exact mechanism for the redistrubiton is unknown. The effects of corticosteroids on circulating lymphocytes are not uniform. T lymphocytes are more depressed than non-T lymphocytes and OKT4 (helper-inducer) lymphocytes decrease to a greater extent than OKT8 (suppressor-cytotoxic) lymphocytes (114). Monocytes are extremely sensitive to corticosteroids and are more depleted than any other cell type. The etiology of this monocytopenia may also be related to cell redistribution.

Corticosteroids induce decreases in eosinophils and basophils. In addition, corticosteroids reversibly inhibit the chemotactic response of eosinophils and decrease eosinophil adherence (115). Most eosinophils reside in the extravascular sites and corticosteroids may disrupt the normal mobilization of eosinophils from the extravascular to intravascular sites (70).

The neutrophilia observed after corticosteroid therapy is multifactorial. There is an accelerated release of neutrophils from the bone marrow and decreased migration out of the circulation. Corticosteroids also increase vascular endothelial integrity, cause direct vasoconstriction, decrease capillary permeability, and decrease the ability of neutrophils to adhere to the endothelium, thus inhibiting the egress of neutrophils to extravascular sites (112).

3. Leukocyte Function

Corticosteroids alter the leukocytes and their recruitment in the inflammatory process. Some of these effects are mediated by the inhibition of the release of lymphokines, interleukin-1 (IL-1), as well as interleukin-2 (IL-2), which profoundly impairs lymphocyte and immune responses (112,113).

Both T and B lymphocytes are affected by corticosteroids (116). In addition to their inhibition of interleukin-2 production, they inhibit the proliferative responses of T cells to antigens and mitogens. This effect is thought to be important in the corticosteroid immunomodulating effect on the cell-mediated immune response. B cells are relatively resistant to the effects of corticosteroids. Only modest decreases in serum immunoglobulin levels occur, and antibody responses to new antigens are not affected (112). Some effects of corticosteroids on B cells may be mediated by their effect on other accessory cells.

Corticosteroids also alter macrophage and monocyte functions. Monocyte chemotaxis is inhibted and bactericidal action is suppressed (117). There are decreases in Fc-mediated immune clearance and expression of monocyte Fc receptors, and perhaps a decrease in the expression of DR antigens on monocytes which inhibits their ability to present antigen (118,119). There is a decrease in the release of interleukin, as noted previously, as well as an inhibition of the release by macrophages of nonlyzosomal enzymes such as elastase, collagenase, and plasminogen activator (120).

The effects on mast cells are variable with either no effect or a decrease in number and/or histamine release (121). They may also decrease antigen-induced histamine release from basophils. Further study in these areas is required.

Finally, natural killer cell activity is gnerally decreased by corticosteroids (122). Antibody-dependent cellular cytotoxicity has been reported to be reactively resistant to corticosteroids, but suppression may occur (123).

B. Prostaglandins and Leukotrienes

Corticosteroids inhibit prostaglandin and leukotrienes, both of which are potent mediators of inflammation and have been postulated to be important in IBD (14,24–127). Increased levels of prostaglandins and leukotrienes are produced in the inflamed mucosa with inflammatory bowel disease (126,127). Mononuclear cells have been shown to produce both mediators and they have been implicated in the increased local production (127). Inhibition occurs through the increased synthesis of lipocortin, a natural inhibitor of phospholipase A_2, the enzyme well known to cleave membrane phospholipids to arachidonic acid (128).

The role of prostaglandins in IBD is controversial (127). In active disease there is an increased production of prostaglandins, which is proportional to the disease activity (129,130). However, clinical trials have shown no benefit of the prostaglandin inhibitors, indomethacin (131) or flurbiprofen (132), which casts doubt on their etiologic role. Indeed it is possible that these agents themselves can potentiate IBD (133).

The role of the leukotrienes and their inhbitiion is also controversial but may be even more important than that of prostaglandins. Leukotriene B4 has been shown in increased amounts in the colonic mucosa of patients with ulcerative colitis; it correlated with disease activity and decreased toward control values in patients responding to therapy (127,129,130).

C. Bowel Water and Electrolyte Transfer

Studies have shown that IBD results in marked impairment of colonic sodium and water absorption (134-136). Inability of the colonic mucosa to absorb normal amounts of fluid and electrolytes may therefore contribute to the diarrhea. In vitro studies indicate that pharmacological doses of glucocorticoids increase sodium and water absorption in the colon, primarily by stimulating electrogenic sodium transport (137-142). In patients with either active or inactive ulcerative colitis the response of the distal colonic fluid and electrolyte transport to glucocorticoids was similar to normal (142). It was suggested that the glucocorticoid-induced decrease in diarrhea in ulcerative colitis reflects stimulation of sodium and water absorption in addition to suppression of the underlying inflammatory process.

IV. ADVERSE REACTIONS

A. General

As with any therapeutic agent, in prescribing corticoids, the physician must weight the potential benefits and risks. In general, the side effects are related to the dose and duration of therapy (143). Since prednisone, prednisolone, and methylprednisolone are the most commonly used corticoid agents, most of the clinical data available on side effects concern these drugs. These agents have the advantage of inducing less mineralocorticoid activity than cortisone and their biological half-lives are 12-36 hr, which would allow once daily doses, if clinically indicated. In contrast, betamethasone is almost totally devoid of mineralocorticoid activity but has a much longer biological half-life, resulting in profound hypothalmic-pituitary-adrenal suppression. The toxicity of ACTH, aside from the rare hypersensitivity reactions, is entirely attributable to the increased rate of secretion of endogenous adrenocorticosteroids. Because it stimulates synthesis and secretion of mineralocorticoids and androgens, ACTH may cause more sodium retention, a greater degree of hypokalemic alkalosis, and more severe acne than do the synthetic congeners of cortisol.

Doses of up to 100 mg of prednisolone daily can be taken for up to three weeks with little risk of adverse effects. However, patients may notice weight gain, fluid retention, hypertension, insomnia, or mood changes (euphoria, depression, or rarely psychosis), especially in patients with pre-existing psychiatric problems (144). However, the absence of a history of psychiatric illness is no guarantee against the development of psychosis during hormonal therapy. Corticosteroid-induced psychiatric disorders occur more frequently in patients receiving daily doses exceeding 40 mg of prednisone or its equivalent, and these reactions appear more often (2:1 ratio) within the first five days of treatment (145, 146). Other effects may include hyperglycemia, hypokalemia, alkalosis, gastric erosions, and bleeding. These effects are reversed when the drugs are discontinued. A rare complication is the development of anaphylactoid reactions (147). Short courses of therapy may cause suppression of the hypothalamic-pituitary-adrenal axis within several days, however, the effect usually disappears rapidly once the therapy is discontinued (148,149).

In the long term, different adverse effects may be seen even when low doses are used. It is likely that daily doses in excess of 10 mg of prednisone will eventually lead to some side effects (150). Even smaller doses are likely to lead to complications in the elderly, who are generally more prone to many of the side effects of corticosteroids (151). There is no safe daily dose at which side effects will not occur with chronic therapy.

Hypernatremia, fluid retention, and hypertension may occur, but are unlikely at low doses of less than 10 mg of prednisone (152). Obesity, striae, delayed puberty, and the development of "Cushing's habitus" also occur. A variety of other cutaneous effects can occur including easy bruising, purpura, and ecchymoses. These are especially common in the elderly and typically involve the face and neck, the extensor surfaces of the arms and the hands and the areas below the knees. Hirsutism has been reported in approximately 10% of patients, and depends on the duration of therapy (153). Acne that affects primarily the face and upper trunk occurs in a minority of patients on long-term therapy (154).

Growth impairment is an important problem in children. There is both inhibition of linear bone growth and epiphysial closure. Growth arrest is usually associated with long-term, high-dose therapy but occasionally can be seen with low doses (155). Fortunately, accelerated growth usually follows the cessation of corticosteroid therapy, as there is also inhbition of epiphysial closure. However, this growth catch-up does not always occur after long term therapy.

Glucocorticoid drugs impair carbohydrate metabolism by increasing hepatic gluconeogenesis and by decreasing the utilization of glucose by various tissues (156). An impaired glucose tolerance test is the most common manifestation of the disturbed carbohydrate metabolism. This impairment is usually greatest when therapy begins and improves considerably during the long term (138). The development of overt diabetes is unusual except in individuals with a pre-existing abnormal glucose tolerance test. The drug-induced diabetic state is frequently reversible upon the cessation of corticoid therapy, although it may take several months (157).

Osteoporosis is thought to be a serious complication of corticoid therapy, although some dispute their association (158). Most physicians agree it is a constant threat during therapy, especially in the elderly, immobilized patients, or postmenopausal women. Ribs, vertebrae, and distal radius, all bones with a high degree of trabecular structure, are most severely affected. Osteoporosis is an indication for the withdrawal of therapy.

Corticosteroids may also predispose a patient to aseptic necrosis of the femoral head. In a 10-year study of pulmonary disease, 1% of the patients receiving corticosteroids developed this complication (159). A typical patient had been receiving greater than physiological doses for more than three months and more often for years. Patients with other disorders such as hyperuricemia or polycythemia, who also take corticosteroids are at a higher risk of developing aseptic necrosis than those without these disorders (159).

Peptic ulceration has been suspected to be an adverse effect of corticoid agents. Support for this therapy has waxed and waned over the years, however, current evidence now suggests a small but significant association (160,161). Symptoms of gastrointestinal intolerance, such as dyspepsia and nausea, are common. If anatacids are used to threat these symptoms, it is important to choose agents such as aluminum hydroxides, magnesium trisilicate, and magnesium hydroxide which do not appear to affect the absorption of the corticosteroid (162). Acute pancreatitis is a rarc but serious gastrointestinal complication. It does not appear to be related to the dosage, duration, or type of corticoid used. Although it is a rare complication, it is one of the more common causes of drug-induced pancreatitis (163).

Myopathy is also a serious complication and is an indication for the withdrawal of therapy. It presents as weakness and wasting of the proximal limbs and girdle musculature. There does not appear to be a good correlation between the total dose, the duration of therapy, the patient's age or sex, and the incidence or severity of the myopathy. The patient usually recovers within weeks of the cessation of therapy, although the process may be very slow and incomplete in some cases. The incidence appears higher with the fluorinated corticosteroid drugs, such as triamcinolone (164). The appearance of Guillain-Barré syndrome is another neuromuscular complication which has been reported in a rare patient, including one with ulcerative colitis (165).

After months or years of treatment, the intraocular pressure may become elevated (166). This risk, which appears to be genetically determined, is greatest in patients with myopia or diabetes. The increased pressure is usually reversible when the corticoid therapy is ceased. Posterior subcapsular cataracts may also occur during long-term therapy. The usual minimum time required for the development of cataracts is one year, with at least 10 mg of prednisone per day (166). This complication may be more common among children and patients with rheumatoid arthritis (167,168).

A small proportion of patients, usually children or young women, develop signs of increased intracranial pressure when their dosage is being reduced. The usual therapy is to increase the dose temporarily and then attempt a more gradual withdrawal (169).

It is well known that corticoids decrease cell-mediated immunity, however, whether there is a real clinical risk of infection remains controversial. Nevertheless, it has been suspected that patients on long-term therapy are predisposed to certain bacterial (mycobacteria, staphylococcus, listeria), viral (herpes, cytomegalovirus), fungal (candida, cryptococcus), and parasitic (toxoplasma, pneumocystis) infections (170). Patients with positive results of Mantoux skin test to intermediate strength tuberculin (5 TU), but normal chest x-ray and receiving only modest doses of a corticoid agent (10–15 mg prednisone) do not appear to carry an increased risk of tuberculosis (171). However, if the chest x-ray shows features of inactive tuberculosis, they warrant treatment with two drugs, such as isoniazid and ethambutol or rifampicin (172).

There is an increasing body of information suggesting that prolonged corticoid therapy accelerates the development of atherosclerosis (173). As yet, however, no long-term epidemiologic or morphologic studies have been performed to elucidate this issue. An important element in the process is that these drugs exacerbate several of the well-known risk factors, including hypertension, hypercholesterolemia, hypertriglyceridemia, and impairment of glucose tolerance.

Therapy with corticosteroid agents results in adrenal suppression. In contrast to the rapid recovery which occurs after 2 or 3 weeks of therapy, long-term use may suppress the hypothalamic-pituitary-adrenal axis for up to 9 months after the cessation of therapy (174). Since recovery of the adrenal cortex lags behind that of the pituitary, one can usually assume that full integrity has been restored when the adrenal gland can mount an adequate response of cortisol to ACTH (174). An alternative to routine extensive testing to assure return of normal function would be to assume a poor response during physiologically stressful periods and administer supplemental corticosteroid therapy for one or two years after the medication has been discontinued. This problem, of course, does not occur after ACTH therapy.

A syndrome called "steroid pseudorheumatism," which is distinct from simple adrenal insufficiency has been recognized in patients who take their corticosteroid therapy erratically or whose dosage is reduced abruptly. It is characterized by fever, anorexia, malaise, myalgia, and arthralgias. These symptoms resolve after increasing the dose of the corticosteroid agent; a more gradual reduction prevents their recurrence (143).

B. Inflammatory Bowel Disease Related

The toxicity of corticoid therapy at the doses used to suppress active inflammatory bowel disease is appreciable, although there is very little quantitative information available. This therapy has even been suggested to increase the overall mortality rate and the need for surgery (13,75).

The NCCDS provided important information regarding the incidence and severity of corticosteroid side effects during the course of therapy for Crohn's disease (175). Contrary to earlier clinical reports, there was not an increased incidence of Crohn's disease complication including perineal disease, intra-abdominal abscess, peritonitis, bowel perforation or fistulas. There were, however, a large number of adverse effects noted among those patients treated for active disease, including facial mooning (47%), acne (30%), ecchymosis (17%), petechial bleeding (6%), and striae (6%). When the lower maintenance doses were evaluated, moon face was seen among 25%, hirsutium 8%, and striae 7%. Other minor side effects reported by the patients occurred with similar frequency among those receiving corticosteroids or placebo. More serious side effects, which were noted more commonly among those receiving prednisone for active disease, included infection (27%) and hypertension (13%). Peptic ulcer and severe emotional disturbances were also frequently seen. These complications generally responded to the withdrawal or reduction of the prednisone dose and specific therapy for the complication. Despite this, perforated ulcers and hypertension associated with cerebrovascular accidents pose life-threatening situations. In this study no patient suffered more than one major adverse effect, in contrast to prior clinical data (75). Corticosteroid toxicity sufficient to result in withdrawal from the NCCDS occurred in 18% of the patients receiving therapeutic doses for active disease over 17 weeks, compared to a 6% withdrawal rate among the corresponding placebo group (175).

The ECCDS also provided valuable information regarding side effects which can be expected during corticosteroid therapy of Crohn's disease (8). The side effects noted were similar to those in the U.S. study (175). Five (4%) patients were withdrawn because of side effects related to 6-methylprednisolone. Three patients who received 6-methylprednisolone died of septic complications, two during the course of the study, and one a few months after withdrawal. All three of these patients had a palpable abdominal mass. Thus, the presence of such a mass, with its usually associated suppuration, might increase the potential risk associated with corticosteroid therapy.

The bone mineral content in spinal trabecular and peripheral cortical bone has been specifically measured in 75 patients with inflammatory bowel disease (176). Osteoporosis was present in a high percentage (30.6%) of this relatively young group of patients. Three women with amenorrhea had severe clinical osteoporosis and a further three patients had one or more vertebral crush fractures. Of the 23 patients, 18 had disease of the small intestine with one or more prior resections and the mean lifetime steroid dose was significantly higher than in patients with normal bone mineral content. Bone mineral content of spinal travecular bone showed a significant negative correlation with the lifetime steroid dose. The pathogenesis of the osteoporosis was probably multifactorial; corticosteroid therapy is likely to have been an important contributory factor.

REFERENCES

1. Truelove, S. C., L. J. Witts, Cortisone in ulcerative colitis. Final report on a therapeutic trial, Br. Med. J., 2:1041–1048 (1955).
2. Lennard-Jones, J. E., A. J. Longmore, A. C. Newel, C. W. E. Wilson, F. Avery Jones, An assessment of prednisone, salazopyrine, and topical hydrocortisone hemisuccinate used as outpatient treatment for ulcerative colitis, Gut, 1:217–222 (1960).
3. Truelove, S. C., Treatment of ulcerative colitis with local hydrocortisone hemisuccinate sodium: a report on a controlled therapetuic trial, Br. Med. J., 2:1072–1077 (1958).
4. Watkinson, G., Treatment of ulcerative colitis with topical hydrocortisone hemisuccinate sodium: a controlled trial employing restricted sequential analysis, Br. Med. J., 2:1077–1082 (1958).
5. Matts, S. G. F., Local treatment of ulcerative colitis with prednisolone-21-phosphate enemata, Lancet, 1:517–519 (1960).
6. Lennard-Jones, J. E., J. H. Baron, A. M. Connell, F. Avery Jones, A double-blind trial of prednisone-21-phosphate suppositories in the treatment of idiopathic proctitis, Gut, 3:207–210 (1962).
7. Summers, R. W., D. M. Switz, J. T. Sessions, Jr., et al., National cooperative Crohn's disease study: results of drug treatment, Gastroenterology, 77: 847–869 (1979).
8. Malchow, H., K. Ewe, J. W. Brandes, et al., European cooperative Crohn's disease study (ECCDS): results of drug treatment, Gastroenterology, 249–266 (1984).
9. Gray, S. J., R. W. Reiffenstein, J. A. Benson, J. C. Gordon-Young, Treatment of ulcerative colitis and regional enteritis with ACTH, Arch. Intern. Med., 87:646–662 (1951).
10. Kirsner, J. B., W. L. Palmer, J. A. Spencer, R. D. Bicks, C. F. Johnson, Corticotropin (ACTH) and the adrenal steroids in the management of

ulcerative colitis: observations in 240 patients, Ann. Intern. Med., 50: 891-927 (1959).

11. Truelove, S. C., L. J. Witts, Cortisone and corticotropin in ulcerative colitis, Br. Med. J., 1:387-394 (1959).
12. Jones, J. H., J. F. Lennard-Jones, Corticosteroids and corticotropin in the treatment of Crohn's disease, Gut, 7:181-187 (1966).
13. Cooke, W. T., J. F. Fielding, Corticosteroid or corticotropin therapy in Crohn's disease, Gut, 11:921-297 (1970).
14. Gray, C. H., M. A. Green, N. J. Holness, Urinary metabolic products of prednisone and prednisolone, J. Endocrinol., 14:146-154 (1956).
15. Jenkins, J. S., P. A. Sampson, Converstion of cortisone to cortisol and prednisone to prednisolone, Br. Med. J., 1:205-207 (1967).
16. Meikle, A. W., J. A. Weed, F. H. Tyler, Kinetics and innerconversion of prednisolone and prednisone studied with new radioimmunassays, J. Clin. Endocrinol., 41:717-721 (1975).
17. Sullivan, T. J., E. Sakmar, K. S. Elbert, et al., In vitro and in vivo availability of commercial prednisone tablets, j. Pharm. Sci., 64:1723-1725 (1975).
18. Sullivan, T. J., M. R. Hallmark, K. S. Sakmar, et al., Comparative bioavailability: eight commercial prednisone tablets, J. Pharmacokinet. Biopharm., 64:157-172 (1976).
19. Uribe, M., S. W. Schlam, W. H. Summerskill, et al., Oral prednisone for chronic active liver disease: dose responses and bioavailability studies, Gut, 19:1131-1135 (1978).
20. Powell, L. W., E. Axlsen, Corticosteroids in liver disease: studies on the biological conversion of prednisone to prednisolone and plasma protein binding, Gut, 13:690-696 (1972).
21. Hulme, B., V. H. James, R. Rault, Absorption of enteric and non-enteric coated prednisolone tablets, Br. J. Clin. Pharmacol., 2:257-270 (1975).
22. Henderson, R. G., T. Wheatly, J. English, et al., Variation in plasma prednisolone concentrations in renal transplant recipients given enteric coated prednisolone, Br. Med. J., 1:1534-1136 (1979).
23. Tembo, A. V., M. R. Hallmark, E. Sakmar, Bioabailability of prednisone tablets, J. Pharmacokinet. Biopharm., 5:912-916 (1977).
24. Blackwell, G., R. Carnuccio, M. DiRosa, et al., Macrocortin: a polypeptide causing the antilipase effect of glucorticoids, Nature, 287:147-149 (1980).
25. Swartz, S. L., R. G. Dluhy, Corticosteroids: clinical pharmacology and therapeutic use, Drugs, 16:238-255 (1978).
26. Pickup, M. E., Clinical pharmacokinetics of prednisone and prednisolone, Clin. Pharmacokinet., 4:111-128 (1979).
27. Al-Habet, S., H. J. Rogers, Pharmacokinetics of intravenous and oral prednisolone, Br. J. Clin. Pharmacol., 10:503-511 (1980).
28. Kaplan, H. P., B. Portnoy, H. J. Binder, T. Amatruda, H. Spiro, A controlled evaluation of intravenous adrenocorticotropic hormone and hydrocortisone in the treatment of acute colitis, Gastroenterology, 69:91-95 (1975).

29. Powell-Tuck, J., N. A. Buckell, J. E. Lennard-Jones, A controlled trial of corticotropin and hydrocortisone in the treatment of severe proctocolitis, Scand. J. Gastroenterol., 12:971–975 (1977).
30. Meyers S., D. B. Sachar, J. D. Goldberg, H. D. Janowitz, Corticotropin versus hydrocortisone in the intravenous treatment of ulcerative colitis. A prospective, randomized, double-blind clinical trial, Gastroenterology, 85: 351–357 (1983).
31. Brien, T. G., Human corticosteroid binding globulin. Review, Clin. Endocrinol., 14:193–212 (1981).
32. Steele, W. H., G. M. Hawksworth, H. E. Barber, The binding of prednisolone to human serum and to recrystalized human albumin in vitro, Br. J. Clin. Pharmacol., 14:667–672 (1982).
33. Lewis, G. P., W. J. Jusco, C. W. Burke, L. Graves, Prednisone side-effects and serum-protein levels, Lancet, 2:778–780 (1971).
34. Shaffer, J. A., Absorption of prednisolone in patients with Crohn's disease, Gut, 24:182–186 (1983).
35. Tanner, A. R., J. W. Halliday, L. W. Powell, Serum prednisolone levels in Crohn's disease or celiac disease following oral prednisone administration, Digestion, 21:310–315 (1981).
36. Elliot, P. R., J. Powell-Tuck, P. E. Gillespie, et al., Prednisolone absorption in acute colitis, Gut, 21:49–51 (1980).
37. Berghouse, L. M., P. R. Elliot, J. E. Lennard-Jones, J. English, V. Marks, Plasma prednisolone levels during intravenous therapy in acute colitis, Gut, 23:980–983 (1982).
38. Begg, E. J., H. C. Atkinson, N. Gianarakis, The pharmacokinetics of corticosteroid agents, Med. J. Aust., 146:37-41 (1987).
39. Rose, J. Q., A. M. Jurchak, W. J. Jusko, Dose dependent pharmacokinetics prednisone and prednisolone in man, J. Pharmacokinet. Biopharm., 9:389–415 (1981).
40. Tanner, A., R. F. Bochne, J. Caffin, et al., Dose-dependent prednisolone kinetics, Clin. Pharmacol. Ther., 25:571–578 (1979).
41. McKenzie, S. A., J. A. Selly, J. E. Agnew, Secretion of prednisolone into breast milk, Arch. Dis. Child., 50:894–896 (1975).
42. Stjernholm, M. R., F. H. Katz, Effects of diphenylhydantoin, phenobarbital and diazepam on the metabolism of methylprednisolone and its sodium succinate, J. Clin. Endocrinol. Metab., 55:762–767 (1982).
43. Bergrem, H., I. J. Grottum, H. E. Rugstad, Pharmacokinetics and protein binding of prednisolone after oral and intravenous administration, Eur. J. Clin. Pharmacol., 24:415–419 (1983).
44. Legler, U. R., F. J. Frey, L. Z. Benet, Prednisolone clearance at steady state in man, J. Endocrinol. Metab., 55:762–767 (1982).
45. Meffin, P. J., L. M. Wing, B. C. Sallustio, et al., Marked alterations in prednisolone disposition as a result of oral contraceptive use and dose, Br. J. Clin. Pharmacol., 17:655–664 (1984).
46. Gambertoglio, J. G., W. J. Amend, L. Z. Benet, Pharmacokinetics and bioavailability of prednisone and prednisolone in healthy volunteers and patients: a review, J. Pharmacokinet. Biopharm., 8:1–52 (1980).

47. Petereit, L. B., A. W. Meikle, Effectiveness of prednisolone during phenytoin therapy, Clin. Pharmacol. Ther., 22:912-916 (1977).
48. Kozower,M., L. Veatch, M. M. Kaplan, Decreased clearance of prednisolone, a factor in the development of corticosteroid side effects, J. Clin. Endocrinol. Metab., 38:407-412 (1974).
49. Legler, U. F., L. Z. Benet, Marked alterations in prednisolone elimination for women taking oral contraceptives, J. Clin. Pharmacol. Ther., 31:243 (1982).
50. Lewis, G. P., W. J. Jusko, C. W. Burke, L. Graves, Prednisone side-effects and serum-protein levels, Lancet, 2:778-780 (1971).
51. Powell-Tuck, J., R. L. Brown, J. E. Lennard-Jones, A comparison of oral prednisolone given as single or multiple daily doses for active proctocolitis, Scand. J. Gastroenterol., 13:833-837 (1978).
52. Powell-Tuck, J., R. L. Brown, J. E. Lennard-Jones, F. A. Jones, Outpatient treatment of ulcerative colitis, Br. Med. J., 2:441-443 (1962).
53. Heazelwood, V. J., J. P. Galligan, G. R. Cannel, et al. Plasma cortisol delivery from oral cortisol and cortisone acetate: relative bioavailability, Br. J. Clin. Pharmacol., 17:55-59 (1984).
54. Toothakere, R. D., W. A. Craig, P. G. Pelling, Effect of dose size on the pharmacokinetics of oral hydrocortisone suspension, J. Pharm. Sci., 71: 1182-1185 (1982).
55. Thakker, K. M., Predicting the dose-dependent bioavailability of hydrocortisone and chlorothiazide in humans, J. Pharm. Sci., 72:577-578 (1983).
56. Florini, J. R., D. A. Buyske, Plasma protein binding of triamcinolone-H3 and hydrocortisone-4-C14, J. Biol. Chem., 236:247-250 (1961).
57. Toothaker, R. D., P. G. Welling, Effect on dose size on the pharmacokinetics of intravenous hydrocortisone during endogenous hydrocortisone suppression, J. Pharmacokinet. Biopharm., 10:147-156 (1982).
58. Peterson, R. E., C. E. Pierce, J. B. Wyngaarden, et al., The physiological disposition and the metabolic fate of cortisone in man, J. Clin. Invest., 36: 1301-1312 (1957).
59. Peterson, R. E., Metabolism of adrenalcorticosteroids in man, Ann. NY Acad. Sci., 82:846-853 (1959).
60. Choi, Y., K. Thrasher, E. E. Werk, et al., Effect of diphenylhydantoin on cortisol kinetics in humans, J. Pharmacol. Exp. Ther., 176:27-34 (1971).
61. Narang, P. K., R. Wilder, D. C. Chatterji, et al., Systemic bioavailability and pharmacokinetics of methylprednisolone in patients with rheumatoid arthritis following "high-dose" pulse administration, Biopharm. Drug Dispos., 4:233-248 (1983).
62. Antal, E. J., C. E. Wright, W. R. Gillespie, et al., Influence of route of administration on the pharmacokinetics of methylprednisolone, J. Pharmacokinet. Biopharm., 11:561-576 (1983).
63. Loo, J. C., I. J. McGilveray, Jordon, et al., Pharmacokinetic evaluation of betamethasone and its water soluble phosphate ester in humans, Biopharm. Drug Dispos., 2:265-272 (1981).

64. Truelove, S. C., E. G. Lee, C. P. Willoughby, M. G. W. Kettlewell, Further experience in the treatment of severe attacks of ulcerative colitis, Lancet, 2:1068–0000 (1978).
65. Meyers, S., H. D. Janowitz, Corticosteroid therapy of ulcerative colitis, Gastroenterology, 89:1189–1191 (1985).
66. Jewell, D. P., Diagnosis and medical treatment of ulcerative colitis, Br. Med. J., 27:456–462 (1982).
67. Chapman, R. W., W. S. Selby, D. P. Jewel, Controlled trial of intravenous metronidazole as an adjunct to corticosteroids in severe ulcerative colitis, Gut, 27:1210–1212 (1986).
68. Meyers, S., H. D. Janowitz, The place of steroids in the therapy of toxic dilation of the colon, Gastroenterology, 75:729–731 (1978).
69. Meyers, S., H. D. Janowitz, The management of toxic megacolon, J. Clin. Gastroenterol., 1:345–347 (1979).
70. Bondy, P. K., Disorders of the adrenal cortex. In: Textbook of Endocrinology. (Wilson, J. D., Foster, D., Foster, D. W., eds.) Philadelphia, W.B. Saunders, pp. 816–890 (1985).
71. Haynes, R. C., F. Murad, Adrenocorticotropic hormone; adrenocortical steroids and their synthetic analogs; inhibitors of adrenocortical steroid synthesis. In: The Pharmacological Basis of Therapeutics. (Gilman, A. G., Goodman, L. S., Gilman, A., eds.) New York, MacMillan, pp. 1466–1496 (1980).
72. Meyers, S., P. K. Lerer, E. J. Feuer, J. W. Johnson, H. D. Janowitz, Predicting the outcome of corticoid therapy for acute ulcerative colitis. Results of a prospective, randomized, double-blind clinical trial, J. Clin. Gastroenterol., 9:50–54 (1987).
73. Spencer, J. A., J. B. Kirsner, P. Mlynaryk, P. I. Reed, W. L. Palmer, Immediate and prolonged therapeutic effects of corticotropin and adrenal steroids in ulcerative colitis, Gastroenterology, 42:113–128 (1962).
74. Powell-Tuck, J., R. L. Brown, T. J. Chambers, J. E. Lennard-Jones, A controlled trial of alternate day prednisolone as a maintenance treatment for ulcerative colitis in remission, Digestion, 22:263–267 (1981).
75. Sparberg, M., J. B. Kirsner, Long-term corticosteroid therapy for regional enteritis: an analysis of 58 courses in 54 patients, Am. J. Dig. Dis., 11:865–880 (1966).
76. Goldstein, F., H. Menduke, J. J. Thornton, J. Abramson, Anti-inflammatory treatment of Crohn's disease: a prospective evaluation of 100 consecutively treated patients, J. Clin. Gastroenterol., 2:77–85 (1980).
77. Whittington, P. F., H. V. Barnes, T. M. Bayles, Medical management of Crohn's disease in adolescence, Gastroenterology, 72:1338–1344 (1977).
78. Harris, D. M., Properties and therapeutic uses of some corticosteroids with enhanced topical potency, J. Steroid Biochem., 6:711–716 (1975).
79. Harris, D. M., Some properties of beclomethasone dipropionate and related steroids in man, Postgrad. Med. J., 51(Suppl):20–25 (1975).
80. Kumana, C. R., T. Seaton, M. Meghji, M. Castelli, R. Benson, T. Sivakumaran, Beclomethasone dipropionate enemas for treating inflammatory

bowel disease without producing Cushing's syndrome or hypothalmic-pituitary-adrenal suppression, Lancet, 1:579–583 (1982).

81. Levine, D. S., C. E. Rubin, Topical beclomethasone dipropionate enemas improve distal ulcerative colitis and idiopathic proctitis without systemic toxicity (abstr), Gastroenterology, 88:1473 (1985).
82. Singleton, J. W., Drug therapy of inflammatory bowel disease. In: Inflammatory Bowel Diseases. (Rachmilewitz, D., ed.) The Hague, Martinus Nijhoff, pp. 235–243 (1982).
83. Bansky, G., H. Buhler, B. Stamm, W. Hacki, P. Buchman, J. Muller, Treatment of distal ulcerative colitis with beclomethasone enemas: high therapeutic efficacy without endocrine side effects, Dis. Colon. Rectum., 30: 288–292 (1987).
84. Levine, D. S., V. A. Raisys, V. Ainardi, Coating of oral beclomethasone dipropionate with cellulose acetate phthalate enhances delivery of topically active drug to the terminal ileum, Gastroenterology, 92:1037–1044 (1987).
85. Bergman, L., U. Krause, Postoperative treatment with corticosteroids and salazosulphapyridine (Salazopyrin) after radical resection for Crohn's disease, Scand. J. Gastroenterol., 11:651–656 (1976).
86. Truelove, S. C., D. P. Jewell, Intensive intravenous regimen for severe attacks of ulcerative colitis, Lancet, 1:1067–1070 (1974).
87. Jarnerot, G., P. Rolny, H. Sandberg-Gertzen, Intensive intravenous treatment of ulcerative colitis, Gastroenterology, 89:1005–1013 (1985).
88. Shepherd, H. A., G. D. Barr, D. P. Jewel, Use of an intravenous steroid regimen in the treatment of acute Crohn's disease, J. Clin. Gastroenterol., 8:154–159 (1986).
89. Mekhjan, H. S., D. M. Switz, H. D. Watts, J. J. Deren, R. M. Katon, F. M. Berman, National cooperative Crohn's disease study: factors determining recurrence of Crohn's disease after surgery, Gastroenterology, 77:907–913 (1979).
90. Smith, R. C., J. Rhodes, R. V., Heatley, et al., Low dose steroids and clinical relapse in Crohn's disease: a controlled trial, Gut, 19:606–610 (1978).
91. Murphy, B. E. P., S. J. Clark, I. R. Donald, M. Pinsky, D. Vedady, Coversion of maternal cortisol to cortisone during placental transfer to the human fetus, Am. J. Obstet. Gynecol., 118:538–541 (1974).
92. Beitins, I. Z., F. Bayard, I. G. Ances, A. Kowarski, C. J. Migeion, The transplacental passage of prednisolone and prednisone in pregnancy near term, J. Pediatr., 81:936–945 (1972).
93. Eriksson, M., C. S. Catz, S. J. Yaffee, Drugs and pregnancy, Clin. Obstet. Gynecol., 16:199–224 (1973).
94. Kenny, M. J., C. Preeyasombat, J. S. Spaulding, C. J. Migeon, Cortisol production rate. IV. Infants born of steroid treated mothers and of diabetic mothers. Infants with trisomy syndrome and with anencephaly, Pediatrics, 37:960–966 (1966).
95. Peterson, M. C., C. B. Collier, J. J. Ashley, W. G. McBride, R. L. Nation, Disposition of betamethasone in parturient woman after intravenous administration, Eur. J. Clin. Pharmacol., 25:803–810 (1983).

96. Beely, L., Adverse effects of drugs in later pregnancy, Clin. Obstet. Gynecol., 13:197-214 (1986).
97. DeCosta, E. J., M. A. Abelmann, Cortisone and pregnancy, Am. J. Obstet. Gynecol., 64:746–747 (1952).
98. Warrell, D. W., R. Taylor, Outcome for the fetus of mothers receiving prednisolone during pregnancy, Lancet, 1:117-118 (1968).
99. Reinisch, J., N. G. Simon, W. G. Karow, R. Candelman, Prenatal exposure to prednisone in humans and animals retards intrauterine growth, Science, 202:436–438 (1978).
100. Miller, J. P., Inflammatory bowel disease in pregnancy: a review, J. R. Soc. Med., 79:221-225 (1986).
101. Fielding, J. F., W. T. Cooke, Pregnancy and Crohn's disease, Br. Med. J., 2:76–77 (1970).
102. Willoughby, C. P., S. C. Truelove, Ulcerative colitis and pregnancy, Gut, 21:469–474 (1980).
103. Vender, R. J., H. M. Spiro, Inflammatory bowel disease and pregnancy, J. Clin. Gastroenterol., 4:231-249 (1982).
104. Mogadam, M. J., W. O. Dobbins, B. I. Korelitz, S. W. Ahmed, Pregnancy in inflammatory bowel disease: effect of sulfasalazine and corticosteroids on fetat outcome, Gastroenterology, 80:7506 (1981).
105. Khosla, R., C. P. Willoughby, D. P. Jewell, Crohn's disease and pregnancy, Gut, 25:52–56 (1984).
106. Baiocco, P. J., B. I. Korelitz, The influence of inflammatory bowel disease and its treatment on pregnancy and fetal outcome., J. Clin. Gastroenterol., 6:211-216 (1984).
107. Morrison, J., N. Kilpatrick, Low urinary estriol excretion in pregnancy with oral prednisone therapy, J. Obstet. Gynecol. Br. Cwlth., 76:719–720 (1969).
108. McKenzie, S. A., J. A. Selley, J. E. Agnew, Secretion of prednisolone into breast milk, Arch. Dis. Child., 50:894–896 (1975).
109. Lan, N. C., M. Karin, T. Nguyn, et al., Mechanisms of glucocorticoid hormone action, J. Steroid Biochem., 20:77–88 (1984).
110. Pauwells, R., Mode of action of corticosteroids in asthma and rhinitis, Clin. Allergy, 16:281-288 (1986).
111. Fauci, A. S., Mechanisms of corticosteroid action on lymphocyte subpopulations. Redistribution of the circulating T and B lymphocyte to the bone marrow, Immunology, 28:669–680 (1975).
112. Claman, H. N., Corticosteroids; anti-inflammatory mechanisms, Hosp. Pract., 18:123–151 (1983).
113. Cupps, T., A. S. Fauci, Corticosteroid-mediated immunoregulation in man, Immunol. Rev., 65:133–155 (1982).
114. Cupps, T., L. C. Edgar, C. A. Thomas, A. S. Fauci, Multiple mechanisms of B cell immunoregulation in man after administration of in vivo corticosteroids, J. Immunol., 132:170–175 (1984).
115. Altman, A. C., J. S. Hill, W. M. Hairfield, M. F. Mullarkey, Effect of corticosteroids on eosinophil chemotaxis and adherence, J. Clin. Invest., 67: 28–41 (1981).

116. Tsokos, G. C., J. E. Balow, Immunosuppressive agents and plasmapheresis in immunological disorders. J. Immunopharmacol., 1-15 (1985).
117. Rinehart, J. J., S. P. Balcerzak, A. L. Sagone, A. F. LoBuglio, Effects of corticosteroids on human monocyte function, J. Clin. Invest., 54:1337-1343 (1974).
118. Fries, L. F., C. M. Brickman, M. M. Frank, Monocyte receptors for the Fc portion of IgG increase in number in autoimmune hemolytic states are decreased glucocorticoid therapy, J. Immunol., 131:1240-1245 (1983).
119. Gerrard, T. L., T. R. Cupps, C. H. Jurgensen, A. S. Fauci, Hydrocortisone-mediated inhibition of monocyte antigen presentation; dissociation of inhibitory effect and expression of DR antigens, Cell Immunol., 85:330-339 (1984).
120. Werb, Z., Biochemical actions of glucortcoids on macrophages in culture. Specific inhibition of elastase, collagenase, and plasminogen activation, secretion and effects on other metabolic functions, J. Exp. Med., 447: 1695-1712 (1978).
121. Schleimer, R. P., E. S. Schulman, D. W. MacGlashan, et al., Effects of dexamethasone on mediator release from human lung fragments and purified lung mast cell, J. Clin. Invest., 71:1830-1835 (1983).
122. Onsrud, M., E. Thorsby, Influence of in vivo hydrocortisone on some human lymphocyte populations. Effect on natural killer cell activity, Scand. J. Immunol., 13:573-579 (1981).
123. Routes, J., H. N. Claman, Corticosteroids in inflammatory bowel disease. A review, J. Clin. Gastroenterol., 9:529-535 (1987).
124. Samuelsson, B., Leukotrienes, mediators of immediate hypersensitivity reactions and inflammation, Science, 220:568-575 (1983).
125. Lewis, G. P., Immunoregulatory activity of metabolites of arachidonic acid and their role in inflammation, Br. Med. Bull., 39:243-248 (1983).
126. Rampton, D. S., C. J. Hawkey, Prostaglandins and ulcerative colitis, Gut, 25:1399-1413 (1984).
127. Sharon, P., W. F. Stenson, Enhanced synthesis of leukotriene B4 by colonic mucosa in inflammatory bowel disease, Gastroenterology, 86: 453-460 (1984).
128. DiRosa, M., R. J. Flower, F. Hirata, L. Parente, F. Russo-Marrie, Nomenclature announcement. Anti-phosphilipase proteins, Prostaglandins, 28: 441-442 (1984).
129. Lauritsen, K., L. S. Laursen, K. Bukhave, J. Rask-Madsen, Effects of topical 5-aminosalicylic acid and prednisolone on prostaglandin E2 and Leukotriene B4 levels determined by equilibrium in vivo dialysis of rectum in relapsing ulcerative colitis, Gastroenterology, 91:837-844 (1986).
130. Lauritsen, K., L. S. Laursen, K. Bukhave, J. Rask-Madsen, In vivo effects of orally administered prednisolone on prostaglandin and leukotreiene production in ulcerative colitis, Gut, 28:1095-1099 (1987).
131. Campieri, M., G. A. Lanfranchi, G. Bazzochi, et al. Prostaglandins, indomethacin and ulcerative colitis (Abstr), Gastroenterology, 78:193 (1980).

132. Rampton, D. S., G. E. Sladen, Prostaglandin synthesis inhibitors in ulcerative colitis: Flurbioprofen compared with conventional treatment, Prostaglandins, 21:417-425 (1981).
133. Kaufman, H. J., H. L. Taubin, Nonsteroidal anti-inflammatory drugs activate quiescent inflammatory bowel disease, Ann. Intern. Med., 107: 513–516 (1987).
134. Rask-Madsen, J., Simultaneous measurement of electrical polarization and electrolye transport by the entire normal and inflammed colon during in vivo perfusion, Scand. J. Gastroenterol., 8:327–336 (1973).
135. Rask-Madsen, J., P. B. Jensen, Electrolyte transport capacity and electrical potentials of the normal and the inflammed human rectum in vivo, Scand. J. Gastroenterol., 8:169–175 (1973).
136. Edmonds, C. J., D. Pilcher, Electrical potential difference and sodium and potassium fluxes across rectal mucosa in ulcerative colitis, Gut, 14:784–789 (1973).
137. Binder, H. J., Effect of dexamethasone on electrolyte transport in the large intestine of the rat, Gastroenterology, 75:212–217 (1978).
138. Charney, A. N., M. D. Kinsey, L. Meyers, R. A. Giannella, R. E. Gots, Na+–K+ activated adenosine triphosphatase and intestinal electrolyte transport. Effects of adrenal steroids, J. Clin. Invest., 56:653–660 (1975).
139. Charney, A. N., J. Wallach, S. Ceccarelli, M. Donowitz, C. L. Costenbader, Effects of spironolactone and amiloride on corticosteroid-induced changes in colonic function, Am. J. Physiol., 241:G300–G305 (1981).
140. Foster, E. S., T. W. Zimmerman, J. P. Hayslett, H. J. Binder, Corticosteroid alteration of active electrolyte transport in rat distal colon, Am. J. Physiol., 245:G668–G675 (1983).
141. Sandle, G. L., S. A. Lewis, J. P. Hayslett, H. J. Binder, Dexamethasone induces amiloride-sensitive Na transport in rat distal colon (abstr), Clin. Sci., 62:30 (1982).
142. Sandle, G. I., J. P. Hayslett, H. J. Binder, Effect of glucocorticoids on rectal transport in normal subjects and patients with ulcerative colitis, Gut, 27:309–316 (1986).
143. Thorn, G. W., Clinical considerations in the use of corticosteroids, N. Engl. J. Med., 274:775–781 (1966).
144. Dujorne, C. A., D. L. Azarnoff, Clinical complications of corticosteroid therapy, Med. Clin. North Am., 57:1331-1342 (1973).
145. Hall, R. C. W., M. K. Popkin, S. K. Sticheney, E. R. Gardner, Presentation of steroid psychosis, J. Nerv. Metn. Dis., 167:229-236 (1979).
146. Glaser, G. H., Psychotic reactions induced by corticotropin (ACTH) and cortisone, Psychosom. Med., 15:280–891 (1953).
147. Chan, C. S., I. G. Brown, W. A. Oliver,P. V. Zimmerman, Hydrocortisone-induced anaphylaxis, Med. J. Aust., 141:444–446 (1984).
148. Streck, F., H. Lockwood Dean, Pituitary adrenal recovery following short-term suppression with corticosteroids, Am. J. Med., 66:910–914 (1979).

149. Webb, J., T. J. H. Clark, Recovery of plasma corticotrophin and cortisol levels after a three-week course of prednisolone, Thorax, 36:22–24 (1981).
150. Cochrane, G. M., Systemic steroids in asthma. In: Steroids in Asthma. (Clark, T. J. H., ed.) Balgowlah, Adis Press, pp. 103–120 (1983).
151. Thomas, T. P. L., The complications of systemic corticosteroid therapy in the elderly, Gerontology, 30:60–65 (1984).
152. Jackson, S. H. D., D. G. Beevers, K. Myers, Does long-term low-dose corticosteroid therapy cause hypertension?, Clin. Sci., 6(Supp 7):381–383 (1981).
153. Shubin, H., Long-term (five or more years) administration of corticosteroids in pulmonary diseases, Dis. Chest, 48:287–290 (1965).
154. David, D. S., M. H. Greico, P. Cushman, Adrenal glucocorticoids after 20 years: a review of their clinically relevant consequences, J. Chronic Dis., 22:637–711 (1970).
155. Morris, H. G., Growth and skeletal maturation in asthmatic children: effect of corticosteroid treatment, Pediatr. Res., 9:579–583 (1975).
156. Olefsky, J. M., G. Kimmerling, Effects of glucocorticoids on carbohydrate metabolism, Am. J. Med. Sci., 271:202–210 (1976).
157. Miller, S. E., J. M. Neilson, Clinical features of the diabetic syndrome appearing after steroid therapy, Postgrad. Med. J., 40:660–664 (1964).
158. Guyatt, C. H., C. E. Webber, A. A. Mewa, D. L. Sackett, Determing causation—a case study: adrenocorticosteroids and osteoporosis, J. Chron. Dis., 37:343–352q (1984).
159. Richards, M., M. Santiago, B. Klaustermeyer, Aseptic necrosis of the femoral head in corticosteroid-treated pulmonary disease, Arch. Intern. Med., 140:1473–1475 (1980).
160. Conn, H. O., B. L. Blitzer, Nonassociation of adrenocoticosteroid therapy and peptic ulcer, N. Engl. J. Med., 294:472–479 (1976).
161. Messer, J., D. Reitman, H. S. Sacks, et al., Association of adrenosorticosteroid therapy and peptic-ulcer disease, N. Engl. J. Med., 309:21–24 (1983).
162. Tanner, A. R., J. A. Caffin, J. W. Halliday, et al., Concurrent administration of antacids and prednisone: effect on serum levels of prednisolone, Br. J. Clin. Pharmacol., 7:397–400 (1979).
163. Nakashima, Y., J. M. Howard, Drug-induced acute pancreatitis, Surg. Gynecol. Obstet., 145:105–109 (1977).
164. Golding, D. N., T. B. Begg, Dexamethasone myopathy, Br. Med. J., 2: 1129–1130 (1960).
165. Steiner, I., I. Wirguin, O. Abramsky, Appearance of Guillain-Barré syndrome patients during corticosteroid treatment, J. Neurol., 233:221–223 (1986).
166. David, D. S., J. S. Berkowitz, Occular effects of topical and systemic corticosteroids, Lancet, 2:149–159 (1969).
167. Dikshit, S. K., P. N. Avasthi, Posterior lenticular opacities in children on corticosteroid therapy, Ind. J. Pediatr., 32:93–96 (1965).

168. Loredo, A., R. S. Rodriguez, L. Murillo, Cataracts after short-term corticosteroid treatment, N. Engl. J. Med., 286:160 (1972).
169. Anonymous, Intracranial hypertension and steroids, Lancet, 2:1052–1053 (1964).
170. Dale, D. C., R. G. Petersdorf, Corticosteroids and infectious disease, Med. Clin. North Am., 57:1277–1287 (1973).
171. Shatz, M., R. Patterson, R. Kloner, J. Falk, The prevalence of tuberculosis and positive tuberculin skin tests in a steroid-treated population, Ann. Intern. Med., 84:261–265 (1976).
172. Treatment of tuberculosis. Recommendations of National Tuberculosis Advisory Council. Canberra: Commonwealth Department of Health, (1982).
173. Nashel, D. J., Is atherosclerosis a complication of long-term corticosteroid treatment?, Am. J. Med., 80:925–929 (1986).
174. Chamberlin, P., W. J. Meyer, Management of pituitary-adrenal suppression secondary to corticosteroid therapy, Pediatrics, 67:245–251 (1981).
175. Singleton, J. W., D. H. Law, M. L. Kelly, H. S. Mikhgian, A. L. Sturdevant, National cooperative Crohn's disease study: adverse reactions to study drugs, Gastroenterology, 77:870–882 (1979).
176. Compston J. E., D. Judd, E. O Crawley, et al., Osteoporosis in patients with inflammatory bowel disease, Gut, 28:410–415 (1987).

2
Topical Steroids

Gerald Friedman

Mount Sinai School of Medicine of the City University of New York, New York, New York

Corticosteroids and/or sulfasalazine continue to be the cornerstones of anti-inflammatory therapy for inflammatory bowel disease (IBD). Intermediate and long-term toxicity and side effects for both of these compounds have prompted the search for newer agents with lesser toxicity. Efforts at increasing the concentration of specific anti-inflammatory agents as well as decreasing toxic side effects have resulted in the introduction of unique rectally instilled therapeutic agents.

The rationale for the use of rectally instilled therapeutic agents is, in part, based upon the natural history of left-sided ulcerative colitis. Compared with pancolitis, in left-sided colitis the symptoms are mildly to moderately severe. In addition, complications and extracolonic manifestations of the disease are uncommon. The relatively benign nature of left-sided disease allows time for considered judgment in the selection of appropriate agents to suppress inflammatory activity and ameliorate symptoms.

The ideal rectally instilled agents for the treatment of left-sided colitis should have the following qualities:

1. Rapid onset of action
2. Provide a high concentration of medication at the site of inflammatory activity
3. Produce sustained anti-inflammatory activity
4. Prevent or reduce recurrent inflammatory activity

5. Provide penetrating flow covering areas from the rectum to the splenic flexure or beyond

I. CLINICAL INVESTIGATIONS

A. Standard Preparations

Rectal instillation of steroids has been employed for the treatment of left-sided ulcerative colitis since the late 1950s. Double-blind, placebo-controlled studies have demonstrated the beneficial effects of rectally administered steroids (1). Formulations of hydrocortisone alcohol, hemisuccinate, and acetate, as well as prednisolone-21-phosphate, methyl prednisolone, and betamethasone 17-valerate have been used successfully to suppress inflammatory activity in both left-sided colitis and as adjunctive therapy for patients with pancolitis (2–8). Clinical observations and controlled studies over the past 30 years suggest the beneficial effects are largely related to local topical activity with a possible lesser contribution from absorbed steroids. The bioavailability of steroids administered as retention enemas is largely related to the total duration of retention, dose, formulation of the vehicle, fecal bacterial degradation, and total volume of the administered agent (9). Early studies with rectally instilled steroids employed a rectal drip method instilled over a period of 30 minutes to several hours (2). The anatomic penetration of such preparations achieved levels to the splenic flexure and beyond. A convenient disposable plastic container for easy rectal administration was introduced by Matts (10). Short- and long-term therapy with rectally administered steroids provide evidence that this form of therapy produces a prompt salutary clinical response in most patients with left-sided and pancolitis (11). The favorable response consists of improvement in the number and appearance of bowel movements, reduced bleeding, and amelioration of tenesmus. Such improvement may occur within the first 48 hours. Patients with mild to moderate activity respond more dramatically than those with severe inflammation. Endoscopic reversal of inflammatory activity may not be evident for two weeks after onset of therapy.

Response rates vary from 40 to 80% in patients with left-sided disease and 40 to 50% in patients with pancolitis. Steroid enema therapy has been continued in some patients for more than three years, either alone or combined with other agents. The relapse rate after discontinuation of therapy within 6 months after initial treatment varies between 50 and 70%. In more than half of these patients, a second course of rectal steroids produces a beneficial response.

The side effects and toxicity of rectally administered steroids vary with the total dose, duration of administration, and extent of absorption. Short-term studies reveal no serious side effects. Edema, acne, and muscle weakness are commonly noted with short-term therapy. Patients on long-term therapy are subject to the same potentially serious side effects noted with oral or parenteral steroids. Hypokalemic alkalosis, edema, increased susceptibility to infection, peptic ulceration, myopathy, behavioral disturbance, posterior subcapsular cataracts, osteoporosis, and vertebral compression, as well as growth disturbances in children, are possible complications.

B. Newer Formulations

Efforts to minimize the short- and long-term side effects and toxicity of absorbable systemic steroids have resulted in the introduction of several steroids with unique characteristics. Two major classes of compounds are currently under study: (1) Poorly absorbed steroids with low systemic activity and high mucosal concentration exemplified by prednisolone-21-metasulphobenzoate sodium; and (2) absorbable steroids with no systemic side effects, exemplified by beclomethasone dipropionate and tixocortol pivalate.

1. *Prednisolone-21-Metasulphobenzoate*

Prednisolone-21-metasulphobenzoate (Predenema, Pharmax, Forest Laboratories, Inc.) has been used in Great Britain in both the liquid form (Predenema) and as a rectal foam (Predfoam). This compound contains 20 mg of prednisolone-21-metasulphobenzoate administered rectally nightly. McIntyre et al. (12) conducted a double-blind controlled trial in 40 patients comparing the therapeutic effects of prednisolone-21-metasulphobenzoate, rectally administered, with prednisolone-21-phosphate enemas in patients with distal ulcerative colitis. Both enemas resulted in symptomatic improvement in more than 70% of patients treated. Diarrhea, rectal bleeding, and tenesmus were observed to decrease. Sigmoidoscopic improvement was noted in both groups in this 2-week study. The major difference between these two agents appears to be in the rate of absorption. While prednisolone-21-phosphate was readily absorbed from the colonic mucosa, prednisolone-21-metasulphobenzoate accumulated in mucosal tissue and produced a lower serum level of steroid. The short-term side effects of these compounds were comparable. The study of long-term effects of prednisolone-21-metasulphobenzoate, as well as dose–response curve, may provide more information regarding the value of this agent in the therapy of distal ulcerative colitis.

2. *Beclomethasone Dipropionate*

Beclomethasone dipropionate (Schering) in a dosage of 0.5 mg/cc in 100 ml of diluent suppresses inflammatory activity in patients with distal ulcerative colitis without suppressing the hypothalamic–pituitary axis (13). This steroid may be completely inactivated by first-pass liver metabolism or it may be rapidly metabolized in the colonic mucosa. Clinical studies have compared beclomethasone enemas with betamethasone (5 mg) enemas. Both enemas had similar beneficial effects, but only beclomethasone failed to affect hypothalamic-pituitary-adrenal function. The enema form is unavailable for clinical use at this time.

3. Tixocortol Pivalate

Tixocortol pivalate (Sandoz) is a derivative of cortisol in which a 21-thiol group esterified with pivalic acid replaces a 21-hydroxyl group on ring D. This compound is devoid of systemic activity. Its anti-inflammatory activity when topically administered is its sole steroid-related property. The local anti-inflammatory activity is equal to or greater than that of hydrocortisone. In normal subjects no systemic glucocorticoid activity was demonstrated after oral, rectal, or intranasal administration. By these three routes tixocortol did not induce changes in plasma cortisol, leukocyte counts, blood glucose, or the 24-hr excretion of sodium or potassium. The rapid transformation of the rectally administered compound appears to occur initially within red blood cells. The rapid elimination of tixocortol pivalate, indicating first-pass liver effect, is noted by short initial and terminal disposition, a lower systemic availability than hydrocortisone, rapid plasma clearance, and higher volume distribution in plasma clearance than hydrocortisone. The metabolic pathway of tixocortol is rapid transformation into tixocortol and S-methylation, S-oxidation, and A-ring reduction.

Tixocortol pivalate has been available in France for the past several years, and is currently under investigation in the United States. The initial multicenter trial in the United States compared the efficacy and safety of rectally instilled tixocortol pivalate and hydrocortisone (14) A group of 108 patients with documented distal ulcerative colitis were randomized to receive either tixocortol pivalate (250 mg/10-ml diluent) or hydrocortisone (100 mg/60-ml diluent) for 21 days. At the end of 22 days, 51% of the patients treated with tixocortol pivalate no longer had evidence of ulcerative colitis based upon the results of endoscopic examinations compared with 40% in the hydrocortisone group (no statistical difference). However, after 2 weeks, a statistically significant difference in the reduction of abdominal pain, rectal pain, severity of symptoms, feeling of illness, improvement of appetite, and reduction in rectal bleeding was noted with tixocortol pivalate compared with hydrocortisone. Hematologic parameters for hydrocortisone revealed a statistically significant increase in white blood cell count, a decrease in lymphocyte count, an increase in neutrophils, and a decrease in eosinophils. This pattern was not observed with patients on tixocortol. Local anal reactions occurred in about 5.5% of the patients on tixocortol. The hydrocortisone patient group experienced nausea (5.5%), rectal burning (3.6%), peptic ulcer (1.8%), and polyuria, ankle edema, and fluid retention (1.8%). This study demonstrated that tixocortol pivalate is a rapidly effective local anti-inflammatory steroid comparable to hydrocortisone, but without undesirable systemic activity.

A second clinical trial found that nightly tixocortol pivalate retention enemas were equally effective as hydrocortisone in the treatment of ambulatory patients with left-sided colitis (15). This 3-week, double-blind, randomized, multicenter trial involved 19 investigators who enrolled 125 pateints. Both tixocortol and hydrocortisone produced statistically significant decreases in endoscopic findings, severity of ulceration, and hyperemia at day 14. Both agents improved rectal tenderness by day 7 and reduced the number of bowel movements and rectal bleeding. Complete endoscopic healing was noted in 25% of tixocortol pivalate patients and 35% of hydrocortisone patients at the end of 3 weeks.

An open study in the United States included patients with refractory left-sided colitis who had not responded to treatment with hydrocortisone enemas, sulfasalazine, or both (16). These patients were treated with 250 mg or 500 mg of tixocortol pivalate rectal suspension nightly for 2 to 4 weeks. All patients had a rapid reduction in both diarrhea and rectal bleeding with a parallel endoscopic reduction in mucosal inflammatory activity. No adverse side effects were noted during this limited study.

These newer topical steroid preparations are not as yet commercially available in the United States. If subsequent clinical trials further establish their efficacy and toxicity, one or more of these agents could replace the currently used standard forms.

II. RECOMMENDATIONS FOR THERAPY

Certain aspects of topical steroid therapy are of critical importance to prescriber and patient: (1) Efficient therapeutic activity is, in part, related to the total anatomic area of the colon involved with disease. The extent of macroscopic inflammatory bowel disease is best determined by total colonscopy. Photographic documentation of extent of disease is valuable for follow-up determination of the efficacy of the therapeutic agent employed, as well as following the natural history of the disease in the individual patient. In selected circumstances, biopsies at the limits of macroscopic inflammatory activity and beyond may be of additional value in noting effective therapetuic activity. It has been noted that the visually normal appearing mucosa of the right colon may be the seat of microscopic inflammatory activity in many patients with "left-sided" disease. The implications of this finding of the natural history of left-sided disease remain to be determined; (2) the method of instillation is vitally important if effective therapeutic results are to be obtained. The medication should be at room temperature, the enema tip should be well lubricated, and the patient should be physically able to instill the enema tip properly. Since all patients with left-sided disease have significant rectal involvement, the ability to retain rectally instilled medication will be related to the severity of the rectal ampulla. The latter will be of relatively small capacity in cases of long-standing colitis, where cicatrization has occurred. The usual method of rectal instillation requires the patient to lie on the left side with knees drawn up. Medication is instilled slowly over a period of 5-10 min. Following instillation, the patient should lie on his left side for 15 min, on his right side for 15 min, and then on his back for 15 min. Employing this technique, anatomic penetrations of the rectally instilled medication may achieve levels to the splenic flexure or beyond. The usual volume of diluent used is 60 cc. It has been demonstrated that total volumes of 100 cc may achieve further anatomic penetrations; (3) retention is of vital importance if effective therapeutic action is to be attained. A minimum of 2 hr of retention is necessary for therapeutic activity. Ideally, the rectally instilled medication should be retained overnight. When extreme rectal irritability or intense rectal inflammatory activity is present, the use of rectal foam preparations 1 hr before instilling the liquid preparation may be helpful; (4) the usual frequency of rectal administration is once daily at night. Under certain circumstances, twice daily administrations may be required to suppress intense inflammatory activity. (5) The response time in terms of days or weeks varies from patient to patient. In general, if a patient fails to respond to rectally instilled medication following effective nightly administration for 2 weeks, another agent should be substituted, or the dosage should be increased. A clinical response demonstrated by reduced rectal bleeding, reduced tenesmus, and diminished diarrhea is commonly evident within 5 days. Endoscopic improvement may not be clearly evident for 10–14 days; (6) once effective clinical and endoscopic results are obtained, efforts must be instituted to sustain anti-inflammatory activity and prevent recurrent disease. A reduced frequency of rectal instillation every other night may be employed. As the dose of rectally instilled medication is being reduced, oral sulfasalazine or oral 5-aminosalicylic acid should be introduced. Once effective dosages of the oral preparations have been achieved, the rectal medication may be discontinued.

III. SUMMARY

The natural history of left-sided ulcerative colitis, including proctitis, proctosigmoiditis, and disease extending to the splenic flexure follows a relatively benign course, making it particularly amenable to treatment with rectally instilled steroid medication. Absorbable steroids, such as hydrocortisone, prednisolone-21-phosphate, methyl prednisolone, and betamethasone-17-valerate have been used successfully to suppress inflammatory mucosal disease for more than 30 years. To obviate intermediate and long-term side effects, new congeners of hydrocortisone have been introduced. Two major classes of compounds under study include poorly absorbed steroids, such as prednisolone-21-metasulphobenzoate and absorbable steroids with no systemic side effects such a beclomethasone dipropionate and tixocortol pivalate. These agents possess effective topical anti-inflammatory activity without producing the significant side effects or long-term toxicity commonly associated with absorbable systemic corticosteroids.

REFERENCES

1. Truelove, S. C., Treatment of ulcerative colitis with local hydrocortisone, Br. Med. J., 2:1267–1272 (1956).
2. Truelove, S. C., Systemic and local corticosteroid therapy in ulcerative colitis, Br. Med. J., 1:464–467 (1960).
3. Truelove, S. C., Local corticosteroid treatment of ulcerative colitis, Postgrad. Med., 37:76–82 (1961).
4. Brown, C. H., M. Merlo, Topical steroid therapy for ulcerative colitis, Am. J. Gastroenterol., 36:343–354 (1961).
5. MacDougall, I., Treatment of ulcerative colitis with rectal steroids, Lancet, 1:826–827 (1963).
6. Matts, S. G. F., Intrarectal treatment of 100 cases of ulcerative colitis with prednisolone-21-phosphate retention enemata, Br. Med. J., 3:165 (1961).
7. Lennard-Jones, J. E., Betamethasone 17-valerate and prednisolone-21-phosphate retention enemata in proctocolitis, Br. Med. J., 3:84–86 (1971).
8. Sparberg, N., J. Fennessy, J. B. Kirsner, Ulcerative proctitis and mild ulcerative colitis: A study of 220 patients, Medicine, 45:391 (1966).
9. Lima, J. J., J. Giller, J. J. Mackichan, W. J. Jusko, Bioavailability of hydrocortisone retention enemas in normal subjects, Am. J. Gastroenterol., 73: 232–237 (1980).
10. Matts, S. G., Local treatment of ulcerative colitis with prednisolone-21-phosphate enemata, Lancet, 517 (1960).
11. Spencer, J. S., J. B. Kirsner, Experience with short and long term courses of local adrenal steroid therapy for ulcerative colitis: Report of 98 cases, Gastroenterology, 42:669 (1962).
12. McIntyre, P. B., F. A. Macrae, L. Berghouse, J. English, J. E. Lennard-Jones, Therapeutic benefits from a poorly absorbed prednisolone enema in distal colitis, Gut, 822–824 (1985).
13. Kumana, C. R., M. Meghi, T. Seaton, M. Castelli, R. Benson, T. Sivakumaran, Beclamethasone dipropionate enemas for treating inflammatory bowel disease without producing cushings syndrome or hypothalamic pituitary adrenal suppression, Lancet, 1:579–583 (1982).
14. Levinson, P., Tixocortol pivalate versus hydrocortisone enemas in ulcerative colitis: A multicenter comparative clinical trial. Presented at symposium on idiopathic inflammatory bowel disease, April 12, 1985, Phoenix, AZ.
15. Hanauer, S. B., J. B. Kirsner, W. E. Barrett, The treatment of left-sided ulcerative colitis with tixocortol pivalate (TP), Gastroenterology, 90:1449 (1986).
16. Friedman, G., Treatment of refractory proctosigmoiditis and left-sided colitis with a rectally instilled non-glucocorticoid, non-mineralocorticoid steroid, Gastroenterology, 88:1388 (1985).

3

Sulfasalazine

Mark A. Peppercorn

Beth Israel Hospital, Harvard Medical School, Boston, Massachusetts

In the 1930s, rheumatoid arthritis was known to respond to salicylate therapy and thought to be of bacterial etiology. Sulfasalazine, which combines one of the first sulfonamides, sulfapyridine with 5-aminosalicylic acid, a salicylate analogue, linked by an azo bond was designed to treat the disorder (Fig. 1). Although the drug proved useful in patients with rheumatoid arthritis, and, in Europe, continues to be utilized in the therapy of rheumatologic disorders, when used in a group of patients with inflammatory bowel disease (IBD) the results were striking. Since that initial use over 45 years ago, sulfasalazine has become the most widely prescribed agent for the therapy of inflammatory bowel disease. Clinical studies beginning in the 1950s have provided evidence of the drug's efficacy in the treatment of both ulcerative colitis and Crohn's disease. Studies of sulfasalazine's pharmacology have offered insight into its possible mechanism of action and toxicity and have led to the development of new agents based on sulfasalazine's structure which are now providing a new generation of drugs for the treatment of inflammatory bowel diseases.

I. PHARMACOKINETICS

One quarter to one third of the ingested drug is absorbed from the upper gastrointestinal tract with detectable blood levels obtained within 1 to 2 hr after oral intake and steady-state serum levels achieved within 24 hr (1,2). A portion of the absorbed drug, usually less than 10% of the total administered dose, is

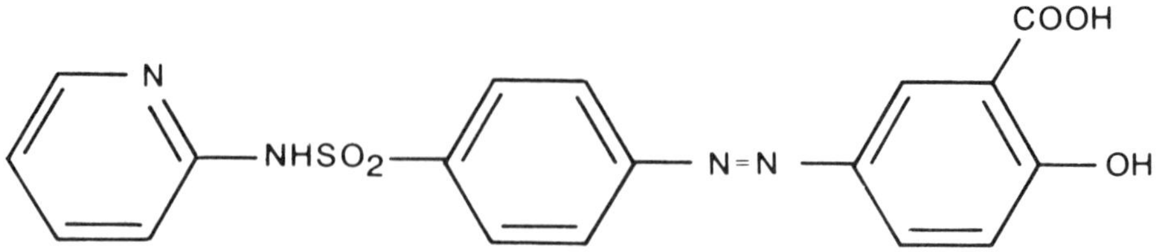

Figure 1 Structural formula of sulfasalazine.

excreted unchanged in the urine, imparting to the urine a strong yellow or light orange color. The remainder of the absorbed sulfasalazine is excreted unchanged in the bile and together with the nonabsorbed portion of the drug traverses the intestinal tract, reaching the distal small intestine and colon (2).

Studies in germ-free and conventional rats have shown that intestinal bacteria are solely responsible for the azo bond reduction, the initial step of sulfasalazine metabolism (3). Conventional rats given sulfasalazine excrete 5-aminosalicylate and sulfapyridine (and their respective conjugates) in urine and feces, whereas germ-free rats show no evidence of sulfasalazine degradation. A study of a wide variety of intestinal bacteria found in the gastrointestinal tracts of humans and experimental animals reveals that these bacteria possess an intracellular azo reductase inhibitable by oxygen that reduces the azo bond of sulfasalazine, releasing 5-aminosalicylate and sulfapyridine (3,4). In humans, this reduction takes place largely in the colon as is strongly suggested by the findings of studies comparing the metabolism of the drug in patients with ileostomies and those with intact colons (5,6). In patients with colons, little intact drug is found in the feces. In patients with ileostomies, most of the drug is recovered unchanged in ileostomy effluent. Moreover, the administration of broad-spectrum antibiotics and an acceleration of intestinal transit time result in a decrease in the breakdown of sulfasalazine (7,8).

After azo bond reduction, most sulfapyridine is absorbed from the colon, partially metabolized, and excreted in the urine as the free sulfonamide or as its metabolites the acetyl and glucuronide derivatives (7). Sulfapyridine is detected in the blood 3–5 hr after oral administration of sulfasalazine, a time consistent with the transit time of the parent drugs to sites of azo bond reduction in the colon (1). Sulfapyridine, like isoniazid and hydralazine, is subject to polymorphic acetylation. Persons who are slow acetylators tend to have higher serum levels of total sulfapyridine (9). 5-Aminosalicylate, however, remains largely in the colon. Only a small portion of this metabolite is absorbed and excreted in the urine, as the acetylated derivative. Most 5-aminosalicylate is recovered unchanged in the feces, but some may be found in the acetylated form (7). Studies suggest that 5-aminosalicylate may be subject to gut wall as well as systemic acetylation (10).

When 5-aminosalicylate and sulfapyridine are administered as single agents orally, both are absorbed promptly in the proximal gastrointestinal tract, metabolized by the liver, and excreted in the urine (1).

Distribution studies showing that sulfasalazine is almost fully metabolized in the colon suggested that the parent drug may act as a vehicle for delivery of one or more of its metabolites to distal disease sites (7). Recovery of the drug primarily as 5-aminosalicylate in the feces raised the possibility that this metabolite is the therapeutically active moiety of sulfasalazine, whereas the demonstration that sulfapyridine is the principal portion of the drug found in serum suggested that the sulfonamide component of sulfasalazine may be responsible for most of the drug's toxicity.

II. CLINICAL INVESTIGATIONS

A. Ulcerative Colitis

The first report of a randomized controlled trial of sulfasalazine in 1962 fully supported prior anecdotal observations of the drug's efficacy in the treatment of ulcerative colitis (11,12). Patients with mild symptoms with a variable extent of disease were treated for 3 weeks with sulfasalazine (4 g/day for 1 week and then 2 g/day for 2 weeks), placebo, or salicylazosulfadimidine (a compound similar to sulfasalazine but with substitution of the sulfonamide). Improvement was defined as diminution in symptoms and improvement in sigmoidoscopic appearance. Of 20 patients on the drug, 16 compared with 7 of 20 given placebo and 3 of 10 given the salicylazosulfadimidine improved.

In a subsequent study, patients with ulcerative proctitis and colitis with mild to moderate symptoms were treated for 1 month with sulfasalazine (4-6 g/day or placebo) (13). As in the prior study, 78% of patients given sulfasalazine improved, compared with only 30% who received placebo. In a study with a different design, sulfasalazine was compared with low-dose prednisone and hydrocortisone retention enemas used in combination (14). Response to the steroid therapy was judged to be more rapid and overall more effective than that of sulfasalazine. These authors suggested the combined use of sulfasalazine and corticosteroids, but no controlled trials of the role of sulfasalazine as an adjunct to steroid therapy in patients with ulcerative colitis have been reported. The place of sulfasalazine in the treatment of patients with severe ulcerative colitis also has not been studied, although early use of the drug in such patients once a response to systemic steroids has been shown has been advocated (15).

Further studies have established an important role for sulfasalazine in maintaining remissions of ulcerative colitis. This role is especially important since corticosteroids in both oral and enema forms are not effective in preventing disease relapse (16). Patients who had a well-documented episode of ulcerative colitis within the preceding year and who were in remission according to clinical and sigmoidoscopic criteria were studied for 1 year, while they were given either sulfasalazine (2 g/day) or placebo. In the sulfasalazine-treated group, 24 of 34 patients (70%) remained symptom free compared with only 8 of 33 patients (24%) given placebo (17).

Whether sulfasalazine therapy given for more than 1 year continues to provide prophylaxis against remissions of ulcerative colitis was initially unclear, because of conflicting results obtained from two studies. In one, the criterion for entry was only that a patient have a history of ulcerative colitis with no symptoms for 1 year while on a regimen of 2 g of sulfasalazine (18). Patients were randomly assigned to receive either further sulfasalazine therapy or placebo. At the end of 6 months, 6 of 25 patients given sulfasalazine and 7 of 24 patients given placebo had a recurrence of symptoms. The authors concluded that 75% of patients in remission after 1 year on a regimen of sulfasalazine would remain symptom free for at least 6 months once therapy with the drug was stopped and that the use of the drug beyond 1 year was no more effective than the use of the placebo.

These results contrasted with those of a similar study wherein 64 patients in remission for at least 1 year on treatment with 2 g of sulfasalazine were randomly assigned to receive either placebo or further sulfasalazine therapy (19). Unlike the earlier study (18), criteria for admission included a normal sigmoidoscopic appearance and no significant inflammation on rectal biopsy samples, as well as a lack of symptoms. At the end of 6 months, 17 of 31 patients (55%) given placebo had a relapse (clinical symptoms, plus sigmoidoscopic and biopsy evidence of inflammation) but only 4 of 33 patients (12%) given the sulfasalazine had evidence of disease activity.

Several subsequent studies of patients with ulcerative colitis compared the prophylactic effect of sulfasalazine with that of a high-fiber diet or mast cell stabilizers such as cromoglycate. Each study has shown convincingly that the relapse rate is significantly higher in patients going off sulfasalazine therapy regardless of the length of the previous remission while on drug therapy (20-23). Therefore, sulfasalazine therapy continued beyond 1 year seems likely to provide continued prophylaxis against relapses of the disease. The optimum dose of sulfasalazine for maintenance therapy has been studied as well. The relapse rate over a 6-month period was significantly greater in patients maintained on 1 g/day than in those given the conventional 2 g/day dose (24). Patients had fewer relpases on 4 g/day than 2 g/day, but more than one-third of the patients maintained on the higher dose had intolerable side effects.

B. Crohn's Disease

As was the experience with ulcerative colitis, initial uncontrolled observations suggested that sulfasalazine was useful in the therapy of Crohn's disease (25-27).

In 1974 a controlled double-blind study involving a small number of patients found sulfasalazine (3 g/day) to be significantly more effective than placebo in patients with active Crohn's disease who had no prior surgery (28). However, in patients with a prior resection and recurrent disease, no benefit of the drug was noted. No comment was made about disease distribution in this group of patients.

Subsequently, three randomized controlled trials have confirmed the efficacy of sulfasalazine in Crohn's disease. Results from the National Cooperative Crohn's Disease Study showed that over a 4-month period sulfasalazine was effective in treating patients with Crohn's colitis and ileocolitis; however, no benefit of the drug could be shown in patients with ileitis alone (29). A subsequent European cooperative study confirmed these findings (30). These studies used both subjective and objective parameters to define disease activity. The third study that used primarily objective parameters of disease activity such as fever, sedimentation rate, and serum albumin levels found that 8 of 13 patients given sulfasalazine (4-6 g/day) had a favorable response compared with 1 of 13 patients given placebo (31). Improvement generally occurred in the first 4-8 weeks of the 6-month study and was then maintained throughout the study. In contrast to the results of the other two investigations (29,30), patients with ileitis alone, as well as colitis and ileocolitis responded to sulfasalazine treatment. However, the small number of patients studies who had ileitis alone makes it difficult to derive a conclusion from the data. A more recent retrospective review of 23 years of therapy of ileitis with sulfasalazine suggested that 25% of patients will respond at times with total regression of clinical and radiologic abnormalities (32).

An investigation of the role of sulfasalazine as adjunctive therapy found the combination of sulfasalazine and prednisone to be less effective than prednisone alone in the treatment of patients with active Crohn's disease (33). Moreover, sulfasalazine was not effective as a steroid-sparing agent in allowing a more rapid or complete withdrawal of prednisone treatment in patients with quiescent disease. Unfortunately, unlike the case in ulcerative colitis, sulfasalazine has not been shown to be beneficial in maintaining remission in Crohn's disease regardless of distribution (29,30,34). In the National Crohn's Study (29), a 25% flare-up rate occurred in one year and a 40% flare-up rate in two years, regardless of whether the patients were on placebo or drug treatment. The doses used in these studies were 2-3 g/day. Higher maintenance doses may have been more beneficial, but are generally less well tolerated.

Three other studies have evaluated the effect of sulfasalazine in preventing recurrence of Crohn's disease in patients after surgery. In one study, the combination of sulfasalazine and prednisone had no effect on the recurrence of Crohn's disease over a 33-week postoperative period (35). The National Crohn's Disease Study found similar results in a one- to two-year follow-up (29).

However, in a study with an 18-month follow-up, 9 of 34 patients given placebo had a recurrence postoperatively compared with 4 of 32 patients given sulfasalazine at a dose of 3 g/day (36). This study suggested a trend in favor of sulfasalazine therapy but the results were not significant statistically.

C. Use During Pregnancy and Nursing

Concern over the use of sulfasalazine during pregnancy has been fostered by findings of high concentrations of the drug and its metabolites in the mature placenta and fetal tissues of experiemtnal animals (37,38).

Although both sulfasalazine and sulfapyridine also appear in the milk of nursing mothers, both have poor bilirubin-displacing capabilities, likely accounting for the lack of reported cases of kernicterus (39,40). The accumulated evidence suggests that sulfasalazine therapy can be continued throughout pregnancy as maintenance in women with ulcerative colitis and that in pregnant women not taking the medication, the drug can be used to treat flareups of both ulcerative colitis and Crohn's disease in the same manner as the drug would be used if the women were not pregnant (41,42). There is no evidence to indicate that the medication should be stopped as the date of delivery nears due to the possible risk of neonatal hyperbilirubinemia or that use of the drug by a nursing mother will harm the newborn. Chapter 11 goes into more detail on these issues in the therapy of inflammatory bowel disease during pregnancy and nursing.

D. Use in Other Disorders

Sulfasalazine has been reported in a uncontrolled trial to be useful in patients with severe radiation bowel disease (43) as well as in collagenous colitis (44). The drug also has been used with success in scleroderma (45) and dermatitis herpetiformis (46). There has been a reawakening of interest in the use of the drug in rheumatologic disorders. Recent controlled trials in patients with rheumatoid arthritis and ankylosing spondylitis indicate improvement in clinical as well as laboratory parameters (47,48).

Knowledge of the pharmacokinetics of sulfasalazine has led to its use as a method of measuring mouth to cecum transit time in humans. Because sulfapyridine normally is detected in the serum at 3-5 hr after sulfasalazine administration, a delayed or rapid intestinal transit time can be determined by analyzing the time course of serum sulfapyridine levels (49). Similarly, the early detection of sulfapyridine in blood and urine has been shown both in experimental animals with blind loops (50) and in patients with jejunal diverticula (51) to correlate with the presence of bacterial overgrowth in the proximal small intestine. Use of this pharmacokinetic data provides another method for the detection of bacterial overgrowth syndromes.

E. Sulfasalazine Analogues

Since 1977 several randomized controlled trials have established the efficacy and safety of topical 5-aminosalicylate in enema and suppository form for the therapy of distal ulcerative colitis (52-55). An analogue of 5-aminosalicylate, 4-aminosalicylate also has been shown to be effective in topical form (56,57). Moreover, topical 5-aminosalicylate is effective prophylactically in preventing relapses of distal ulcerative colitis in remission (58).

More recently, several oral formulations of 5-aminosalicylate have been shown to be effective in the therapy of active ulcerative colitis and as prophylactic agents to prevent relapses (59-62). Studies of both topical and oral aminosalicylates in Crohn's disease are underway and early results are encouraging (63). Moreover, about 80% patients intolerant or allergic to sulfsalazine are able to take the topical or oral aminosalicylates without adverse effect (64). The status of these new sulfasalazine-based aminosalicylate drugs is discussed in detail in Chapter 4.

The trials with 5-aminosalicylte have renewed interest in the delivery of sulfasalazine by enema. Enemas containing sulfasalazine were effective in inducing clinical and sigmoidoscopic remission in patients with proctitis or left-sided colitis, including patients who had a prior subtotal colectomy or ileostomy. Sulfasalazine enemas were well tolerated by all patients, even those who had previously displayed intolerance to the oral preparation (65,66). Scintiscan studies of technetium-labeled sulfasalazine have shown the homogeneous distribution of the drug beyond the rectum in enema form which spreads as far as the ascending colon in several patients (67).

F. Recommendations for Therapy

Based on the accumulated experience, sulfasalazine can be recommended as the initial therapeutic choice in patients with ulcerative colitis who have mild to moderate symptoms. Although 4 g/day is the maximum dose tolerated by most patients, a few patients will tolerate higher levels and respond better to doses of up to 6 g/day. Therapy with the drug can be continued indefinitely with benefit as prophylaxis in such patients who have gone into remission. In patients whose disease flares up on the standard maintenance dose of 2 g/day, it is reasonable to try the drug at a higher dose for subsequent prophylaxis as long as it is tolerated.

In the same manner, sulfasalazine is a reasonable initial choice in patients with active Crohn's disease. The decision to use the drug in patients with ileitis alone is not fully supported by the existing data. Nevertheless, because a subpopulation of such patients may respond to the drug, and because corticosteroids are the major treatment alternative, an initial therapeutic attempt with sulfasalazine seems warranted. The drug does not appear to have a prophylactic role in patients with Crohn's disease once remission has been achieved, although in clinical practice, the drug is often continued for patients who do go into the remission, as is the case with ulcerative colitis. Until more information is available, routine use of the drug to prevent recurrences of Crohn's disease postoperatively is not indicated.

The ultimate role of the new topical and oral aminosalicylate preparations as alternatives to sulfasalazine or in conjunction with the drug is not clear. These considerations are dealt with in detail in Chapter 4.

III. MECHANISM OF ACTION

Although the pharmacokinetics of sulfasalazine has been clarified and its clinical efficacy proved, the mechanism of action of the drug remains unclear. Early speculations on sulfasalazine's mechanism of action focused on studies of histologic changes in the connective tissue associated with ulcerative colitis as well as observations in experimental animals showing that the drug and its metabolite 5-aminosalicylate have a strong affinity for connective tissue (68,69).

A possible antibacterial mode of action of the drug has been suggested because of the sulfonamide component. Moreover, uncontrolled data in patients with rheumatoid arthritis suggest the sulfapyridine moiety, but not 5-ASA is therapeutically active (70). Initial studies were not able to show any change in fecal flora ascribable to sulfasalazine (71), but a subsequent investigation using improved isolation techniques has shown that patients taking sulfasalazine have a significant diminution in the population of certain clostridial organisms, nonsporing anaerobes, and aerobic enterobacteria (72). However, the decrease in levels of these bacteria did not correlate with the patients' disease activity.

Because immunologic mechanisms may be important in the pathogenesis of inflammatory bowel disease, the possible effects of sulfasalazine on systemic and local immunity have been studied. Previously, sulfasalazine, and to a lesser extent sulfapyridine, had been shown to inhibit mitogen-induced in vitro cytotoxicity by human lymphocytes (73). Studies of patients with both ulcerative colitis and Crohn's disease, however, have shown that neither sulfasalazine nor either of its metabolites alters several subpopulations of circulating mononuclear cells in vivo or in vitro (74). Moreover, no inhibition of antibody-dependent cellular cytotoxicity or change in skin test reactivity was seen. Further data indicate that sulfasalazine does not exert a benefical action by effects on suppressor T-cell activity (75). Neither the drug nor its metabolites alter immunoglobulin production by peripheral blood mononuclear cells (76).

Much investigation has focused on sulfasalazine's possible effect on prostaglandin synthesis and metabolism. Compared with normal persons and patients with ulcerative colitis in remission, patients with active ulcerative colitis have increased levels of various prostaglandins in feces, colorectal venous plasma, urine, and cultures of rectal mucosal biopsy specimens (77,78). Moreover, sulfasalazine, 5-aminosalicylate, and N-acetyl-5-aminosalicylate have been shown to be inhibitors of prostaglandin biosynthesis in vitro through inhibitory effects on prostaglandin synthetase (cyclo-oxygenase). The observed effects of sulfasalazine in vitro in converting net sodium and water secretion in diseased colon to net absorption could relate to an effect on local prostaglandin production, although one study suggests an independent mechanism (79,80).

Although many aspects of this model fit, some important observations argue against inhibition of prostaglandin synthesis as the mechanism of action of sulfasalazine. Indomethacin and fluriboprofen are considerably more potent prostaglandin inhibitors than sulfasalazine and 5-aminosalicylate (81). When patients with inflammatory bowel diseases are treated with nonsteroidal anti-inflammatory drugs, the prostaglandin levels in their serum and rectal mucosa decline, but their clinical condition does not improve (82,83). Indeed, evidence is emerging that indicate such nonsteroidal anti-inflammatory drugs may exacerbate inflammatory bowel disease (84). These findings suggests that prostaglandins may not be important mediators of inflammation in IBD and that the mode of action of sulfasalazine or 5-aminosalicylate is not inhibition of prostaglandin synthesis.

An alternative hypothesis has used data showing that sulfasalazine inhibits prostaglandin F_2 breakdown and that 5-aminosalicylate in low concentrations actually enhances prostacycline formation (85). These data have led to speculation that sulfasalazine or 5-aminosalicylate may work by increasing local levels of prostaglandins which may act in a cytoprotective manner in the colon as has been suggested in the stomach. Problems with this proposal include the observation that the levels of 5-aminosalicylate found in the feces of patients with inflammatory bowel disease inhibit prostaglandin production, consistent with the finding that the prostaglandin levels decline after administration of therapeutic doses of sulfasalazine.

Another area of investigation has focused on the possible effects of sulfasalazine and its metabolites on the contribution of polymorphonuclear leukocytes to the inflammatory reaction. Both sulfasalazine and sulfapyridine inhibit the random migration of polymorphonuclear leukocytes as well as inhibiting superoxide production by them; 5-aminosalicylate and sulfapyridine inhibit myeloperoxidase-mediated iodination and cytotoxicity (86).

Some of these effects have been proposed to occur through inhibition of the lipoxygenase pathway. Although almost all mammalian cells contain cyclo-oxygenase, some cells, especially inflammatory cells, contain an alternate pathway of arachidonic acid metabolism, the lipoxygenase pathway. The major products of this pathway are the leukotrienes and certain hydroxy fatty acids, potent chemotactic agents which recruit inflammatory cells into sites of inflammation.

Sulfasalazine and 5-aminosalicylate block the synthesis of these products of the lipoxygenase pathway which are elevated in patients with active ulcerative colitis (87-89). Inhibition of the synthesis of these agents may account for some of the anti-inflammatory effects of sulfasalazine in inflammatory bowel disease. Awaited are clinical studies utilizing specific inhibitors of the lipoxygenase pathway.

A new area of investigation has focused on the interactions of sulfasalazine and 5-ASA with oxygen-derived free radicals. The "respiratory burst" of polymorphonuclear leukocytes and other phagocyte cells involved in the inflammatory response releases oxygen-derived species such as O_2 and H_2O_2 which are cytotoxic. Accumulating evidence suggests that sulfasalazine and 5-ASA, but not sulfapyridine may be cytoprotective by absorbing or scavenging oxygen-derived free radicals (90,91).

IV. DRUG INTERACTIONS

Several studies have shown an interaction between sulfasalazine and folic acid. In a group of patients with quiescent ulcerative colitis, the mean serum folate level was significantly lower in patients taking the drug than in those not taking it (92). An explanation for this finding, as shown in preparations of rat gut, has been that the absorption of folic acid is inhibited by sulfasalazine but not by either of its metabolites (93). Impairment of folic acid absorption by sulfasalazine was also noted both in patients with inflammatory bowel disease and in normal volunteers. Studies have also shown that sulfasalazine is a competitive inhibitor of the jejunal brush-border enzyme folate conjugase, which hydrolizes polyglutameal folate to the monoglutamate form for intestinal transport (94). This interference with dietary folate metabolism as well as the effect on folate transport provide mechanisms for folate malabsorption in patients taking sulfasalazine. Although not a major clinical problem, patients on sulfasalazine should take folic acid 1 mg/day.

Some patients with Crohn's disease involving the ileum may be on a regimen of both cholestyramine, a nonabsorbable anion exchange resin that binds bile acids, and sulfasalazine. Studies in rats have shown that the metabolism of sulfasalazine is markedly reduced by the concurrent administration of cholestyramine (95). In vitro data suggest that the mechanism of the decreased azo bond reduction of sulfasalazine relates to direct binding of sulfasalazine to cholestyramine in the gut lumen; in the bound state, the azo bond of sulfasalazine apparently is inaccessible to bacterial metabolism. Although no information is available about any effect of cholestyramine on sulfasalazine's clinical efficacy, this interaction should be considered in patients taking both agents.

A somewhat similar interaction has been reported between ferrous sulfate and sulfasalazine. Administration of both agents in healthy volunteers has resulted in decreased concentrations of intact sulfasalazine in serum, but has no effect on overall sulfasalazine metabolism (96). This effect can be attributed to a physical interaction between sulfasalazine and the iron. Although iron absorption would seem likely to be similarly affected, there are no studies of the possible influence of simultaneous administration of sulfasalazine on the bioavailability of iron. Because many patients take both iron and sulfasalazine, administering the drugs separately may be prudent.

Another agent with a possible interaction with sulfasalazine is digoxin. Studies in volunteers have shown that sulfasalazine interferes with the bioavailability of digoxin, causing a mean decrease of approximately 25% in serum digoxin levels (97). The reason for this apparent effect is not clear. No adsorption of digoxin by sulfasalazine in vitro has been shown.

Finally, in experimental animals and a few patients, sulfasalazine metabolism has been shown to be diminished by the concurrent administration of broad-spectrum antibiotics (7). This effect is not surprising, given the studies on metabolism of the drug. The effect is presumably related to a diminution in gut flora responsible for azo bond reduction. To date, however, there are no data as to whether the concurrent administration of antibiotics with sulfasalazine in patients with inflammatory bowel disease has any influence on the effectiveness of sulfasalazine.

V. ADVERSE REACTIONS

One limitation of the use of sulfasalazine has been the high incidence of complications in patients taking the drug. One review has found that 28 of 133 patients (21%) taking sulfasalazine had one or more side effects (98). The most common but least severe adverse reactions include nausea, vomiting, anorexia, and headache. Heartburn, epigastric distress, and diarrhea are occasionally seen as well (98,99).

Although serious adverse reactions involving almost every organ system have been noted, they are, in fact, uncommon. Various skin eruptions related to the use of sulfasalazine have been recognized, including urticaria, maculopapular lesions, and a blue discoloration resembling cyanosis not related to the development of methomoglobinemia or a diminished oxygen-carrying capacity of hemoglobin (100). The most serious skin reaction reported is toxic epidermal necrolysis (101,102). Studies of one patient with this disorder have shown that the patient's serum contained antibodies that reacted with his skin and monocytes only in the presence of sulfasalazine (102).

Bloody diarrhea in conjunction with fever and rash resembling an acute flare-up of ulcerative colitis has been reported in two children (103), and a sulfasalazine-associated relapse of ulcerative colitis and the development of iridocyclitis have been described in an adult patient (104). Reversible pancreatitis has been noted with sulfasalazine as with other drugs containing a sulfa moiety (105). Recently, a spectrum of hepatotoxicity related to sulfasalazine has emerged. The clinical and histologic features of liver disease reported include a reaction similar to acute viral hepatitis with very high serum transmission levels (106), cholestasis with high bilirubin and alkaline phosphatase levels (107), granulomatous hepatitis (108,109), and a mixed picture with mild to moderate elevations of transaminase, alkaline phosphatase, and bilirubin levels (110), and massive hepatic necrosis (111). Most patients with sulfasalazine-related hepatitis also have had fever and associated skin eruptions. Although corticosteroids have been used to treat some patients, most patients have had a total resolution of the hepatitis upon withdrawal of the sulfasalazine.

Pulmonary complications include one report of subacute fibrosing alveolitis that proved fatal (112), tracheolaryngitis with bronchospasm (113), and a clinical and radiologic picture resembling eosinophilic pneumonia (114–117). In these latter patients the onset of symptoms occurred 2 to 5 months after the patients began taking the drug, and dyspnea, cough, fever, and weight loss were the predominant symptoms and signs. Peripheral infiltrates on chest roentgenogram and eosinophilia completed the clinical picture. Cessation of sulfasalazine treatment led to resolution of the lung abnormalities and eosinophilia. Although patients with sulfasalazine-induced lung disease have had various abnormal pulmonary functions (118), no effect of the drug on diffusion capacity could be shown in a group of patients with inflammatory bowel disease (119).

A report has confirmed previous observations on the effects of sulfasalazine on heart rate (120). The mean resting heart rate in a group of patients with ulcerative colitis who received 3 to 6 g/day of sulfasalazine was 94 beats/min. This rate contrasted with that in matched controls on no therapy who had a mean rate of 77 beats/min. The salicylate moiety has been postulated to be directly responsible for the accelerated heart rate.

Effects of sulfasalazine on the hematopoietic system have been described repeatedly. Neutropenia and agranulocytosis are potentially devastating adverse reactions (121–123). Thrombocytopenia secondary to megakaryocytic aplasia also has been described (124). The effects on erythrocytes are the most frequently reported abnormalities and include red cell aplasia (124), megaloblastic anemia secondary to folic acid deficiency (125), and hemolytic anemia associated with glucose-6-phosphate dehydrogenase deficiency (126), as well as with Heinz bodies, methemoglobinemia, and sulfhemoglobinemia (127). At times, the hemolysis may be compensated, with only reticulocytosis evident. Pancytopenia caused apparently by interference with dietary folate absorption also has been noted (128).

Several patients taking sulfasalazine have had a generalized allergic reaction with fever, skin rash, arthralgias, and lymphadenopathy (129–131). In one patient, low complement levels and evidence of circulating immune complexes were present, whereas in others elevated titers of antinuclear antibodies and antibodies to double-stranded DNA were seen, consistent with a drug-induced lupus syndrome. Another patient had reversible Raynaud's phenomena without other evidence of a collagen vascular abnormality (132). Reversible neurotoxicity manifested as numbness, paresthesias, and ataxia also has been reported (133).

Finally, an additional potentially important adverse effect is male infertility. Several men with inflammatory bowel disease given sulfasalazine have had documented low sperm counts, abnormal sperm motility, and a higher number of sperm with abnormal morphology. To date, these changes have been reversible within weeks of stopping sulfasalazine treatment, with subsequent return of fertility (134-139). Aminosalicylates can be substituted for sulfasalazine in such cases without occurrence of the sperm defects (140,141). The incidence of this side effect is unknown, although in one study of 25 patients with inflammatory bowel disease (sulfasalazine dose, 2-4 g/day) 18 patients had a lower than normal sperm count within two months of beginning drug therapy (142). It has been speculated that sulfasalazine may produce a maturation arrest in spermatogenesis, and it is possible that an antifolate action of the drug suppresses the rapid turnover of cells that occurs in normal spermatogenesis. In addition, because prostaglandins can increase sperm motility in vitro, a possible antiprostaglandin effect of the drug in semen also has been suggested (137,139).

As has been the case in defining the possible mechanism of action of sulfasalazine, studies of the drug's metabolism and distribution have provided insights into the way in which adverse reactions are produced. The common side effects, including nausea, vomiting, and headache, have been directly related to the level of sulfapyridine in serum (98). Because patients who are slow acetylators and who are given large doses of sulfasalazine will tend to have the highest serum levels of sulfapyridine, it is not surprising that most side effects have been described in patients who are slow acetylators and who are taking doses of 4 g/day or greater (98). Side effects have not been correlated with serum levels of intact sulfasalazine or 5-aminosalicylate. In addition to the more common side effects, the occurrence of hemolysis in many patients also seems directly related to serum sulfapyridine levels and to the acetylator status of the patient (143).

Several investigators have shown that patients intolerant or allergic to sulfasalazine may tolerate the drug when it is reintroduced gradually in small doses. In 26 of 28 patients who had an adverse reaction to suflasalazine, including nausea, vomiting, and headache, as well as evidence of hemolysis, the drug treatments could be continued by lowering the daily dose by about 50% (98). These authors advocate discontinuance of sulfasalazine treatments for one to two weeks in patients who have nausea, vomiting, abdominal pain, headache, reticulocytosis, and mild rash; treatment then can be restarted at a dose of 0.125 to 0.25 g/day for 1 week, with a gradual increase by 0.125 g/week to a maintenance dose of 2 g/week (144). The dyspeptic side effects may be overcome by the use of enteric-coated tablets (145).

Desensitization to sulfasalazine has been successful in several patients who had fever and rash attributed to the drug. Treatment was begun at a dose of 1 mg/day which can be administered in a concentrated liquid form or 1/8 of a tablet per day and slowly advanced to the usual therapeutic doses over 2-4 weeks (146,147). The knowledge that minor side effects and mild allergic reactions can be overcome by dosage reduction or desensitization, along with the observations that the serious adverse reactions are rare, has added to the utility of sulfasalazine in therapy for inflammatory bowel disease.

REFERENCES

1. Schroder, H., D. E. S. Campbell, Absorption, metabolism, and excretion of salicylazosulfapyridine in man, Clin. Pharmacol. Ther., 13:539-551 (1972).
2. Das, K. M., J. R. Chowdhury, B. Zapp, J. W. Fara, Small bowel absorption of sulfasalazine and its hepatic metabolism in human beings, cats and rats, Gastroenterology, 77:280-284 (1979).
3. Peppercorn, M. A., P. Goldman, The role of intestinal bacteria in the metabolism of salicylazosulfapyridine, J. Pharm. Exp. Ther., 181:555-562 (1972).
4. Azad Khan, A. K., G. Guthrie, H. H. Johnston, S. C. Truelove, D. H. Williamson, Tissue and bacterial splitting of sulphasalazine, Clin. Sci., 64: 349-354 (1972).
5. Schroder, H., R. M. Lewkonia, D. A. Price Evans, Metabolism of salicylazosulfapyridine in healthy subjects and in patients with ulcerative colitis: Effects of colectomy and of phenobarbital, Clin. Pharmacol. Ther., 14: 802-809 (1973).
6. Das, E. M., M. A. Eastwood, J. P. McManus, W. Sircus, The role of the colon in the metabolism of salicylazosulfapyridine, Scand. J. Gastroenterol., 9:137-141 (1974).
7. Peppercorn, M. A., P. Goldman, Distribution studies of salicylazosulfapyridine and its metabolites. Gastroenterology, 64:240-245 (1973).
8. Van Hees, P. A. M., J. H. M. Tuinte, J. M. Van Rossum, J. H. Van Tongeren, Influence of intestinal transit times on azo-reduction of salicylazosulphapyridine (Salazopyrin), Gut, 20:300-304 (1979).
9. Das, K. M., M. A. Eastwood, Acetylation polymorphism of sulfapyridine in patients with ulcerative colitis and Crohn's disease, Clin. Pharmacol. Ther., 18(5 pg. 1):514-520 (1975).
10. Pieniaszer, H. J., Jr., T. R. Bates, Capacity-limited gut wall metabolism of 5-aminosalicylic acid, a therapeutically active metabolite of sulfasalazine, in rats, J. Pharm. Sci., 68:1323-1325 (1979).
11. Svartz, N., The treatment of ulcerative colitis, Gastroenterologia, 86:683 (1956).

12. Baron, J. H., P. M. Connell, J. E. Lennard-Jones, et al., Sulphasalazine and salicylazosulphadimidine in ulcerative colitis, Lancet, 1:1094–1096 (1962).
13. Dick, A. P., M. J. Grayson, R. G. Carpenter, et al., Controlled trial of sulphasalazine in the treatment of ulcerative colitis, Gut, 5:437–442 (1964).
14. Truelove, S. C., G. Watkinson, G. Draper, Comparison of corticosteroid and sulphasalazine therapy in ulcerative colitis, Br. Med. J., 2:1708–1711 (1962).
15. Truelove, S. C., C. P. Willoughby, E. G. Lee, M. G. Kettlewell, Further experience in the treatment of severe attacks of ulcerative colitis, Lancet, 2:1086–1088 (1978).
16. Lennard-Jones, J. E., J. J. Misiewicz, A. M. Connell, Prednisone as maintenance treatment for ulcerative colitis in remission, Lancet, 1:188–189 (1965).
17. Misiewicz, J. J., J. E. Lennard-Jones, A. M. Connell, Controlled trial of sulphasalazine in maintenance therapy for ulcerative colitis, Lancet, 1: 185–188 (1965).
18. Riis, P., P. Anthonisen, H. R. Wulff, O. Folkenborg, O. Bonnevie, V. Binder, The prophylactic effect of salazosulphapyridine in ulcerative colitis during long-term treatment: a double-blind trial on patients asymptomatic for one year, Scand. J. Gastroenterol., 8:71–74 (1973).
19. Dissanayake, A. S., S. C. Truelove, A controlled therapeutic trial of long-term maintenance treatment of ulcerative colitis with sulphasalazine, Gut, 14:923–926 (1973).
20. Davies, P. S., J. Rhodes, Maintenance of remission in ulcerative colitis with sulphasalazine or a high-fibre diet: A clinical trial, Br. Med. J., 1:1524–1525 (1978).
21. Dronfield, M. W., M. J. S. Langman, Comparative trial of sulphasalazine and oral sodium cromoglycate in the maintenance of remission in ulcerative colitis, Gut, 19:1136–1139 (1978).
22. Willoughby, C. P., M. F. Heyworth, J. Piris, S. C. Truelove, Comparison of disodium cromoglycate and sulphasalazine as maintenance therapy for ulcerative colitis, Lancet, 1:119–122 (1979).
23. Davies, P. S., J. Rhodes, B. Counsell, B. K. Evans, Maintenance of remission in ulcerative colitis: Effect of an orally absorbed mast cell stabilizer, Am. J. Gastroenterol., 74:150–153 (1980).
24. Azad Khan, A. K., D. T. Howes, J. Piris, S. C. Truelove, Optimum dose of sulphasalazine for maintenance treatment in ulcerative colitis, Gut, 21: 232–240 (1980).
25. Goldstein, F., M. G. Murdock, Clinical and radiologic improvement of regional enteritis and enterocolitis after treatment with salicylazosulfapyridine, Am. J. Dig. Dis., 16:421–431 (1971).
26. Goldstein, F., J. J. Thornton, Objective and subjective improvement with drug treatment in Crohn's disease (abstract), Gastroenterology, 66:702 (1974).

27. Goldstein, F., J. J. Thornton, J. Abramson, Anti-inflammatory drug treatment in Crohn's disease, Am. J. Gastroenterol., 66:251–258 (1976).
28. Anthonisen, P., F. Barany, O., Folkenborg, et al., The clinical effect of salazosulphapyridine (Salazopyrin) in Crohn's disease: a controlled double-blind study, Scand. J. Gastroenterol., 9:549–554 (1974).
29. Summers, R. W., D. M. Switz, J. T. Sessions, et al., National Cooperative Crohn's Disease Study: Results of drug treatment, Gastroenterology, 77(4 pt. 2):847–869 (1979).
30. Malchow, H., K. Ewe, J. W. Brandes, et al., European Cooperative Crohn's Disease Study: Results of drug treatment: Gastroenterology, 86:249–266 (1984).
31. Van Hees, P. A. M., H. J. J. Van Lier, P. H. Van Eltern, et al., Effect of sulphasalazine in patients with active Crohn's disease: A controlled double-blind study, Gut, 22:404–409 (1981).
32. Goldstein, F., S. Farquhar, J. J. Thornton, J. Abramson, Favorable effects of sulfasalazine on small bowel Crohn's disease: A long-term study, Am. J. Gastroenterol., 82(9):848–853 (1987).
33. Singleton, J. W., R. W. Summers, F. Kern, Jr., A trial of sulfasalazine as adjunctive therapy in Crohn's disease, Gastroenterology, 77(4 pt 2):887–897 (1979).
34. Lennard-Jones, J. E., Sulphasalazine in asymptomatic Crohn's disease: A multicentre trial, Gut, 18:69–76 (1977).
35. Bergman, L., U. Krause, Postoperative treatment with corticosteroids and salazosulphapyridine (Salazopyrin) after radical resection for Crohn's disease, Scand. J. Gastroenterol., 11:651–656 (1976).
36. Wenkert, A., M. Kristensen, A. E. Eklund, The long-term prophylactic effect os salazosulphapyridine (Salazopyrin) in primarily resected patients with Crohn's disease: A controlled double-blind trial, Scand. J. Gastroenterol., 13:161–167 (1978).
37. Hanngren, A., E. Hansson, N. Svartz, Distribution and metabolism of salicyl-azo-sulfapyridine: 1. A study with C^{14} salicyl-azo-sulfaypridine and C^{14} 5-aminosalicylic acid, Acta Med. Scand., 173:61–72 (1963).
38. Gluckmann, R. F., Sulfasalazine, IBD, and pregnancy (letter), Gastroenterology, 81:194 (1981).
39. Azad Khan, A. K., S. C. Truelove, Placental and mammary transfer of sulphasalazine, Br. Med. J., 11:1553 (1979).
40. Jarnerot, G., M. B. Into-Malmberg, Sulphasalazine treatment during breast feeding, Scand. J. Gastroenterol., 14:869–871 (1979).
41. Mogadam, M., W. O. III. Dobbins, B. I. Korelitz, S. W. Ahmed, Pregnancy in inflammatory bowel disease: Effect of sulfasalazine and corticosteroids on fetal outcome, Gastroenterology, 80:72–76 (1981).
42. Willoughby, C. P., S. C. Truelove, Ulcerative colitis and pregnancy, Gut, 21: 469–474 (1980).
43. Goldstein, F., J. Khoury, J. J. Thornton, Treatment of chronic radiation enteritis and colitis with salicylazosulfapyridine and systemic corticosteroids: A pilot study, Am. J. Gastroenterol., 65:201–208 (1976).

44. Weidner, N., J. Smith, B. PaHee, Sulfasalazine in treatment of collagenous colitis. Case report and review of the literature, Am. J. Med., 77:102–106 (1984).
45. Dover, N., Salazopyrin (azulfidine) treatment in scleroderma, Isr. J. Med. Sci., 7:301–303 (1971).
46. Andreozzi, R. J., D. D. Nuss, Dermatitis herpetiformis: Treatment with azulfidine, Cutis, 13:366–370 (1974).
47. Pinals, R. S., S. B. Kaplan, J. G. Lawson, B. Hepburn, Sulfasalazine in rheumatoid arthritis. A double-blind placebo-controlled trial, Arthritis Rheum., 29:1427–1434 (1986).
48. Dougados, M., P. Boumier, B. Amor, Sulphasalazine in ankylosing spondylitis: A double-blind controlled study in 60 patients, Br. Med. J., 293:911–914 (1986).
49. Kennedy, M., P. Chinwah, D. N. Wade, A pharmacological method of measuring mouth caecal transit time in man, Br. J. Clin. Pharmacol., 8: 372–373 (1979).
50. Peppercorn, M. A., T. Amnway, D. Fromm, P. Goldman, Detection of bacterial overgrowth by analysis of drug metabolites, Gastroenterology, 70: 926 (1976).
51. Thithapandha, A., Detection of human intestinal bacterial overgrowth by sulfasalazine, J. Clin. Pharmacol., 18:549–555 (1978).
52. Azad Khan, A. K., J. Piris, S. C. Truelove, An experiment to determine the active therapeutic moiety of sulphasalazine, Lancet, 2:892–895 (1977).
53. Van Hees, P. A. M., J. H. Bakker, J. H. M. Van Tongeren, Effect of sulfphapyridine, 5-aminosalicylic acid, and placebo in patients with idiopathic proctitis: A study to determine the active therapeutic moiety of sulphasalazine, Gut, 21:632–635 (1980).
54. Klotz, U., K. Maier, G. Fischer, K. Heinkel, Therapeutic efficacy of sulfasalazine and its metabolites in patients with ulcerative colitis and Crohn's disease, N. Engl. J. Med., 303:1499–1502 (1980).
55. Campieri, M., G. A. Lanfranchi, G. Bazzocchi, Treatment of ulcerative colitis with high-dose 5-aminosalicylic acid enemas, Lancet, 2:270–271 (1981).
56. Campieri, M., G. A. Lanfranchi, F. Bertoni, 4-Aminosalicylic acid and 5-aminosalicylic acid in topical treatment of ulcerative colitis patients (abstract), Gastroenterology, 86:1039 (1984).
57. Ginsberg, A. L., W. M. Steinberg, L. E. Nochomovitz, Evaluation of 4-aminosalicylate enemas in patients with left sided ulcerative colitis (abstract), Gastroenterology, 86:1089 (1984).
58. Biddle, W. L., N. J. Greenberger, J. T. Swan, N. S. Mephee, P. B. Jr. Miuer, 5-aminosalicylic acid enemas: Effective agent in maintaining remission in left-sided ulcerative colitis, Gastroenterology, 94:1075–1079 (1988).
59. Peppercorn, M. A., Sulfasalazine: Pharmacology clinical use, toxicity and related new drug development, Ann. Intern. Med., 3:377–386 (1984).

60. Schroeder, H. W., W. J. Tremaive, D. M. Listore, Coated oral 5-aminosalicylic acid: Therapy for mildly to moderate active ulcerative colitis, N. Engl. J. Med., 284:1291-1292 (1987).
61. Dew, M. J., A. D. Harris, N. Evans, B. K. Evans, J. Rhodes, Maintenance of remission in ulcerative colitis with 5-aminosalicylic acid in high doses by mouth, Br. Med. J., 287:23-24 (1983).
62. Riley, S. A., V. Mani, M. J. Goodman, M. G. Herd, L. A. Turnberg, Comparison of delayed release 5-aminosalicylic acid and sulfasalazine as maintenance treatment for patients with ulcerative colitis, Gastroenterology, 94: 1383-1389 (1988).
63. Rasmussen, S. N., V. Binder, K. Maier, Treatment of Crohn's disease with peroral 5-aminosalicylic acid, Gastroenterology, 85:1350-1353 (1983).
64. Rao, S. S., P. A. Cann, C. D. Holdsworth, Clinical experience of the tolerance of mesalazine and olsalazine in patients intolerant of sulphasalazine, Scand. J. Gastroenterol., 22:332-336 (1987).
65. Palmer, K. R., J. R. Goepei, C. D. Holdsworth, Sulphasalazine retention enemas in ulcerative colitis: A double-blind trial, Br. Med. J. (Clin. Res.), 282:1571-1573 (1981).
66. Gallone, L., L. Olmi, U. Marchetti, Use of topical rectal therapy to preserve the rectum in surgery of ulcerative colitis, World J. Surg., 4:609-613 (1980).
67. Kruis, W., U. Bull, Eisenburg, G. Paumgartner, Retrograde colonic spread of sulphasalazine enemas, Scand. J. Gastroenterol., 17:933-938 (1982).
68. Levine, M. D., J. B. Kirsner, A. P. Klotz, A new concept of the pathogenesis of ulcerative colitis, Science, 114:552-553 (1951).
69. Hanngren, A., E. Hansson, N. Svartz, Distribution and metabolism of salicyl-azo-sulfapyridine. Acta Med. Scand., 173:391-399 (1963).
70. Neumann, V. C., A. J. Taggart, P. LeGallez, C. Astburg, J. Hill, H. A. Bird, A study to determine the active moiety of sulphasalazine in rheumatoid arthritis, J. Rheumatol., 13:285-287 (1986).
71. Cooke, E. M., Faecal flora of patients with ulcerative colitis during treatment with salicylazosulfapyridine, Gut, 10:565-568 (1969).
72. West, B., R. Lendrum, M. J. Hill, Effects of sulphasalazine on faecal flora in patients with inflammatory bowel disease, Gut, 15:960-965 (1974).
73. Holm, G., P. Perlmann, Cytotoxicity of lymphocytes and its suppression, Antibiot. Chemother., 15:295-309 (1969).
74. Thayer, W. R. Jr., C. Charland, C. E. Field, Effects of sulfasalazine on selected lymphocyte subpopulations in vivo and in vitro, Dig. Dis. Sci., 24:672-679 (1979).
75. Holdstock, G., E. F. Chastenay, E. L. Krawitt, Functional suppressor T cell activity in Crohn's disease and the effects of sulphasalazine, Clin. Exp. Immunol., 48:619-624 (1982).
76. Holdstock, G., W. B. Ershler, E. L. Krawitt, Defective lymphocyte IgA production in inflammatory bowel disease, Clin. Immunol. Immunopathol., 24:47-54 (1982).

77. Sharon, P., M., Ligumsky, D. Racmilewitz, U. Zor, Role of prostaglandins in ulcerative colitis: Enhanced production during active disease and inhibition by sulfasalazine, Gastroenterology, 75:638–640 (1978).
78. Smith, P. R., D. J. Dawson, C. H. J. Swan, Prostaglandin synthetase activity in acute ulcerative colitis: effects of treatment with sulphasalazine, codeine phosphate and prednisolone, Gut, 20:802–805 (1978).
79. Harris, J., E. Q. Archampong, C. G. Clark, The effect of salazopyrin on water and electrolyte transport in the human colon measured in vivo and in vitro, Gut, 13:855 (1972).
80. Rampton, D. S., G. E. Sladen, The effects of sulphasalazine withdrawal on rectal mucosal function and prostaglandin E2 release in inactive ulcerative colitis, Scand. J. Gastroenterol., 16:157–159 (1981).
81. Hawkey, C. J., M. Lo Casto, Inhibition of prostaglandin synthetase in human rectal mucosa, Gut, 24:213–217 (1983).
82. Gilat, T., J. Ratan, Y. Peled, Prostaglandins and ulcerative colitis (letter), Gastroenterology, 76(5 pt. 1):1083 (1979).
83. Rampton, D. S., G. E. Sladen, Prostaglandin synthesis inhibitors in ulcerative colitis: flurbiprofen compared with conventional treatment, Prostaglandins, 21:417–425 (1981).
84. Kaufman, H. J., H. L. Taubin, Nonsteroidal anti-inflammatory drugs activate quiescent inflammatory bowel disease, Ann. Intern. Med., 107:513–516 (1987).
85. Kolassa, N., R. Becher, H. Weiner, Influence of sulfasalazine, 5-aminosalicylic acid and sulfapyridine on prostanoid synthesis and metabolism in rabbit colonic mucosa, Prostaglandins, 1:133–142 (1985).
86. Molin, L., O. Stendahl, The effect of sulfasalazine and its active components in human polymorphonuclear leukocyte function in relation to ulcerative colitis, Acta Med. Scand., 206:451–457 (1979).
87. Nielsoen, O. H., K. Bukhave, J. Elmgreen, J. Ahufelt-Rovne, Inhibition of 5-lipoxygenase pathway of arachadonic acid metabolism in human neutrophils by sulfasalazine and 5-aminosalicylic acid, Dig. Dis. Sci., 6:577–582 (1987).
88. Stenson, W. F., E. Lobos, Sulfasalazine inhibits the synthesis of chemotactic lipids by neutrophils, J. Clin. Invest., 69:494–497 (1982).
89. Sircar, J. C., C. F. Schwender, M. E. Carethers, Inhibition of soybean lipoxygenase by sulfasalazine and 5-aminosalicylic acid: a possible mode of action in ulcerative colitis, Biochem. Pharmacol., 32:170–172 (1983).
90. Craven, P. A., J. Planstiel, R. Saito, F. R. DeRubertis, Actions of sulfasalazine and 5-aminosalicylic acid as reactive oxygen scavengers in the suppression of bile acid-induced increases in colonic epithelial cell loss and proliferative activity, Gastroenterology, 92:1998–2008 (1987).
91. Dull, B. J., K. Salata, A. Van Langenhove, P. Goldman, 5-Aminosalicylate: Oxidation by activated leukocytes and protection of cultured cells from oxidative damage, Biochem. Pharmacol., 36:2467–2472 (1987).

92. Halsted, C. H., G. Gandhi, T. Tamura, Sulfasalazine inhibits the absorption of folates in ulcerative colitis, N. Engl. J. Med., 305:1513–1517 (1981).
93. Franklin, J. L., I. H. Rosenberg, Impaired folic acid absorption in inflammatory bowel disease: effects of salicylazosulfapyridine (azulfidine), Gastroenterology, 64:517–525 (1973).
94. Reisenauer, A. M., C. H. Halsted, Human jejunal brush border folate conjugase: Characteristics and inhibition by salicylazosulfapyridine, Biochem. Biophys. Acta, 659:62–69 (1981).
95. Pieniaszek, H. J., T. R. Bates, Cholestyramine-induced inhibition of salicylazosulfapyridine (sulfasalazine) metabolism by rat intestinal microflora, J. Pharmacol. Exp. Ther., 198:240–245 (1976).
96. Das, K. M., M. A. Eastwood, Effect of iron and calcium on salicylazosulfapyridine metabolism, Scot. Med. J., 18:45-50 (1973).
97. Juhl, R. P., R. W. Summers, J. K. Guillory, S. M. Blaug, F. H. Cheng, D. D. Brown, Effect of sulfasalazine on digoxin bioavailability, Clin. Pharmacol. Ther., 20:387–394 (1976).
98. Das, K. M., M. A. Eastwood, J. P. McManus, W. Sircus, Adverse reactions during salicylazosulfapyridine therapy and the relation with drug metabolism and acetylator phenotype, N. Engl. J. Med., 289:491–495 (1973).
99. Singleton, J. W., D. H. Law, L. M. Kelly, Jr., H. S. Mehkjian, R. A. Sturdevant, National Cooperative Crohn's Disease Study: Adverse reactions to study drugs, Gastroenterology, 77(4 pt. 2):870–882 (1979).
100. Das, K. M., I. Sternlieb, Salicylazosulfapyridine in inflammatory bowel disease, Am. J. Dig.Dis., 20:971–976 (1975).
101. Strom, J., Toxic epidermal necrolysis (Lyell's syndrome), Scand. J. Infect. Dis., 1:209–216 (1969).
102. Hensen, E. J., F. H. Class, B. J. Vermeer, Drug-dependent binding of circulating antibodies in drug-induced toxic epidermal necrolysis (letter), Lancet, 2:151–152 (1981).
103. Werlin, S. L., R. J. Grand, Bloody diarrhea—a new complication of sulfasalazine, J. Pediatr., 92:450–451 (1978).
104. Schwartz, A. G., S. R. Targan, A. Saxon, W. M. Weinstein, Sulfasalazine-induced exacerbation of ulcerative colitis, N. Engl. J. Med., 306:409–412 (1982).
105. Block, M. B., H. K. Genant, J. B. Kirsner, Pancreatitis as an adverse reaction to salicylazosulfapyridine, N. Engl. J. Med., 282:380–382 (1970).
106. Kanner, R. S., F. J. Tedesco, M. H. Kalser, Azulfidine- (sulfasalazine)-induced hepatic injury, Am. J. Dig. Dis., 23:956–958 (1978).
107. Jacobs, E., P. Paulet, J. Rahier, Hypersensitivity reaction to sulfasalazine-another case (letter), Gastroenterology, 75:1193 (1978).
108. Callen, J., R. M. Soderstrom, Granulomatous hepatitis associated with salicylazosulfapyridine therapy, South. Med. J., 71:1159–1160 (1978).
109. Namias, A., R. Bhalotra, M. Donowitz, Reversible sulfasalazine-induced granulomatous hepatitis, J. Clin. Gastroenterol., 3:193–195 (1981).

110. Gulley, R. M., A. Mirza, C. E. Kelly, Hepatotoxicity of salicylazosulfapyridine: A case report and review of the literature, Am. J. Gastroenterol., 72:561-564 (1979).
111. Ribe, J., K. J. Benkov, S. N. Thung, S. C. Shen, N. S. Leleiko, Fatal massive hepatic necrosis: A probable hypersensitivity reaction to sulfasalazine, Am. J. Gastroenterol., 81:205-208 (1986).
112. Davies, D., A. MacFarlane, Fibrosing alveolitis and treatment with sulphasalazine, Gut, 15:185-188 (1974).
113. Jones, G. R., D. N. S. Malone, Sulphasalazine-induced lung disease, Thorax, 27:713-717 (1972).
114. Constantinidis, K. A., Eosinophilic pneumonia: An unusual side effect of therapy with salicylazosulfapyridine (letter), Chest, 70:315 (1976).
115. Berliner, S., A. Neeman, Y. Schoenfeld, et al., Salazopyrin-induced eosinophilic pneumonia, Respiration, 39:119-120 (1980).
116. Tydd, T. R., Sulphasalazine lung, Med. J. Aust., 1:570-573 (1976).
117. Valche, Y., R. Pauwels, M. Van der Straeteu, Bronchoalveolar lavage in acute hypersensitivity preumonitis caused by sulfasalazine, Chest, 92: 572-573 (1987).
118. Sulfasalazine-induced lung disease (editorial), Lancet, 2:504-505 (1974).
119. Eade, O. E., C. L. Smith, J. R. Alexander, P. J. Whorwell, Pulmonary function in patients with inflammatory bowel disease, Am. J. Gastroenterol., 73:154-156 (1980).
120. Neeman, A., S. Berliner, K. Schoenfeld, U. Kadish, J. Pinkham, Salazopyrine-induced tachycardia (letter), Biomedicine, 33:1-2 (1980).
121. Jamshidi, K., T. Arlander, M. C. Garcia, H. W. Windschitl, W. R. Swaim, Azulfidine agranulocytosis with bone marrow, megakaryocytosis, histiocytosis, and plasmacytosis, Minn. Med., 55:545-548 (1972).
122. Mitrone, M. P., A. Singh, J. R., Seibold, Cholestestasis and fatal agranulocytosis complicating sulfasalazine therapy: Case report and review of the literature, J. Rheumatol., 13:969-972 (1986).
123. Jacobson, I. M., P. B. Kelsey, G. T. Bladeau, Z. N. Demirjian, K. J. Isselbacher, Sulfasalazine-induced agranulocytosis, Am. J. Gastroenterol., 80:118-121 (1985).
124. Davies, G. E., J. Palek, Selective erythroid and megakaryocytic aplasia after sulfasalazine administration (letter), Arch. Intern. Med., 140:1122 (1980).
125. Schneider, R. E., L. Beeley, Megaloblastic anaemia associated with sulphasalazine treatment, Br. Med. J., 1:1638 (1977).
126. Cohen, S. M., D. S. Rosenthal, P. J. Karp, Ulcerative colitis and erythrocytic G6PD deficiency: salicylazosulfapyridine-provoked hemolysis, JAMA 205:528-530 (1968).
127. Gabor, E. P., Hemolytic anemia as adverse reaction to salicylazosulfapyridine (letter), N. Engl. J. Med., 289:1372 (1973).
128. Logan, E. C., L. M. Williamson, D. R. Ryrie, Sulphasalazine associated pancytopenia may be caused by acute folate deficiency, Gut, 27:868-872 (1986).

129. Griffiths, I. D., S. P. Kane, Sulphasalazine-induced lupus syndrome in ulcerative colitis, Br. Med. J., 2:1188–1189 (1977).
130. Mihas, A. A., D. J. Goldenberg, R. L. Slaughter, Sulfasalazine toxic reactions: hepatitis, fever, and skin rash with hypocomplementemia and immune complexes, JAMA 239:2590–2591 (1978).
131. Clementz, G. L., B. J. Dolin, Sulfasalazine-induced lupus erthematosis, Am. J. Med., 84:535–538 (1988).
132. Reid, J., S. Holt, E. Housley, D. J. Snedden, Raynaud's phenomenon induced by sulphasalazine, Postgrad. Med. J., 56:106–107 (1980).
133. Wallace, I. W., Neurotoxicity associated with a reaction to sulphasalazine, Practitioner, 204:850–851 (1970).
134. Levi, A. J., A. M. Fisher, K. Hughes, W. F. Hendry, Male infertility due to sulphasalazine, Lancet, 2:276–278 (1979).
135. Toth, A., Male infertility due to sulphasalazine (letter), Lancet, 2:904 (1979).
136. Toth, A., Reversible toxic effect of salicylazosulfapyridine on semen quality, Fertil. Steril., 31:538–540 (1979).
137. Grieve, J., Male infertility due to sulphasalzine (letter), Lancet, 2:464 (1979).
138. Traub, A. I., W. Thompson, J. Carville, Male Infertility due to sulphasalazine (letter), 2:639–640 (1979).
139. Collen, M. J., Axulfidine-induced oligospermia, Am. J. Gastroenterol., 74:441–442 (1980).
140. Rile, S. A., J. Lecarpentier, V. Mani, M. J. Goodman, B. K. Mandal, L. A. Tumberg, Sulphasalazine induced seminal abnormalities in ulcerative colitis: results of mesalazine substitution, Gut, 28:1008–1012 (1987).
141. Chatzinoxx, M., J. M. Guarino, S. L. Corson, F. R. Batzer, L. S. Friedman, Sulfasalazine-induced abnormal sperm penetration assay reversed in changing to 5-aminosalicylic acid enemas, Dig. Dis. Sci., 33:108–110 (1988).
142. Levi, A. J., S. Toovey, E. Hudson, Male infertility due to sulphasalazine (abstract), Gastroenterology, 80:1208 (1981).
143. Fan Hees, P. D., L. W. Van Elferen, J. M. Van Rossum, J. H. Van Tongeren, Hemolysis during salicylazosulfapyridine therapy, Am. J. Gastroenterol., 70:501–505 (1978).
144. Taffet, S. L., K. M. Das, Sulfasalazine: adverse effects and desensitization, Dig. Dis. Sci., 28:833–842 (1983).
145. Nielsen, O. H., Sulfasalazine intolerance: a retrospective survey of the reasons for discontinuing treatment with sulfasalazine in patients with chronic inflammatory bowel disease, Scand. J. Gastroenterol., 17:389–393 (1982).
146. Holdsworth, C. D., Sulphasalazine desensitization, Br. Med. J. (Clin. Res.), 282:110 (1981).
147. Korelitz, B. I., D. H. Present, P. H. Rubin, S. E. Fochios, Desensitization to sulfasalazine in allergic patients with IBD: an important therapeutic modality (abstract), Gastroenterology, 82:1104 (1982).

4

Topical and Oral Aminosalicylates

Stephen B. Hanauer

University of Chicago Medical Center, Chicago, Illinois

I. INTRODUCTION

The landmark clinical studies by Azad Khan et al. (1), Van Hees et al. (2), and Klotz et al. (3), which identified 5-aminosalicylic acid (5-ASA) as the active moiety of sulfasalazine have opened the door to the first real advancement in therapy of inflammatory bowel disease (IBD) in several decades. Not only has the potential for improved efficacy with reduced adverse effects been realized, but the pharmacologic delivery of 5-ASA to specific sites along the digestive tract has created new possibilities for "targeted delivery" of topically active, nonsystemic agents which may be applicable to future medical advancements for IBD and other conditions.

Once the pharmacology of sulfasalazine was clarified (see Chap. 3), it became apparent that the majority of sulfapyridine was absorbed from the gastrointestinal tract and accounted for the preponderance of adverse consequences which have limited therapy with sulfasalazine. Although sulfasalazine's effectiveness has been shown to have a significant dose-response relationship (at least for prevention of relapse), many patients cannot tolerate sufficient doses for an optimal therapeutic response. The requirement for bacterial azoreduction to release 5-ASA would explain the lack of efficacy of sulfasalazine in small bowel Crohn's disease and its reduced effectiveness in severe colitis where 5-ASA may be rapidly transported through the colon. Additionally, the absence of stool in the rectum of patients with active distal colitis may deprive the mucosa of adequate concentrations of 5-ASA derived from orally ingested sulfasalazine.

Azad Khan et al. (1) designed a simple but elegant clinical trial to assess the efficacy of the individual components of sulfasalazine. Using equimolar concentrations of sulfasalazine (2 g), 5-ASA (700 mg), and sulfapyridine (1400 mg) administered in 100-ml enemas to patients with distal ulcerative colitis, the Oxford group demonstrated equal success in symptomatic relief, mucosal healing, and histologic improvement for sulfasalazine and 5-ASA with minimal responses in patients receiving sulfapyridine. These results were confirmed by Van Hees and colleagues (2), who used even lower doses of 5-ASA, 200 mg twice daily in suppository form, compared with sulfapyridine and placebo, and Klotz et al. who compared the response of patients with distal ulcerative or Crohn's colitis treated with oral sulfasalazine (1 g t.i.d.), oral sulfapyridine (500 mg t.i.d.), or 5-ASA suppositories (500 mg t.i.d.). The latter study not only confirmed the efficacy of locally applied 5-ASA for ulcerative colitis, but was the initial evidence suggesting a role for local therapy in Crohn's disase.

Subsequent to these now classic clinical trials, efforts have focused on: defining the pharmacokinetics of different delivery systems for 5-ASA; further trials to specify clinical utility of various preparations: mechanisms of action of 5-ASA in IBD with hope of further delineating the etiopathogenesis of the inflammatory response in ulcerative colitis and Crohn's disease; and the potential for human toxicity. Additionally, 4-ASA (para-amino-salicylic acid, PAS) also has been shown to have clinical efficacy in ulcerative colitis and affords the opportunity to clarify the mechanisms of action of other similar anti-inflammatory mediators.

II. PHARMACOKINETICS

A. General Properties

5-ASA [5-aminosalicylic acid, mesalamine (U.S. nomenclature), mesalazine (European nomenclature)] is an amphoion with differing pKa values (Fig. 1) which will influence the solubility and absorption depending upon the environmental pH (4). 5-ASA is rapidly and extensively absorbed from the proximal gastrointestinal tract when instilled intrajejunally in a neutral solution (5). Conversely, only a fraction (~10-20%) of 5-ASA is absorbed from a rectally administered dose. The rectal retention time, pH of the solution, volume, and status of the diseased mucosa all influence absorption. Plasma concentrations of 5-ASA and its primary metabolite, acetyl-5-ASA, (Ac-5-ASA) are higher after administration of a neutral enema (pH 7.4) than a slightly acidic enema (pH 4.8) (6), after higher volume enemas, and in patients with less active inflammation (7).

5-ASA is absorbed and rapdily acetylated to Ac-5-ASA. Acetylation appears to be irreversible and takes place within the gut lumen (8), colonic epithelial

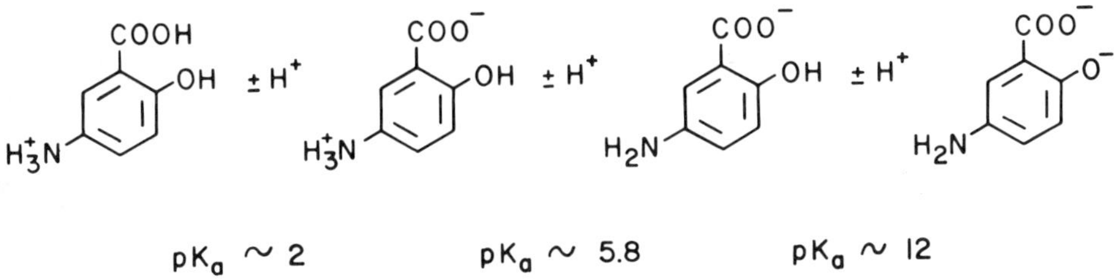

Figure 1 pH dependency of 5-ASA structure.

cells (9,10), and within the liver (11). While some enterohepatic circulation takes place within the gut lumen (8), colonic epithelial cells (9,10), and within the liver (11). While some enterohepatic circulation takes place (12), the hepatic acetylation rate for 5-ASA is not genetically controlled and only small amounts of 5-ASA appear in the bile or breast milk (13). The epithelial acetylation of 5-ASA is similar in the ileum and colon of rats (9), however, human colonic epithelium has a significantly greater uptake for 5-ASA than Ac-5 ASA (14), which may account for different therapeutic responses between 5-ASA and its deriverative (see below).

Approximately 80% of Ac-5-ASA is protein bound compared with 40% of 5-ASA (13). The major route of elimination is renal tubular excretion for both 5-ASA and Ac-5-ASA, although the latter proceeds at a lower rate (200–400 ml/min) (13,15) accounting for the 2–3 times higher plasma concentrations of the acetylated metabolite and the half-life of 6–9 hr for Ac-5-ASA compared to 0.5–1.5 hr for 5-ASA (13,15,16). Plasma concentrations and urinary excretion vary according to specific preparations and dosages (see below). There does not appear to be an accumulation of either metabolite with continuous treatment as average concentrations are <6.5 μmol/1 (1 μg/ml) and 15 μmol/1 (3 μg/ml) for 5-ASA and Ac-5-ASA, respectively. These levels are somewhat higher than those achieved with equimolar concentrations of sulfasalazine (<1.5 μg/ml) (4). It can be assumed that Ac-5-ASA will accumulate in renal failure, and while it is dialyzable, dosage reduction for patients with severe renal insufficiency is probably warranted (17). The only published studies of 5-ASA during pregnancy and lactation refer to sulfasalazine where Ac-5-ASA achieves similar maternal and fetal plasma concentrations while fetal transfer of 5-ASA is negligible. The measured concentrations of Ac-5-ASA from sulfasalazine in breast milk is higher than in plasma compared with only trace amounts of 5-ASA (13,18,19).

The pharmacologic properties of 5-ASA discussed above limit the routes of administration of this topically active agent. Rapid proximal absorption from unprotected 5-ASA necessitates either a delayed-release system or attachment to a carrier molecule for "protected" delivery to the distal small bowel or colon.

Likewise, the solubility and chemical properties of 5-ASA influence potential vehicles for topical delivery per rectum. Of course, a parenteral preparation would not be rational in view of the proposed mechanisms of mucosal action and the low plasma concentrations achieved.

B. Topical 5-ASA Preparations

5-ASA is poorly soluble in water and is easily oxidized with exposure to increased light, temperature, or changes in pH. Hence, for most pharmaceutical preparations, a suspension of 5-ASA protected with antioxidants (including metasulfites) has been utilized (Rowasa). In the commercially available preparations of 5-ASA enemas (see Table 1), 5-ASA has been buffered to an acidic pH to minimize absorption and the stability has been enhanced with antioxidants and protective packaging. While recipes for proprietary preparations do exist in the literature (20), the purity and stability depend upon the chemical (vs. pharmaceutical) grade of the compound and the solution in which it is suspended. The influence of 5-ASA oxidation products has not been studied in humans or animals, nor have their potential beneficial/harmful effects on the mucosa been ascertained. In the United States, the FDA has not approved the use of such proprietary preparations.

The distribution of 5-ASA enemas depends upon the volume administered and, as previously discussed, the absorption is influenced by pH. Campieri and colleagues have demonstrated that 100-ml suspensions reach the splenic flexure in the majority of patients with distal colitis; increasing the volume to 200 ml increases the proximal spread into the transverse colon (21). In practice, the appropriate volume will depend upon the commercial packaging and the tolerance of the individual patient. We have found the 60 ml preparation available in the United States (Rowasa) to be well tolerated by the great majority of our patients, with only 2 of 75 initial patients not able to retain the enema for at least several hours. The average retention time in the large U.S. clinical trial was 10 hr (Lowell Borgen, personal communication).

5-ASA remains stable suspended in a wax matrix formulated as a suppository. Indeed, some of the original studies on the efficacy of 5-ASA utilized suppositories (2,3). The extent of spread of 500-mg suppositories is limited to the rectum (22) and the mean retention time in studies using t.i.d. dosing was 3 hr.

Pharmaceutical development is currently underway to formulate 5-ASA as a rectal foam, but it is necessary to overcome the biochemical antifoaming properties.

C. Oral 5-ASA Preparations

There are two methods of delivering 5-ASA beyond the jejunum. Formulations have been developed which link 5-ASA as a prodrug requiring bacterial reduction

Table 1 New Salicylates

Product	Preparation	Dose (mg)	Delivery
Oral			
Pentasa Marion, US Ferring, Abroad	Mesalamine encapsulated in ethylcellulose microgranules	250	Time/pH release, 30–55% urinary recovery
Asacol Norwich-Eaton, US Tillots, UK	Mesalamine coated with Eudragit-S	400	Release at pH >7, 20–35% urinary recovery
Claversal/Salofalk Smith Kline/Falk	Mesalamine in sodium/glycine buffer coated with Eudragit-L	250,500	Release at pH >6, 25–45% urinary recovery
Rowasa Reid-Rowell	Mesalamine in enteric-coated compressed, coated with coteric opadry	250,500	Release at pH > ~4.5, 60% urinary recovery
	Mesalamine in enteric-coated tablet coated with Eudragit L100	250,500	Release at pH >5, ~30% urinary recovery
4-ASA Reed and Carnrick	Enteric coated with Eudragit compound	500	Time/pH release
Dipentum Pharmacia	Olsalazine (azodisalicylate)	250	Two molecules of 5-ASA released into colon ~25% 5-ASA urinary recovery
Balsalazide Brorek	4-aminobenzoyl-B-alanine-5-ASA	500	Inert carrier delivers 5-ASA into colon
Rectal			
Rowasa/Salofalk/ Claversal	Enemas, 4 g/60 ml buffered suspension, pH 4.5		
Reid-Rowell, US Interfalk, Canada Smith Kline, International	Suppository 0.5 g/1 g		
Pentasa Marion, US Ferring, Abroad	Enema 1, 2, 4 g/100 ml Buffered suspension, pH 4.8		
4-ASA Reed and Carnrick	Enema, 2 g Na-4-ASA requires reconstitution		

similar to sulfasalazine or delayed release of 5-ASA from an inert coating. There are several delayed-release preparations which slowly deliver 5-ASA in a time- and pH-dependent manner or more rapidly release 5-ASA once a pH-dependent capsule has dissolved. Both of these systems will depend upon the intestinal transit time and pH in IBD which have yet to be adequately studied. Hence, measurements of the absorption, serum levels, and urinary excretion of 5-ASA defined in normal or quiescent IBD patients under controlled conditions may not predict values in patients with active disease and varying disease distributions (e.g., ileitis vs. distal colitis). Moreover, these results may be influenced by varying diets and concurrent medications (antacids, H_2 receptor antagonists, cholestyramine). Nevertheless, the concept of targeted delivery of a locally active therapeutic agent to specific sites along the digestive tract is appealing and the 5-ASA compounds are models which will test this principle over time as further pharmaceutical development and clinical studies evolve.

1. Azo-Bond Prodrugs

Olsalazine (azodisalicylate, Dipentum) is a dimer of two 5-ASA molecules linked by the same azo bond present in sulfasalazine. Hence, olsalazine is a new compound with its own chemical properties, which upon reaching the colon, provides twice the molar quantity of 5-ASA per mole of parent compound as sulfasalazine (23). Olsasalazine requires an intact gastrointestinal tract with a normal bacterial flora for effective splitting of the azo bond (24,25). In normal volunteers there is minimal absorption of the intact molecule (serum levels < 2.7 μg/ml with a dose of 250 mg; < 12 μg/ml after 2 g/day) and because of colonic delivery, serum concentrations of 5-ASA (0.8 mg/ml) and Ac-5 ASA (1.1 mg/ml) also are low. The majority (34%) of the compound is recovered as 5-ASA or Ac-5 ASA in the feces (26). In the setting of extensive colitis or rapid colonic transit, the splitting may not be effective, corresponding to increased fecal excretion of unsplit olsalazine and diminished clinical efficacy (27). A small portion of olsalazine is absorbed and is slowly metabolized with a serum half-life of 6–10 days and detectable serum levels for up to 3 weeks (26). However, long-term administration does not produce accumulating serum levels of olsalazine or its metabolites (24).

Olsalazine is a unique molecule with different properties from 5-ASA. One major clinical effect of olsalazine is the induction of small intestine secretion which is manifest as diarrhea in up to 20% of patients. Diarrhea was first observed as a complication in patients receiving olsalazine on an open basis (27) and subsequently confirmed in a placebo-controlled trial (28). Ileostomy output also was increased in a dose-dependent manner in patients receiving olsalazine (29), corresponding to increased small bowel secretion observed in animals (30, 31), not associated with changes in luminal prostaglandins. Utilizing Ussing chambers in experiments, we have shown the secretion to be due to a unique mechanism of bicarbonate secretion which is accompanied by sodium and water transport (32).

While other azo-bond prodrugs of 5-ASA have been developed (33), the only additional preparation which continues to receive clinical attention is balsalazide (Fig. 2). Again, the pharmacokinetics are similar to sulfasalazine with nondetectable serum concentrations of the parent or carrier molecules (34). Recently, clinical trials have been completed which support the predicted clinical efficacy (35,35a).

2. *Oral Nonlinked 5-ASA*

As previously discussed, 5-ASA in an unprotected formulation is rapdily absorbed after jejunal instillation (5) or administration in a gelatin capsule (36). Higher serum concentrations oɪ ɔ-ASA and Ac-5 ASA are present compared with delayed-release preparations and approximately 50% of the dose is recoverable in the urine, mainly as Ac-5-ASA.

Oral preparations of 5-ASA can be conceptually divided into delayed-release versus slow-release formulations. Despite differing pharmacokinetics properties, no significant clinical differences, as yet, have been identified and the distinction between products may be diluted by individual patterns of disease location, disease activity, transit time, diet, intestinal pH, indigenous intestinal bacterial populations, and concurrent medications. Thus, while one may postulate that a slow-release formulation which provides higher fecal and lower serum and urinary 5-ASA recovery due to gradual release and increased intraluminal acetylation of 5-ASA has advantages over preparations which are rapidly released and absorbed to a greater degree with lower fecal and higher urinary recovery, a clinical benefit has yet to be proven (15,37). Likewise, the concept of targeted delivery of high doses of 5-ASA released at designated sites along the intestine to treat specific clinical scenarios needs to be tested and confirmed by comparing various preparations in similar clinical situations. As the immediate priority of the competing pharmaceutical companies remains that of obtaining FDA approval, it is not likely that such extensive and costly clinical comparisons will be available. This will allow clinical researchers and marketing directors to continue speculating through the immediate future.

Unfortunately, because no direct comparisons of equimolar preparations of the various protected formulations are available in the literature, the following comparisons based upon separate clinical studies require cautious interpretation.

Delayed-Release Preparations.

Asacol. This delayed-release formulation of 5-ASA coated with an acrylic-based resin, Eudragit-S, was designed to deliver 5-ASA into the colon in a comparable fashion to sulfasalazine (38). The tablet core is composed of 400 mg of 5-ASA (equal to 1 g sulfasalazine) and the coating remains intact until the luminal pH reaches 7. In healthy volunteers, approximately 80% of the 5-ASA is

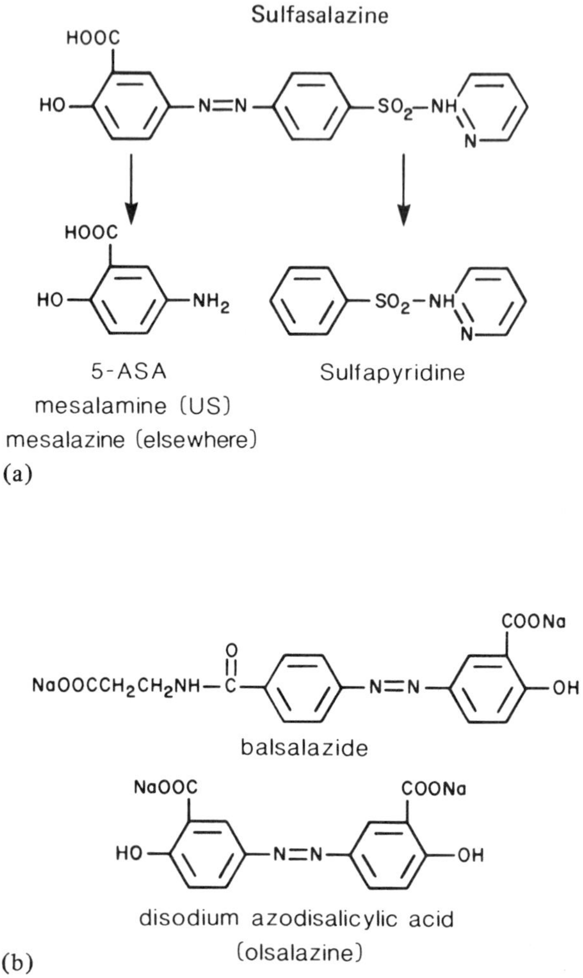

Figure 2 (a) Structural formula and metabolism of sulfasalazine. (b) Structural formulas of balsalazide and olsalazine.

released in the colon after 12 hr (3) with 20-30% of the drug excreted in the urine (36,37). Likewise, in patients with ulcerative colitis in remission the 25% urinary recovery approximated that of sulfasalazine (38), and in patients with active ulcerative colitis and severe diarrhea the tablets were reported to have broken down reliably with peak serum levels attained after 6 hr (39), although the release is quite variable in individual patients and intact tablets have been noted to pass per rectum in many anecdotal circumstances. Conversely, Christensen et al. have measured higher urinary recovery with Asacol from normal subjects (36%), but only 6% from ileostomates as may be expected from the formulation (40). Plasma concentrations of 5-ASA and Ac-5-ASA vary depending on the dose, but do not appear to accumulate over time (4) and are generally within the range of plasma levels attained with sulfasalazine.

Salofalk/Claversal/Mesasal. In this preparation, 5-ASA is finely dispersed, buffered with sodium carbonate and glycine and coated with Eudragit-L, a polymer which dissolves at pH > 6 (16). In healthy volunteers and in patients with Crohn's disease the urinary recovery range was 35-45% (16,37,40) and peak plasma level range was 3-10 mmol/l (16) at a dose of 500 mg t.i.d. Gamma scin tigraphy studies have demonstrated in vivo protection against gastric breakdown of the tablet with release of the 5-ASA core within the distal small bowel (41).

Rowasa. 5-ASA in a composite, delayed-release capsule is currently under investigation in the United States, although the eventual formulation for marketing has yet to be determined (Lowell Borgen, personal communication).

Sustained-Released 5-ASA-Pentasa. Pentasa is a formulation of 5-ASA microgranules coated with a semipermeable membrane of ethylcellulose produced according to granule size to release 5-ASA in a time- and pH-dependent manner through the entire gut (15). In ileostomy patients, approximately 50% of 5-ASA is released from the granules permitting the delivery of the residual dose to the colon. As would be expected, the urinary recovery of 5-ASA and Ac-5-ASA was approximately 60% in normal controls (15), although in subsequent studies by the same (40) and other (37) investigators, the urinary recovery was considerably lower (~25-30%), similar to the delayed-release preparations. Neither transit time (42) nor an ileorectal anastomosis (43) significantly reduce the delivery of 5-ASA to the colon or altered systemic absorption. Plasma levels of Ac-5-ASA in healthy subjects and patients with Crohn's disease receiving 500 mg t.i.d. range between 4-9 mmol/l (4).

III. CLINICAL STUDIES

A. Topical Agents

As noted above, Azad Khan et al. was the first to demonstrate the short-term efficacy of 5-ASA enemas in distal ulcerative colitis (1). They administered 700 mg of 5-ASA in 100-ml isotonic solution buffered to pH 7. The topical application of an equivalent to 2 g of sulfasalazine produced clinical sigmoidoscopic, and histologic improvement after 2 weeks in 75%, 64%, and 30%, respectively; these results were comparable to those attained with sulfasalazine enemas and significantly superior to the results with topical sulfapyridine.

Campieri and his Bolognese colleagues investigated varying dosages of 5-ASA enemas in patients with distal colitis. After pilot studies using 1–6 g 5-ASA enemas, they randomized patients into a controlled study comparing 4 g 5-ASA enemas to 100 mg hydrocortisone enemas over 2 weeks. Again, they observed excellent results in patients treated with 5-ASA: 93% achieved a clinical remission compared to 57% of patients randomized to hydrocortisone (20). The same group summarized their four-year experience involving 144 patients who were treated with 2–4-week therapeutic cycles with 2–4 g of 5-ASA in 100 ml. Clinical improvement was noted after 88% of the treatments (44,45). Of 44 patients previously allergic to or intolerant of sulfasalazine, only 5 were not able to tolerate 5-ASA enemas due to skin rash or diarrhea (46).

Additional controlled trials have confirmed these preliminary findings regarding the "high dose" 4-g enemas. In the United States and Canada, a 6-week, double-blind, randomized trial involving 153 patients with distal colitis compared 4-g 5-ASA enemas buffered to pH 4.8 (Rowasa) to a placebo enema (47). Most of the patents had previously received either sulfasalazine and/or rectal corticosteroids with about half of these patients reporting no prior response to treatment. At the conclusion of the 6-week study, 63% of patients were considered to be "much improved" and life-table analysis revealed that patients were continuing to improve at the end of the study. The response was not influenced by concurrent treatment with sulfasalazine, although the patients treated with concurrent corticosteroids showed a reduced response.

Using the 4-g (Rowasa) enemas, we were able to demonstrate excellent clinical responses in previously "refractory" patients (48,49). Approximately 75% of our patients achieved remission, despite the failure of prior sulfasalazine or corticosteroids as long as the colitis was distal to the splenic flexure. We did find, however, that it took an average of more than 6 weeks of continuous treatment to heal these previously intractable patients (49). Similar efficacy in refractory patients has been described by Barber (50), McPhee (51), Janssens (52), and their colleagues.

We (49), and others (53), have shown that patients who respond to local therapy with 5-ASA enemas tend to flare as the frequency of enema administration is reduced; findings analogous to maintenance trials with sulfasalazine. While formal dosing trials for patients in remission are in progress, either nightly enemas of 1 g (not commercially available in the United States) or administration of 4-g 5-ASA enemas for one week per month have been shown to maintain remissions in up to 75% of patients over one year (54,55).

A number of investigators have studied lower doses of 5-ASA enemas in the acute setting. Controlled trials of nightly 1-g 5-ASA enemas (Pentasa) have shown comparable efficacy to 25-mg prednisolone enemas in a Danish population and superiority over placebo (56,56a). Again, the former study demonstrated the benefit of continuing treatment even if patients do not completely respond by the end of two weeks. Powell-Tuck and Parkins (57) could not demonstrate a difference between 1- or 2-g 5-ASA enemas and a large multicenter, randomized dose-ranging trial in the United States found no difference between patients treated with 1-, 2-, or 4-g Pentasa enemas as single therapy with all doses producing superior results compared to placebo (58).

The issue of dose–response also applies to topical therapy with 4-ASA (59–62). Campieri et al. first compared 2-g doses of 4-ASA enemas to 5-ASA enemas after a pilot study of 4-g 4-ASA enemas showed the dose to be poorly tolerated (59). Both preparations were equally efficacious with clinical improvement in over 75% of patients. However, Gandolfo et al. (62) found the 2-g dose superior to 4 g in a trial, which raises further issues regarding optimal dosing balancing efficacy versus irritation with 4-ASA enemas.

While the Italian group was pioneering the use of 5-ASA enemas, German investigators paved the way for 5-ASA in suppository form. 5-ASA suppositories formulated in a wax matrix have the advantages of stability, concentrated local delivery for proctitis and ease of application allowing multiple daily doses. Williams et al. (22) have demonstrated that ^{99m}Tc-labelled 5-ASA suppositories remain localized to the rectum and sigmoid. In patients with distal colitis Van Hees et al. (63) described healing with 200-mg suppositories administered twice daily over 4 weeks. Klotz et al. (3) have shown that 500-mg suppositories administered t.i.d. were equal to sulfasalazine 1 g t.i.d., and the Italians demonstrated that 1-g suppositories administered b.i.d. were as effective and better tolerated than 2 g nightly enemas (64). Follow-up studies in Germany have confirmed the effectiveness of the 1.5-g daily dose of 5-ASA suppositories for active disease (65) and 250-mg suppositories administered t.i.d.. for maintaining remissions (66). Placebo-controlled studies also have confirmed the effectiveness of 500 mg 5-ASA suppositories administered t.i.d. for active ulcerative proctitis (67), while studies of 500 mg b.i.d. in active disease and maintenance studies of 500 mg nightly to sustain remissions look promising (Lowell Borgen, personal communication).

B. Oral Agents

1. *Ulcerative Colitis: Active Disease*

Clinical trials on both sides of the Atlantic have begun to confirm the efficacy of oral preparations of 5-ASA for both acute ulcerative colitis (UC) and to prevent relapse for UC in remission. The similar pharmacokinetics of azo-linked 5-ASA in olsalazine to sulfasalazine make the 5-ASA dimer an excellent potential alternative to sulfasalazine in intolerant or allergic patients. Meyers et al. (68) studied such a population. They randomized 66 mild to moderate UC outpatients unable to tolerate a minimal (2 g) dose of sulfasalazine to either placebo, 0.75 g, 1.5 g, or 3 g doses of olsalazine divided into three daily doses over three weeks. At the conclusion of the trial, 16% of the placebo group had improved compared with 29%, 27%, and 50% of the 0.75 g, 1.5 g, and 3 g groups, respectively. The results demonstrated the efficacy of olsalazine as well as a trend toward a dose-response, although the study duration was too short to examine "remission rates." The 3-g dose provided almost twice the amount of 5-ASA available from the usual 4-g dose of sulfasalazine (1.6 g). The Oxford group also has demonstrated the efficacy of oral olsalazine in 40 patients with active UC randomized to receive either olsalazine 2 g/day or placebo over 2 weeks. They reported improvement in 13 of 20 olsalazine-treated patients compared with 8 of 20 in the placebo group. Sigmoidoscopic improvement also was confirmed in 45% of the olsalazine patients compared with 35% of the placebo group (69). Another small trial of the 2-g dose also suggested a therapeutic benefit for olsalazine in patients treated over 6 weeks. Although statistical significance was not reached, 6 of 15 patients receiving olsalazine compared with 2 of 15 on placebo had good clinical results ($p = 0.11$) (27). Unpublished trials by Willoughby et al. (70) and Ewe (71), reported at a recent symposium, confirmed the anticipated therapeutic similarity between olsalazine and sulfasalazine with an improved safety profile for the former. Feurle, however, reported on a multicenter German trial which could not demonstrate superiority of 2 g olsalazine versus placebo due to a 60% placebo-response (72).

Oral, nonlinked 5-ASA products have been less well studied in the setting of acute UC and have been utilized primarily for maintenance of UC in remission. However, there are several reports of trials which do support the predicted benefit in acute UC. Asacol 800 mg or 2.4 g, was superior to sulfasalazine, 2 g daily, in a randomized trial involving 61 patients with mild to moderate relapses of UC. Remissions were induced in 30% and 42% of patients on Asacol by 4 weeks compared with 21% of the sulfasalazine group (73). In an open study from Bologna, 72% of patients with mild to moderate UC improved with a mean dose of 2.4 g/day (equivalent to 6 g of sulfasalazine) (74). In the only North American trial, to date, a double blind, randomized trial from the Mayo Clinic demonstrated statistical benefit of Asacol at a dose of 4.8 g/day compared with placebo (75). It is of great interest, however, that patients randomized to receive 1.6 g of Asacol (equivalent to 4 g of sulfasalazine) did not have a statistically greater response than patients treated with placebo. Further dose ranging studies are clearly indicated to ascertain the appropriate dose for Asacol in active UC.

Salofalk (Claversal/Mesasal) has been evaluated for short-term efficacy in patients with active UC at comparable molar doses of 5-ASA as are provided with sulfasalazine. Maier et al. (76) compared 1.5 g Salofalk with 3 g sulfasalazine in 30 patients. Clinical improvement was noted in 86% of both groups by 8 weeks with endoscopic remission in 60% of the 5-ASA group and 53% of the sulfasalazine group. Similar results were obtained in a large multicenter trial comparing Claversal with SASP in acute UC (76a). Open studies have confirmed the clinical utility of this product at doses of 1.5 g/day (77). Again, dose-ranging studies are necessary to assess the optimal dose and the margin of safety versus efficacy.

A recently completed trial has demonstrated a dose-response for Pentasa in acute UC, with 2-g and 4-g daily doses providing superior clinical, endoscopic, and histologic efficacy compared to 1 g of placebo (77a).

2. Ulcerative Colitis: Maintenance Trials

In European trials, the oral 5-ASA compounds have, to date, been used primarily to maintain remissions in patients with UC intolerant to sulfasalazine. Sandberg-Gertzen et al. described 160 patients treated with olsalazine who had been intolerant or allergic to sulfasalazine (25). After 6 months, 100 patients were in remission and were entered into a randomized controlled trial of a 2-g dose compared with placebo. After a 6-month trial, 77% of the olsalazine group remained in remission compared with 55% of the patients randomized to receive placebo. Jewell and Ireland compared the relapse-prevention effects of olsalazine, 1 g daily, with sulfasalazine, 2 g daily, in 164 patients in remission for at least 6 months (78). Both drugs were comparable with 6-month relapse rates of 19.5% for olsalazine and 12.5% for sulfasalazine. The adverse effect profile was equal in the latter study, although most of the patients had previously tolerated sulfasalazine prior to randomization.

Most of the nonlinked 5-ASA compounds also have been evaluated for their relapse-prevention properties. Dew et al. (79) initially studied 72 patients who had been in remission for at least one month and had been taking at least 2 g of sulfasalazine daily. Patients were randomized to continue receiving sulfasalazine at the same dose (minimum 2 g) or an equivalent dose of 5-ASA from Asacol. Nine of 34 patients receiving Asacol and 6 of 33 patients on sulfasalazine relapsed over 4 months. The same investigators subsequently evaluated a higher dose of Asacol (minimum 2.4 g) compared with sulfasalazine (minimum 2 g) in another 67 patients with inactive UC who were followed for 6 months. Despite the higher dose of 5-ASA, there was no significant difference in the 6-month relapse rate between Asacol (22%) and sulfasalazine (20%) (80). In a similar trial, Riley et al. (81) compared maintenance therapy with Asacol or sulfasalazine in 92 patients followed over 48 weeks. Again, equal proportions of patients relapsed; 38% of patients receiving sulfasalazine and 37% of patients randomized to Asacol. The mean times to relapse, cumulative relapse rate, and severity of relapse were comparable in both groups.

Both Pentasa and Claversal also have been tested for their relapse-prevention properties in UC. A Dtuch multicenter randomized trial compared Pentasa, 500 mg t.i.d., to sulfasalazine, 1 g t.i.d., in 75 patients in remission longer than one month who were followed for one year (82). Remission was maintained for 6 months in 63% and 12 months in 54% of the Pentasa group compared with 71% and 45% of patients treated with sulfasalazine. Likewise, a multicenter randomized trial comparing Claversal 0.75 mg with sulfasalazine 1.5 g for patients with quiescent UC has recently confirmed the clinical equivalency (83), and in open studies in Europe, Claversal was well-tolerated at a maintenance dose of 1.5 g/day (77).

In summary, the 5-ASA compounds appear as effective as sulfasalazine in both acute UC and maintenance therapy. The wide variations in populations studied, disease extent and severity, length of follow-up, and doses make exact comparisons between products difficult. It is interesting that the improved tolerance compared with sulfasalazine has not produced evidence of enhanced efficacy nor a clearly delineated dose-response and, as yet, no group of patients who have failed therapy with oral sulfasalazine have been substantiated to improve with oral 5-ASA.

3. Crohn's Disease: Active Disease

As described in Chapter 3, it has been difficult to prove a therapeutic role for sulfasalazine in Crohn's disease when the small bowel alone is involved. Some potential problems have been related to the delivery of an adequate amount of 5-ASA to the site of inflammation, the length of time required to document a therapeutic effect with Crohn's disease, and differences between treatment groups. Furthermore, the local activity of 5-ASA (via sulfasalazine) is likely to have a lesser effect on the transmural inflammation of Crohn's disease compared with the systemic activity of corticosteroids. Rather, one would anticipate a clearer effect from 5-ASA with milder, more superficial disease or in relapse prevention.

One of the first reports suggesting potential efficacy of 5-ASA in Crohn's disease came from Klotz and colleagues as they evaluated the independent activities of sulfasalazine, sulfapyridine, and 5-ASA in patients with distal colitis (3). In the four patients with rectal Crohn's disease who were treated with 500 mg 5-ASA suppositories administered three times daily, the CDAI fell from 263 ± 83 to 165 ± 129 ($p > 0.035$) after 4 to 6 weeks. The same group then performed a randomized trial comparing 5-ASA in a delayed-release preparation (Salofalk 500 mg t.i.d.) to sulfasalazine (1 g t.i.d.) in 30 patients (76). The CDAI fell from 308 to 119 and the ESR from 49 to 20 in the 5-ASA group compared with 310 to 162 and 40 to 32 in the sulfasalazine group. Over the 8-week trial, 87% of patients treated with 5-ASA and 80% treated with sulfasalazine "improved."

Rasmussen and colleagues first published "hopeful" results of an open trial of slow-release 5-ASA in a small group of patients with mild Crohn's disease who received Pentasa, 1.5 g daily, over 6 weeks (84). Although the drug was well tolerated and judged effective in 72% of patients, their subsequent randomized, placebo-controlled trial failed to provide statistical evidence of efficacy despite a trend toward improvement (85). These studies demonstrate the difficulty in evaluating Crohn's disease activity compared to UC, as well as the requisite for placebo-controlled clinical trials. Saverymuttu et al. examined the effect of 1.5 g of Pentasa on the fecal granulocyte excretion in six patients with active Crohn's disease. After 10 days of treatment the indium-labelled leukocyte excretion was reduced in the six patients receiving 5-ASA compared with placebo-treated controls. (86).

Other investigators have evaluated the effectiveness of 5-ASA for active Crohn's disease in open studies utilizing a variety of clinical response criteria. Wellman and colleagues administered 5-ASA along with "whole gut irrigation" and noted an improvement in both the CDAI and plasma endotoxin concentratin in the patients treated with combination therapy compared to controls (87). Barbara et al. (74) reported the response of 32 patients treated with a mean dose of 2.4 g 5-ASA over 7 weeks noting clinical improvement in 72% and laboratory evidence of improvement in 66% (74). We reported the results of therapy with Claversal, 1.5 g daily, in 25 patients with active Crohn's disease (77). Stool frequency, number of diarrheal stools, the percentage of bowel movements with blood, and the CDAI all improved in this 6-week open trial.

4. Crohn's Disease: Maintenance Trials

There also has been preliminary data from a limited number of clinical trials evaluating the role of 5-ASA for the maintenance of Crohn's disease in remission. Brignola et al. (88) followed 46 patients in clinical remission (CDAI <150) with laboratory parameters which predicted a potential relapse. Over a 4-month period of observation, patients receiving 1 g 5-ASA daily fared no better than placebo-treated controls, whereas patients treated with a 2-g dose had fewer relapses. Wellman reported the results of 66 patients with Crohn's disease in remission for more than 3 months who were randomized to receive 5-ASA, 1.5 g daily, or placebo over 12 months (89). While they could not identify a significant difference in the overall relapse rate, there appeared to be more relapses in the patients with "ileocecal" Crohn's treated with placebo compared with those receiving 5-ASA maintenance. These findings were supported by an open study of 221 patients with quiescent Crohn's disease treated with Claversal 500 mg t.i.d. in whom the CDAI, stool frequency, and number of bloody bowel movements continued to decline over 6 weeks of therapy (77).

Recently, a large, multicenter, randomized, controlled trial compared Claversal, 1.5 g/day, to placebo in patients with Crohn's disease in remission (CDAI <150). The estimated 12-month relapse rates were 22% for patients treated with 5-ASA compared with 43% for patients receiving placebo ($p < 0.05$) (90).

The accumulating data are optimistic, if not definitive, regarding the ultimate efficacy of 5-ASA in Crohn's disease. Further controlled clinical trials are necessary to document the role of 5-ASA for active Crohn's disease and relapse prevention, as well as to define the optimal dose, length of therapy, and ability to "target" individual preparations for specific sites of disease. Moreover, clinical trials should be designed to clarify the role of 5-ASA as a primary and/or adjunctive agent in Crohn's disease.

C. Recommendations for Therapy

Based on efficacy and toxicity studies it is appropriate to consider 5-ASA enemas and suppositories in the initial therapy for patients with distal ulcerative colitis and proctitis respectively. However, because of the cost of the enemas (twice that of hydrocortisone enemas and many times the cost of sulfasalazine) the apparent need for maintenance and the very acceptable records of both sulfasalazine and topical corticosteroids, physicians may be reluctant to use topical 5-ASA as the initial drug of choice. It is clear that topical 5-ASA is a valuable addition in the patient with distal colitis refractory or intolerant of other modes of treatment, and should be considered for maintenance in patients with recurrent distal colitis who cannot be maintained on sulfasalazine.

It remains unclear not only which oral agents will emerge as effective and safe, but also what their ultimate role will be in therapy of IBD. They clearly should be important alternatives for most patients intolerant or allergic to sulfasalazine. Moreover, the oral nonlinked 5-ASA forms may prove useful in small bowel Crohn's disease where suflasalazine as noted has limited efficacy. It is possible that oral aminosalicylates will ultimately replace sulfasalazine in active UC and Crohn's disease and as prophylactic therapy for these disorders.

IV. MECHANISMS OF ACTION

Since it appears that 5-ASA is the active therapeutic moiety of sulfasalazine, the mechanism(s) of action are similar to those discussed in Chapter 3, and likely relate to local inhibition of products of arachidonic acid metabolism and the ablity to scavenge oxygen-derived free radicals after inflammatory mediators have been released.

V. ADVERSE EFFECTS

The two advantages of 5-ASA over sulfasalazine are directed delivery to specific sites along the gastrointestinal tract and elimination of the sulfa moiety. The latter has markedly improved the margin of safety for the treatment of IBD and allowed the option of increased dosing without the adverse consequences of sulfapyridine intolerance or allergy. While the overall safety profile for 5-ASA has been significantly enhanced, we are becoming increasingly aware of potential adverse effects which are similar to sulfasalazine or unique to the 5-ASA molecule.

In general, 5-ASA has been very well tolerated in animals. Toxicologic studies have revealed that the kidneys are the primary target organ for 5-ASA damage as predicted by the structural resemblance of 5-ASA to aspirin and phenacetin (91). Initial studies in rats have confirmed proximal tubule necrosis and papillary necrosis after single intravenous doses of 5-ASA above 150 mg/kg (92). Longer-term studies in rats over 6 months and dogs over 12 months produced papillary damage only at doses above 80 mg/kg and 40 mg/kg, respectively, confirming the safety of serum concentrations attained in animals which are at least 10 times the level attained in humans at therapeutic doses (93). Further reassurance from oral dosing studies in animals comes from Bondesson et al., who described minimal glomerular hypercellularity and synecchiae and tubular changes after much higher doses administered to rats compared with humans, but no interstitial changes in rats, rabbits, or pigs (4). Likewise, a 4-week study of rats receiving 30-200 mg/kg of 5-ASA by gastric gavage failed to demonstrate either histologic changes or increased urinary excretion of *N*-acetyl-B-D-glucoaminidase (NAG) or alanineaminopeptidase (AAP) (94). Similarly, patients with Crohn's disease receiving 1.5 g of delayed-release 5-ASA for 4–12 weeks failed to reveal increases in urinary excretion of NAG or AAP (94).

It appears that there is a wide margin of safety for orally administered 5-ASA-induced nephrotoxicity in humans. Rasmussen (personal communication), however, has described reduced creatinine clearances without histological findings at biopsy in two patients receiving 4-g doses of 5-ASA for Crohn's disease. The only report, to date, of human nephrotoxicity related to 5-ASA described a patient with nephrotic syndrome due to minimal change nephropathy (95), which is likely unrelated to the anticipated dose-related salicylate effect. Nevertheless, there is a potential for long-term nephrotoxicity which should be monitored, especially in patients receiving concomitant therapy with other nonsteroidal anti-inflammatory drugs.

Experience from controlled clinical trials has confirmed the general safety of the 5-ASA preparations. In the largest 5-ASA enema trial involving over 150 patients, the number of reported adverse effects were less with active drug than with placebo (47). Rare reports of hair loss (96) have not been confirmed in large clinical trials with 5-ASA enemas or suppositories (48,63,98). A few patients have reported minor anal irritation or pruritis with the topically instilled products (personal observation). Rarely, exacerbation of colitis may occur with topical 5-ASA similar to rare occurrences noted with oral 5-ASA (see below).

Clinical trials of the oral 5-ASA preparations have supported the predicted improved safety profile of 5-ASA compared with sulfasalazine. In trials comparing Claversal (1.5 g/day) with sulfasalazine (3 g/day) for acute UC, the proportions of patients reporting adverse effects were 14% and 24%, respectively (76a). Hypersensitivity reactions (12%) and nausea/vomiting (8%) were four times more frequent with sulfasalazine, while headache and abdominal pain were infrequent (5%) and similarly distributed between treatment groups. Six percent of the Claversal patients and 8% of sulfasalazine patients were withdrawn due to adverse effects. In a relapse prevention study of Claversal 750 mg/day versus sulfasalazine 1.5 g/day in patients who were tolerant of sulfasalazine, adverse effects were similar between treatment groups (83). However, of 37 patients who had previously reported adverse events with sulfasalazine, 38% of those randomized to sulfasalazine reported side effects compared to 8% randomized to 5-ASA. In postmarketing studies of Claversal in Germany, only 3% of patients have spontaneously reported adverse events and fewer than 1% of patients discontinued treatment because of such events (98).

In a similar relapse prevention study of UC patients in remission on sulfasalazine who were randomized to Asacol or sulfasalazine, improvement in baseline headache (from sulfasalazine) was noted in 90% of those randomized to Asacol compared with 55% of patients continued on suflasalazine, and gastrointestinal upset was improved in all patients who changed to Asacol versus 53% continuing with sulfasalazine (81). Asacol has been well tolerated in the majority of patients intolerant to SASP, even when administered in larger molar concentrations (79, 80). Similarly, Pentasa appears to be well tolerated, without significant adverse effects at a 1.5-g daily dose in patients intolerant to sulfasalazine (99).

The majority of patients intolerant or allergic to sulfasalazine have been able to tolerate 5-ASA, however, identical adverse effects have been observed in 10–20% of patients withdrawn from sulfasalazine who initiate therapy with either 5-ASA or olsalazine (100,101). The incidence of dyspepsia, headache, and other nonallergic symptoms is significantly reduced, such that 80% of sulfasalazine-intolerant patients can tolerate a sulfa-free 5-ASA preparation. However, despite the reduced frequency, there is a potential for similar adverse events from 5-ASA as with sulfasalazine. Of most concern may be the exacerbation of colitis that is occasionally recognized and appears to be a rare manifestation of salicylate toxicity (100,101).

Olsalazine has a safety profile similar to the nonlinked 5-ASA product with the singular exception of diarrhea. The reported incidence of diarrhea ranges between 15 and 35%, depending upon the dose and extent of colitis (25) (Pharmacia data on file). The diarrhea appears to be due to ileal secretion (25,32) and, in animal studies, fluid and electrolyte secretion has been demonstrated in isolated small intestinal loops (32,105). Olsalazine is an anion secretagogue (primarily bicarbonate) in the small intestine, with a unique mechanism that does not depend on cyclic nucleotides or prostaglandin synthesis (106). It is possible that 5-ASA has a similar effect, but at much higher concentrations (105). Clinically, it has been observed that the diarrhea improves as the inflammation heals or the normal colon accommodates to the increased fluid load. Thus, it would seem prudent to advise upward titration of olsalazine or higher doses of 5-ASA according to an individual's disease extent and severity (personal observation).

In summary, 5-ASA and non-sulfa derivatives offer a safe alternative to patients who have demonstrated intolerance or allergic reactions to sulfasalazine, although a minority of such patients may react similarly to 5-ASA substitution. Sulfasalazine-induced infertility in males would be a singular indication for replacement with 5-ASA and sulfasalazine, and salicylate-induced toxic diarrhea is a condition where substitution would be contraindicated or is to be attempted with extreme caution.

VI. CONCLUSIONS

The clinical studies which led to the recognition of 5-ASA as the active moiety of sulfasalazine have enhanced both the understanding of mechanisms of inflammation in IBD, as well as the management of patients. While the exact mechanism(s) of action of 5-ASA are still being evaluated, recent pharmaceutical developments allowing innovative mechanisms of drug delivery now provide the ability to formulate preparations which will distribute a topically active agent to specific sites along the digestive tract to maximize efficacy and minimize toxicity.

While therapeutic trials have confirmed the efficacy of 5-ASA in a variety of clinical scenarios, a number of very basic questions still need to be addressed in future studies. Of course, basic research into the mechanisms of action will further enhance our knowledge of pathophysiologic mechanisms and allow more specific manipulation of the immunologic/inflammatory response. Meanwhile, physicians still need to know the dose-response relationship for the various oral or topical preparations for acute UC, maintenance UC, and acute or chronic Crohn's disease. Comparisons of oral versus rectal preparations are needed to clarify optimal therapy for individual patients. Studies are necessary to ascertain the situations in which 5-ASA should be administered as primary therapy and those in which it may have an adjunctive role with corticosteroids, metronidazole, or immunosuppressives. Furthermore, while the safety profile is certainly improved compared with sulfasalazine, we need to evaluate whether the ability to tolerate higher doses of 5-ASA will offer new therapeutic advantages and whether the long-term administration of these salicylates will predispose to chronic nephrotoxicity alone or in conjunction with frequently administered nonsteroidal anti-inflammatory drugs. Finally, comparisons between preparations will be necessary for the physician to logically choose an individual product in specific situations based on clinical data rather than marketing predictions as cost-benefit becomes increasingly important.

REFERENCES

1. Khan, A. K. A., J. Piris, S. C. Truelove, An experiment to determine the active therapeutic moiety of sulphasalazine, Lancet, 2:892–895 (1977).
2. Van Hees, P. A. M., J. H. M. Tuinte, J. M. Van Rossum, J. H. M. Van Tongeren, Influence of intestinal transit time on azo-reduction of salicylazosulphapyridine (Salazopyrin), Gut, 20:300–304 (1979).
3. Klotz, U., K. Maier, C. Fischer, K. Heinkel, Therapeutic efficacy of sulfasalazine and its metabolites in patients with ulcerative colitis and Crohn's disease, N. Engl. J. Med., 303:1499–1502 (1980).
4. Bondeson, S., S. N. Rasmussen, J. Rask-Madsen, O. H. Nielsen, K. Lauritsen, B. Binder, S. H. Hansen, E. F. Hvidberg, 5-aminosalicylic acid in the treatment of inflammatory bowel disease, Acta Med. Scand., 221:227–242 (1987).
5. Nielsen, O. H., S. Bondesen, Kinetics of 5-aminosalicylic acid after jejunal instillation in man, Br. J. Clin. Pharmacol., 16:738–740 (1983).
6. Bondesen, S., O. H. Nielsen, O. Jacobsen, S. N. Rasmussen, S. H. Hansen, S. Halskov, V. Binder, E. F. Hvidberg, 5-aminosalicylic acid enemas in patients with active ulcerative colitis: Influence of acidity on the kinetic pattern, Scand. J. Gastroenterol., 19:677–682 (1984).
7. Campieri, M., G. A. Lanfranchi, S. Boschi, Topical administration of 5-aminosalicylic acid enemas in patients with ulcerative colitis. Studies on rectal absorption and excretion, Gut, 26:400–405 (1985).
8. Allgayer, H., W. Kruis, J. G. Paumgartner, Different acetylation of 5-aminosalicylic acid (5-ASA) in mucosa and feces (abstr.). In: Mesalazine Treatment of Inflammatory Bowel Diseases, Vol. I. Mechanics and Pharmacokinetics. Clinical Controversies in Inflammatory Bowel Disease Symposium, September 9–11, Bologna, Italy, 1987.
9. Otten, H. H., R. A. Van Hogezand, J. H. M. Van Tongeren, Rapid acetylation of 5-aminosalicylic acid in the intestinal mucosa (abstr.). Mesalazine Treatment of Inflammatory Bowel Disease Symposium, September 9–11, Bologna, Italy, 1987.
10. Ireland, A., J. D. Priddle, D. P. Jewell, Acetylation of 5-aminosalicylic acid by human colonic epithelial cells (abstr.), Gastroenterology, 90:1471 (1986).
11. Meese, C. O., C. Fischer, U. Klotz, Is N-acetylation of 5-aminosalicylic acid reversible in man?, Br. J. Clin. Pharmacol., 18:612–615 (1984).
12. Fischer, O., K. Maier, E. Stumpf, U. Von Gaisberg, U. Klotz, Disposition of 5-aminosalicylic acid, the active metabolite of sulphasalazine in man, Eur. J. Clin. Pharmacol, 25:511–515 (1983).
13. Klotz, U., Clinical pharmacokinetics of sulphasalazine, its metabolites, and other prodrugs of 5-aminosalicylic acid, Clin. Pharmacokinet., 10:285–302 (1985).
14. Ireland, A., J. D. Priddle, D. P. Jewell, A comparison of the uptake of 5-aminosalicylic acid (5-ASA) and N-acetylaminosalicylic acid (Ac-ASA) into the isolated colonic epithelial cell (abstr.), Gastroenterology, 92:1447 (1987).

15. Rasmussen, S. N., S. Bondesen, E. F. Hvidberg, S. H. Hansen, V. Binder, S. Halskov, H. Flachs, 5-aminosalicylic acid in a slow release preparation: bioavailability, plasma level, and excretion in humans, Gastroenterology, 83:1062–1070 (1982).
16. Klotz, U., K. E. Maier, C. Fischer, K. H. Bauer, A new slow-release form of 5-aminosalicylic acid for the oral treatment of inflammatory bowel disease: biopharmaceutic and clinical pharmacokinetic characteristics, Arzneim-Forsch/Drug Res., 35(1):636–639 (1985).
17. Klotz, U., Pharmacokinetic properties of 5-aminosalicylic acid (mesalazine). Inflammatory bowel diseases—basic research and clinical implications: Falk Symposium 46, pp. 339–347 (1988). (Proceedings of Falk Symposium 46 held during Gastroenterology Week, Titisee, Federal Republic of Germany, June 7–9, 1987). (Goebell, H., Peskar, B. M., Malchow, H., eds.) Manchester, MTP Press Ltd, (1987).
18. Azad Khan, A. K., S. C. Truelove, Placental and mammary transfer of sulphasalazine, Br. Med. J., 2:1553 (1979).
19. Hvidberg, E. F., S. N. Rasmussen, S. H. Hansen, S. Bondesen, 5-aminosalicylic acid (5-ASA) in amniotic fluid, cord and maternal plasma, and breast milk during sulfasalazine treatment (abstr.). In: Abstract book, Iuphar 9th International Congress of Pharmacology, London (1984) no. 2205.
20. Campieri, M., G. A. Lanfranchi, G. Bazzocchi, A. Brignola, F. Sarti, G. Franzin, A. Battochia, G. Labo, P. R. Dal Monte, Treatment of ulcerative colitis with high-dose 5-aminosalicylic acid enemas, Lancet, 2:270–271 (1981).
21. Campieri, M., G. A. Lanfranchi, C. Brignola, G. Bazzocchi, P. Gionchetti, M. R. Minguzzi, F. Adami, 5-aminosalicylic acid for the treatment of inflammatory bowel disease, Gastroenterology, 89:701-702 (1985).
22. Williams, C. N. G. Haber, J. A. Aquino, Double-blind, placebo-controlled evaluation of 5-ASA suppositories in active distal proctitis and measurement of extent of spread using ^{99m}Tc-Labelled 5-ASA suppositories. Dig. Dis. Sci., 32(12):71S–75S (1987).
23. Van Hogezand, R. A., P. A. M. Van Hees, B. Zwanenberg, J. M. Van Rossum, J. H. M. Tongeren, Disposition of disodium azodisalicylate in healthy subjects. A possible new drug for inflammatory bowel disease, Gastroenterology, 88:717–722 (1985).
24. Lauritsen, K., J. Hansen, M. Ryde, J. Rask-Madsen, Colonic azodisalicylate metabolism determined by in vivo dialysis in healthy volunteers and patients with ulcerative colitis, Gastroenterology, 86:1496–1500 (1984).
25. Sandberg-Gertzen, H., M. Ryde, G. Janerot, Absorption, metabolism and excretion of a single 1 gm dose of azodisal sodium in subjects with ileostomy, Scand. J. Gastroenterology, 18:107–111 (1983).
26. Willoughby, C. P., J. R. Aronson, H. Agback, N. O. Bodin, S. C. Truelove, Distribution and metabolism in healthy volunteers of disodium azodisalicylate, a potential therapeutic agent for ulcerative colitis, Gut, 23:1081–1087 (1982).

27. Sandberg-Gertzen, H., G. Jarnerot, W. Kraaz, Azodisal sodium in the treatment of ulcerative colitis: A study of tolerance and relapse-prevention properties, Gastroenterology, 90:1024–1030 (1986).
28. Hetzel, D. J., F. Bochner, D. M. Imhoff, G. E. Gibson, R. J. Fitch, R. Hecker, J. LeBrooy, D. J. C. Shearman, Azodisalicylate (ADS) in the treatment of ulcerative colitis: A controlled trial and assessment of drug disposition (abstr.), Gastroenterology, 88:1418 (1985).
29. Sandberg-Gertzen, H., G. Jarnerot, K. Bukhave, K. Lauritsen, J. Rask-Madsen, Effect of azodisal sodium and sulphasalazine on ileostomy output of fluid and PGE_2 and PGF_2 in subjects with a permanent ileostomy, Gut, 27:1306–1311 (1986).
30. Goerg K. J., et al., Azodisalicylate (Azodisal sodium) causes intestinal secretion: Comparative study of the effect of azodisalicylate, sulfasalazine, 5-aminosalicylic acid and sulfapyridine on the water and electrolyte transfer and the morphology of the rat ileum and colon in vivo, Digestion, 37: 79–87 (1987).
31. Mohsen, A. Q. M., D. Mulvey, J. D. Priddle, D. S. Parsons, D. P. Jewell, Effects of olsalazine in the jejunum of the rat, Gut, 28:346–352 (1987).
32. Pamukcu, R., S. B. Hanauer, E. B. Chang, Effect of disodium azodisalicylate in electrolyte transport in rabbit ileum and colon in vitro: Comparison with sulfasalazine and 5-aminosalicylic acid. Gastroenterology, 95:975–981 (1988).
33. Hanauer, S. B., J. B. Kirsner, Medical therapies in ulcerative colitis. In: Inflammatory Bowel Disease, 3rd ed., (Shorter, R. G., Kirsner, J. B., eds.) Philadelphia, Lea & Febiger pp. 431–476 (1988).
34. Chan, R. P. D. J. Pope, A. P. Gilbert, P. J. Sacra, J. H. Baron, J. E. Lennard-Jones, Studies of two novel sulfasalazine analogues, Ipsalazide and Balsalazide, Dig. Dis. Sci., 28:609–615 (1983).
35. McIntyre, P. B., C. A. Rodrigues, J. E. Lennard-Jones, I. G. Barrison, J. G. Walker, J. H. Baron, Double-blind controlled comparison of balsalazide and sulphasalazine in maintenance therapy of patients with ulcerative colitis (letter), Gut, 27:1271–1272 (1986).
35a. McIntyre, P. B., C. A. Rodrigues, J. E. Lennard-Jones, I. G. Barrison, J. G. Walker, J. H. Baron, P. C. Thornton, Balsalazide in the maintenance treatment of patients with ulcerative colitis, a double-blind comparison with sulphasalazine, Alimentary Pharm. Therapeut., 2:237–243 (1988).
36. Myers, B., D. N. W. Evans, J. Rhodes, B. K. Evans, B. R. Hughes, M. G. Lee, A. Richens, D. Richards, Metabolism and urinary excretion of 5-aminosalicylic acid in healthy volunteers when given intravenously or released for absorption at different sites in the gastrointestinal tract, Gut, 28(2):196–200 (1987).
37. Rijk, M. C. M., A. Van Schaik, J. H. M. Van Tongeren, Disposition of 5-aminosalicylic acid by 5-aminosalicylic acid-delivering compounds, Scand. J. Gastroenterol. 23:107–112 (1988).
38. Dew, M. J., P. Ebden, N. S. Kidwai, G. I. Lee, B. K. Evans, J. Rhodes, Comparison of the absorption and metabolism of sulphasalazine and

acrylic-coated 5-aminosalicylic acid in normal subjects and patients with ulcerative colitis, Br. J. Clin. Pharmacol., 17:474–476 (1984).

39. Dew, M. J., R. E. J. Ryder, B. K. Evans, J. Rhodes, Colonic release of 5-aminosalicylic acid from an oral preparation in active ulcerative colitis, Br. J. Clin. Pharmacol., 16:185–187 (1983).
40. Christensen, L. A., J. Fallingborg, K. Abilgaard, B. Jacobsen, G. Sanchez, S. H. Hansen, S. Bondesen, E. Hvidberg, S. N. Rasmussen, A comparison of topical and systemic availability of three pure 5-aminosalicylic acid preparations (Asacol, Claversal, and Pentasa) in ileostomy patients and normal human volunteers (abstr.). Clinical Controversies in Inflammatory Bowel Disease Symposium, September 9–11, 1987, Bologna, Italy. In: Mesalazine Treatment of Inflammatory Bowel Diseases, Vol. 1: Mechanisms and Pharmacokinetics, p. 181.
41. Hardy, J. G., J. N. C. Healey, S. W. Lee, J. R. Reynolds, Gastrointestinal transit of an enteric-coated delayed-release 5-aminosalicylic acid tablet, Alimentary Pharmacol. Therapeu., 1(3):209–216 (1987).
42. Christensen, L. A., O. Slot, G. Sanchez, J. Boserup, S. N. Rasmussen, S. Bondesen, S. H. Hansen, E. F. Hvidberg, Release of 5-aminosalicylic acid from Pentasa during normal and accelerated intestinal transit time, Br. J. Clin. Pharmacol., 23(3):365–369 (1987).
43. Bondesen, S., U. Tage-Jensen, O. Jacobsen, S. H. Hansen, S. N. Rasmussen, E. F. Hvidberg, 5-aminosalicylic acid in patients with ileo-rectal anastomosis: A comparison of the fate of sulfasalazine and Pentasa, Eur. J. Clin. Pharmacol., 31(1):23–26 (1986).
44. Campieri, M., G. A. Lanfranchi, C. Brignola, G. Bazzocchi, M. R. Minguzzi, P. Gionchetti, High-dose 5-aminosalicylic acid enemas in the treatment of ulcerative colitis, Intern. Med., 5:164–171 (1984).
45. Lanfranchi, G. A., M. Campieri, C. Brignola, G. Bazzocchi, M. R. Minguzzi, P. Gionchetti, D. Valeri, S. Veggetti, Treatment of ulcerative colitis patients with high dose 5-ASA enemas. Report of 2 years in an outpatient clinic (abstr.), Gastroenterology, 86:1151 (1984).
46. Campieri, M., G. A. Lanfranchi, C. Brignola, G. Bazzocchi, M. R. Minguzzi, M. T. Calari, 5-aminosalicylic acid as rectal enemas in ulcerative colitis in patients unable to take sulphasalazine (letter), Lancet, 1:403 (1982).
47. Sutherland, L. R., F. Martin, S. Greer, M. Robinson, N. Greenberger, F. Saibil, T. Martin, J. Sparr, E. Prokipchuk, L. Borgen, 5-Aminosalicylic acid enemas in the treatment of distal ulcerative colitis, proctosigmoiditis, and proctitis, Gastroenterology, 92:1894–1898 (1987).
48. Hanauer, S. B., P. A. Schultz, Efficacy of 5-ASA enemas for steroid dependent ulcerative colitis (abstr.), Gastroenterology, 90:1449 (1986).
49. Hanauer, S. B., P. A. Schultz, Relapse rates after successful treatment of refractory colitis with 5-ASA enemas (abstr.), Gastroenterology, 92(5): 1424 (1987).
50. Barber, G. B., D. E. Lee, D. A. Antonioli, M. A. Peppercorn, Refractory distal ulcerative colitis responsive to 5-aminosalicylate enemas, Am. J. Gastroenterol., 80:612–614 (1985).

51. McPhee, M. S., J. T. Swan, W. L. Biddle, N. J. Greenberger, Proctocolitis unresponsive to conventional therapy: Responsive to 5-aminosalicylic acid enemas, Dig. Dis. Sci., 32:76S–81S (1987).
52. Janssens, J., K. Geboes, C. Delanote, G. Vantrappen, 5-Aminosalicylic acid (5-ASA) enemas are effective in patients with resistant ulcerative rectosigmoiditis (abstr.), Gastroenterology, 84:1198 (1983).
53. Guarino, J., M. Chatzinoff, T. Berk, L. S. Friedman, 5-Aminosalicylic acid enemas in refractory distal ulcerative colitis: Long-Term results, Am. J. Gastroenterol., 87:732–737 (1987).
54. Biddle, W. L., N. J. Greenberger, J. T. Swan, M. S. McPhee, P. B. Miner, 5-aminosalicylic acid enemas: Effective agent in maintaining remission in left-sided ulcerative colitis, Gastroenterology, 94:1075–1079 (1988).
55. d'Albasco, G., F. Pacini, P.Blanc, S. Innocenti, M. Milla, A. Nucci, A controlled trial with intermittent 5-aminosalicylic acid (5-ASA) enemas (abstr.), 2nd International Symposium on Inflammatory Bowel Diseases, Jerusalem, Israel, September 8–11, 1985.
56. Willoughby, C. P., M. Campieri, G. Lanfranchi, S. C. Truelove, D. P. Jewell, 5-Aminosalicylic acid (Pentasa) in enema form for the treatment of active ulcerative colitis, Ital. J. Gastroenterol., 18:15–17 (1986).
56a. A Danish 5-ASA study group, Topical 5-aminosalicylic acid versus prednisolone in ulcerative proctosigmoiditis, A randomized, double-blind multicenter trial, Dig. Dis. Sci., 32:598-602 (1987).
57. Powell-Tuck, J., R. A. Parkins, Controlled comparison of enemas containing 1 gm and 2 gm 5-aminosalicylic acid in patients with ulcerative proctosigmoiditis (abstr.), Gut, 25:A1143 (1984).
58. Hanauer, S. B., S. V. Kane, B. Guernsey, T. O'Connor, M. Robinson, M. Peppercorn, F. B. Rosenberg, D. Weinberg, A. I. Rogers, J. Singleton, Randomized clinical trial of Mesalamine (5-ASA) enemas in distal ulcerative colitis: A dose-ranging placebo-controlled study, Gastroenterology, 96(5): A247 (1989).
59. Campieri, M., G. A. Lanfranchi, F. Bertoni, C. Brignola, G. Bazzocchi, M. R. Minguzzi, G. Labo, A double-blind clinical trial to compare the effects of 4-aminosalicylic acid to 5-aminosalicylic acid in topical treatment of ulcerative colitis, Digestion, 29:204–208 (1984).
60. Selby, W. S., M. K. Bennett, D. P. Jewell, Topical treatment of distal ulcerative colitis with 4-aminosalicylic acid enemas, Digestion, 29:231 (1984).
61. Ginsberg, A. L., L. S. Beck, T. M. McIntosh, L. E. Nochomovitz, Treatment of left-sided ulcerative colitis with 4-aminosalicylic acid enemas: A double-blind, placebo-controlled trial, Ann. Intern. Med., 108:195–199 (1988).
62. Gandolfo, J., F. Farthing, G. Powers, K. Eagen, M. Goldberg, P. Berman, M. Kaplan, 4-aminosalicylic acid retention enemas in treatment of distal colitis, Dig. Dis. Sci., 32(7):700–704 (1987).
63. Van Hees, P. A., J. H. Bakker, J. H. M. Van Tongeren, Effect of sulphapyridine, 5-aminosalicylic acid, and placebo in patients with idiopathic proctitis: a study to determine the active therapeutic moiety of sulphasalazine, Gut, 21:632 (1980).

64. Campieri, M., G. A. Lanfranchi, C. Brignola, G. Bazzocchi, P. Gionchetti, M. R. Minguzzi, A. Belluzzi, O. Basso, A controlled trial on the efficacy and compliance of 5-ASA enemas vs. 5-ASA suppositories in distal ulcerative sigmoiditis (abstr.), Gastroenterology, 90:1364 (1986).
65. Maier, K., C. Fischer, U. Klotz, K. Heinkel, 5-aminosalcysaure bei colitis ulcerosa und morbus Crohn, Detusch. Med. Wschr., 107:1131 (1982).
66. Maier, K., C. Fischer, U. Klotz, 5-aminosalicyasure - ein neues behand lungsprinzip bei colitis ulcerosa und morbus Crohn, Verdauungskrankheiten, 1:62-65 (1983).
67. Borgen, L. A., S. B. Hanauer, L. Good, C. N. Williams, G. Haber, Mesalamine suppository efficacy in ulcerative proctitis: A multicenter placebo-controlled trial, Gastroenterology, 94(5):A42.
68. Meyers, S., D. B. Sachar, D. H. Present, H. D. Janowitz, Olsalazine sodium in the treatment of ulcerative colitis among patients intolerant of sulfasalazine, Gastroenterology, 93:1255-1262 (1987).
69. Ireland, A., W. S. Selby, G. D. Barr, C.H. Mason, D. P. Jewell, Azodisalicylate for the treatment of active ulcerative colitis (abstr.), Gut, 26:A1157 (1985).
70. Willoughby, C. P., R. E. Cowan, S. R. Gould, R. J. Machell, J. B. Stewart, A comparison of oral olsalazine and sulphasalazine in active ulcerative colitis (abstr.). Dipentum (olsalazine) in the treatment of ulcerative colitis: First International Symposium, Oxford, March 20-21, pp. 20 (1987).
71. Ewe, K, Therapeutic trial of olsalazine in ulcerative colitis (abstr.). Dipentum (olsalazine) in the treatment of ulcerative colitis: First International Symposium, Oxford, March 20-21, pp. 29 (1987).
72. Feurle, G. E., Olsalazine vs placebo in the treatment of mild and moderate ulcerative colitis: A randomized, double-blind trial (abstr.). Dipentum (olsalazine) in the treatment of ulcerative colitis: First International Symposium, Oxford, March 20-21 pp. 18-19 (1987).
73. Riley S. A., V. Mani, M. J. Goodman, L. A. Turnberg, Delayed-release 5-aminosalicylic acid (5-ASA) and sulphasalazine (SSZ) in the treatment of mild to moderate ulcerative colitis (UC) relapse (abstr.). Mesalazine Treatment of Inflammatory Bowel Disease, Vol. 2, Therapy and Recurrence Prophylaxis, pp. 166 (1987).
74. Barbara, L., B. Bianchi Porro, G. Biasco, C. Brignola, M. Campieri, L. Codeluppi, G. A. Lanfranchi, F. Manenti, M. Miglioli, Oral 5-aminosalicylic acid (Asacol) in the treatment of active inflammatory bowel diseases: An Italian Cooperative Study. Clinical Controversies in Inflammatory Bowel Disease Symposium, September 9-11, Bologna, Italy (1987).
75. Schroeder, K. W., W. J. Tremaine, D. M. Ilstrup, Coated oral 5-aminosalicylic acid therapy for mildly to moderately active ulcerative colitis. N. Engl. J. Med., 317:1625-1629 (1987).
76. Maier, K., P. Fruhmorgen, J. C. Bode, T. Heller, U. Von Gaisberg, U. Klotz, Erfolgreiche Akutbehandlung chronischentzundlicher Darmerkrankungen mit oraler 5-aminosalyicysaure, Dtsch. Med. Wochenschr., 10:363-368 (1985).

76a. Rachmielowitz, D., Coated mesalazine (5-aminosalicylic acid) versus sulphasalazine in the treatment of active ulcerative colitis: A randomized trial, Br. Med. J., 298:82–6 (1989).
77. Hanauer, S. B., Claversal, a buffered 5-ASA preparation with reliable, consistent ileal delivery providing effective, safe, well-tolerated therapy for inflammatory bowel disease. Clinical Controversies in Inflammatory Bowel Diseases, September 9–11, pp. 32–34 (1987).
77a. Hanauer, S., J. Schwartz, W. Roufail, M. Robinson, J. Cello, M. Safdi, B. Guernsey, L. Beshears, Dose-ranging study of oral mesalamine capsule Pentasa) for active ulcerative colitis, Gastroenterology, 96(5):A195 (1989).
78. Jewell, D. P., A. Ireland, Controlled trial comparing Olsalazine and sulphasalazine for maintenance treatment of ulcerative colitis, Scand. J. Gastroenterol, 23(suppl 148):45–47 (1988).
79. Dew, M. J., P. Hughes, A. D. Harries, G. Williams, B. K. Evans, J. Rhodes, Maintenance of remission in ulcerative colitis with oral preparation of 5-aminosalicylic acid, Br. Med. J., 295:1012 (1982).
80. Dew, M. J., A. D. Harries, N. Evans, B. K. Evans, J. Rhodes, Maintenance of remission in ulcerative colitis with 5-aminosalicylic acid in high doses by mouth, Br. Med. J., 287:23–24 (1984).
81. Riley, S. A., V. Mani, M. J. Goodman, M. E. Herd, S. Dutt, L. A. Turnberg, Comparison of delayed-release 5-aminosalicylic acid (Mesalazine) and sulfasalazine as maintenance treatment for patients with ulcerative colitis, Gastroenterology, 94:1383–1389 (1988).
82. Mulder, C. J. J., G. N. J. Tytgat, I. T. Weterman, W. Dekker, P. Blok, M. Schrijver, v.d. H. Deide, Double-blind evaluation of slow-release 5-aminosalicylic acid (Pentasa) and slazopyridin (Salazopyrin) in the treatment of patients suffering from ulcerative colitis in remission (abstr.). Clinical Controversies in Inflammatory Bowel Diseases, September 9–11, Italy pp. 172 (1987).
83. Ruetgeerts, P., Efficacy and safety of mesalazine in maintenance treatment of ulcerative colitis: A double-blind, randomized comparison with sulfasalazine, Scand. J. Gastroenterol. (submitted).
84. Rasmussen, S. N., V. Binder, K. Maier, S. Bondesen, C. Fischer, U. Klotz, S. H. Hansen, E. F. Hvidberg, Treatment of Crohn's disease with peroral 5-aminosalicylic acid, Gastroenterology, 85:1350–1353 (1983).
85. Rasmussen, S. N., K. Lauritsen, U. Tage-Jensen, O. H. Nielsen, P. Bytzer, O. Jacobsen, K. Ladefoged, M. Vilien, V. Binder, J. Rask-Madsen, S. Bondesen, S. Honore Hansen, E. F. Hvidberg, 5-Aminosalicylic acid in the treatment of Crohn's disease: A 16-week double-blind, placebo-controlled, multicentre study with Pentasa, Scand. J. Gastroenterol., 27:877–883 (1987).
86. Saverymuttu, S. H., S. Gupta, A. Keshavarzian, B. Donovan, H. J. F. Hodgson, Effect of a slow-release 5-aminosalicylic acid preparation on disease activity in Crohn's disease, Digestion, 33:89–96 (1986).
87. Wellman, W., P. C. Fink, F. Banner, F. W. Schmidt, Endotoxaemia in active Crohn's disease, Treatment with whole gut irrigation and 5-aminosalicylic acid, Gut, 27:814–820 (1986).

88. Brignola, C., P. Farruggie, M. Campieri, G. Bazzocchi, A. Tragnone, P. Iannone, S. Pasquali, G. Sacco, G. A. Lanfranchi, Prevention of relapses in CD in clinical remission with oral 5-ASA. Clinical Controversies in Inflammatory Bowel Disease Symposium, September 9–11, Bologna, Italy (1987).
89. Wellmann, W., Maintenance of remission in Crohn's disease and ulcerative colitis with Mesalazine. Clinical Controversies in Inflammatory Bowel Diseases Symposium, September 9–11, Bologna, Italy (1987).
90. Thompson A. B. R., Mesasal/Claversal (5-ASA) prevents relapse and maintains remission of inactive Crohn's disease. International Study Group (submitted). (1988).
91. Calder, I. C., P. J. Williams, R. A. et al, Nephrotoxicity and molecular structure, Xenobiotica, 5:303–307 (1975).
92. Calder, I. C., C. C. Funder, C. R. Green, K. N. Ham, J. D. Tange, Nephrotoxic lesions from 5-aminosalicylic acid, Br. Med. J. 1:152–154 (1972).
93. Bilyard, K., Mesalazine: An overview of key preclinical studies, Scand. J. Gastroenterolo. (submitted).
94. Diener, U., H. V. Tuczek, C. Fischer, K. Maier, U. Klotz, Renal function was not impaired by treatment with 5-aminosalicylic acid in rats and man, Arch. Pharmacol., 326:278–282 (1984).
95. Novis, B. H., Z. Korzets, P. Chen, J. Bernheim, Nephrotic syndrome after treatment with 5-aminosalicylic acid, Br. Med. J., 296:1442 (1988).
96. Kutty, P. K., K. R. Raman, K. Hawken, J. A. Barrowman, Hair loss and 5-ASA enemas, Ann. Intern. Med., 97:785–786 (1982).
97. Martin, F., Oral 5-aminosalicylic acid preparations in treatment of inflammatory bowel disease: An update, Dig. Dis. Sci., 32(12):57S–63S (1987).
98. Brimblecombe, Mesasal/Claversal: A global safety evaluation, Scand. J. Gastroenterol. (submitted).
99. Mulder, C. J. J., G. N. J. Tytgat, W. Dekker, I. J. Terpstra, Pentasa in lieu of sulfasalazine, Ann. Intern. Med., 106:911–912 (1988).
100. Donald, I. P., S. P. Wilkinson, The value of 5-aminosalicylic acid in inflammatory bowel disease for patients intolerant or allergic to sulphasalazine, Postgrad. Med. J., 61:1047–1048 (1985).
101. Rao, S. S., P. A. Cann, C. D. Holdsworth, Clinical experience of the tolerance of mesalazine and olsalazine in patients intolerant of sulphasalazine, Scand. J. Gastroenterol., 22:332–336 (1987).
102. Austin, C. A., P. A. Cann, T. H. Jones, C. D. Holdsworth, Exacerbation of diarrhoea and pain in patients treated with 5-aminosalicylic acid for ulcerative colitis, Lancet, 1(8382):917–918 (1984).
103. Burke, D. A., A. P. Manning, J. M. S. Williamson, A. T. R. Axon, Adverse reactions to sulphasalazine and 5-aminosalicylic acid in the same patient, Alimentary Pharm. Therapeut., i(3):201–208 (1987).
104. Chakraborty, T. K., D. Bhatia, R. C. Heading, M. J. Ford, Salicylate induced exacerbation of ulcerative colitis, Gut, 28:613–615 (1987).
105. Goerg, K. J., R. Wanitschke, C. Beck, P. Diehl, K. H. Meyer zum Buschenfeld, Secretory effect of azodisalicylate (azodisal sodium) on the short circuited mucosa of the rat ileum in vitro, Gut, 29:336–341 (1988).

5
Metronidazole

Lawrence J. Brandt

Montefiore Medical Center/Albert Einstein College of Medicine, Bronx, New York

I. INTRODUCTION AND HISTORY

Metronidazole was discovered in France in 1957 and was introduced on the European market two years later as the first effective therapy for trichomonas infection. In 1963, Shinn (1) demonstrated the efficacy of the drug against a variety of anaerobic organisms, and in 1971 the drug was first used for the treatment of gram-negative and gram-positive anaerobic infections. Some 10 years later the Food and Drug Administration approved metonidazole for use as an antibacterial agent in the United States.

The history of metronidazole as a treatment for inflammatory bowel disease began in 1975, when Ursing and Kamme from University Hospital in Lund, Sweden, reported their experience in using the drug to treat patients with Crohn's disease (2). Their intention and hope was to reduce the bacterial population in the small intestine, thereby improving absorption and eliminating bacterial antigens that might be contributing to the pathogenesis of the disease. They administered metronidazole to five patients, four of whom responded within 2 to 4 weeks, while the fifth responded at 4 months.

Since this seminal report by Ursing and Kamme, there have been reports of hundreds of patients, including dozens of children and adolescents who have received metronidazole for the treatment of Crohn's disease involving the ileum, colon, and perineum, especially when complicated by a variety of fistulas (2-14). Such reports consist largely of uncontrolled observations, with only one double-blind controlled trial (12). In this cooperative study metronidazole was compared to sulfasalazine in the treatment of Crohn's disease and found to be equal or superior to the latter agent, especially for the treatment of colonic disease. Anecdotally, it is probable that thousands of individuals have received metronidazole as primary or adjunctive therapy for Crohn's disease.

In another study, Demling and Schneider obtained remission in 10 of 10 patients with active Crohn's disease using metronidazole as therapy when steroids and sulfasalazine had failed (14). Closure of fistulas was reported in 12 of 24 patients and included enterocutaneous, perineal, rectovaginal, and postoperative fistulas. Metronidazole was considered of particular value in patients whose disease was resistant to other drugs or complicated by fistulas.

Improvement in the symptoms, disease activity, or objective studies in patients with Crohn's disease treated with metronidazole has been variable, ranging in the literature from 19 to 100%. A more consistent improvement has been observed in the perineal manifestations of the disease, and in our study advanced or complete healing was documented in close to 85% of subjects (10).

II. PHARMACOKINETICS

Metronidazole is a nitroimidazole compound, bearing a free nitro group which is essential for its action against anaerobic organisms. The drug has about the same molecular weight as glucose and is rapidly absorbed after oral administration. Absorption after rectal administration is slower and more variable, reaching peak blood levels in approximately 1 hour. The drug is freely diffusible, and less than 20% is protein bound. It penetrates all body fluids rapidly, including cerebrospinal fluid, bile, milk, and pus, and appears quickly on the mucosal surfaces of the gastrointestinal, genitourinary, and respiratory tracts. It is excreted into the urine along with its metabolites and has a serum half-life of about 8 hours.

Following the passive diffusion of metronidazole into a bacterial or parasitic cell, its free nitro group is sequentially reduced by electron donors of low redox potential. During the reduction, unstable toxic intermediates are formed which bind to bacterial DNA and RNA, effecting death of the organism. These active, shortlived intermediates formed within susceptible organisms have not yet been isolated. This bacteriocidal action persists even in the presence of other agents which inhibit replication or protein synthesis, thereby enabling metronidazole to be used in combination antimicrobial regimens. Unchanged metronidazole is excreted in the urine with the end products of anaerobic bacterial reduction and cleavage, acetamide and ethyl hydroxamic acid. These two products are bacteriologically inactive but do possess some mutagenic activity.

Within the mammalian liver, metronidazole is metabolized via a different pathway than in bacterial systems. Rather than nitroreduction, either of the two side chains of metronidazole can be oxidized, forming an "alcohol" or an "acid" metabolite. These major metabolites, along with metronidazole itself, are found in the urine, but only the alcohol metabolite is found in the serum when renal function is normal. Because the free nitro group of metronidazole must be reduced before the cell harboring the nitroreductase can be killed and because mammalian cells lack this enzyme, metronidazole is not generally toxic to human cells. However, mutagenicity, which will be mentioned later is a property of the parent compound and of both major metabolites of metronidazole and has been observed in some mammalian species, albeit not in humans. In patients with impaired liver function, metronidazole has a prolonged half-life. Drug clearance is not altered in the anuric patient, but is increased in subjects undergoing hemodialysis (15).

III. CLINICAL INVESTIGATIONS

A. Crohn's Disease

Metronidazole was first used in the treatment of Crohn's disease in 1975 in preliminary studies by Ursing and colleagues (2). Currently, our indications for the use of metronidazole based on our experience and the patients reported to date include, in decreasing order of effectiveness: (1) disabling or persistent perineal disease; (2) enterocutaneous fistulas; (3) active colonic disease; (4) resistant small bowel disease; and (5) inadvisability of other agents.

A wide variety of fistulas respond to metronidazole. Probably postoperative fistulas respond best, followed by perineal and enterocutaneous fistulas.

Ursing and co-workers from six hospitals reported the results from a double crossover trial in the Scandinavian cooperative study (12). Metronidazole (800 mg) was compared with 3.0 g of sulfasalazine in the treatment of 78 patients with Crohn's disease over a 4-month period. Equality or a slight edge in favor of metronidazole was noted. No difference in the Crohn's Disease Activity Index or in adverse effects between the two drugs was noted. Both drugs were more effective with colonic disease than small bowel disease. In Ursing's experience, approximately two-thirds of patients with colonic disease achieve a quiescent stage of disease within several months of treatment with metronidazole. In 8 of 17 patients the manifestations of colonic disease (e.g., ulcerations, edema, fistulas, and strictures) improved on barium study after four months on the drug. The clinical response of patients with isolated small bowel involvement is limited and seems to be accounted for simply by the treatment of bacterial overgrowth related to intestinal stasis. Metronidazole was more effective on crossover than sulfasalazine, led to a slightly greater rise in hemoglobin, and may have had a more pronounced regressive effect on barium enema changes. The benignity of sulfasalazine with long-term therapy however, and the great experience with this agent make it preferable as primary therapy is uncomplicated disease when it is tolerated by the patients.

Studies of the use of metronidazole in children are limited. Ursing reports on 20 children, half of whom improved—including normalization of growth in some (16). Daum and colleagues have treated 13 children and have noted a decrease in the Crohn's Disease Activity Index and a steroid-sparing effect (unpublished observations).

Since 1979 we have been using metronidazole in the treatment of chronic perineal manifestations of Crohn's disease (10,11). These manifestations include complex abscesses, metastatic ulcer, the unhealed proctectomy wound, and rectovaginal fistulas. In subjects maintained on therapy for more than two months, advanced or complete healing was observed in more than 80% (11).

B. Ulcerative Colitis

Metronidazole is effective in treating carageen-induced "ulcerative colitis" in guinea pigs, a disease not identical with ulcerative colitis in humans and one in which anaerobic bacteria play an important causative role (17). In a double-blind placebo-controlled crossover trial performed by Davies and colleagues, 22 patients with chronic proctitis were treated for 28 days with metronidazole suppositories without beneficial effect (18). In a less rigorous open trial by the same authors in which patients were treated with varying regimens of metronidazole orally and by enema, some beneficial effect was shown. In a more recent study comparing metronidazole with sulfasalazine in the management of acute and active, but not severe ulcerative colitis, metronidazole was shown to be ineffective (19). Metronidazole has also been evaluated as a adjunct to corticosteroids in treating patients with severe ulcerative colitis and was not shown to be of any additional benefit (20). When given to patients with ulcerative colitis on long-term sulfasalazine therapy, metronidazole induced no significant change in sulfapyridine levels, suggesting the split of the azo bond of sulfasalazine by bacterial azoreductase is not inhibited by metronidazole (21).

C. Recommendations for Therapy

1. What Is the Recommended Dose of Metronidazole?

Ursing's original studies employed a dose of almost 40 mg/kg, which resulted in clinical benefit, but was associated with an intolerable incidence of nausea, dizziness, fatigue, and paresthesia. The dose of metronidazole used in our studies of perineal Crohn's disease was 20 mg/kg, a dose we continue to recommend at the present. However, some investigators have found that a 10–15 mg/kg dose is much better tolerated and is still effective (16). Dosage should be increased slowly to the desired level which usually can be reached in several days. Reduction in dosage by 250 mg a day for several days is usually sufficient to minimize intolerance. Dosage recommendation for long-term therapy is arbitrary. I maintain full dosage (20 mg/kg) of the drug for a minimum of 6 months if such can be tolerated. I then begin to decrease the daily amount given by 250 mg (one pill) each month, attempting to discontinue therapy after approximately one year. The optimal dose for long-term maintenance therapy has yet to be established.

2. When Will Patients Show a Response to Metronidazole Therapy?

Some patients with colonic or ileocolonic disease will show signs of improvement within two weeks to one month after beginning therapy (16). Most intestinal responses will manifest after one to two months of treatment.

Some patients with perineal manifestations of Crohn's disease, especially those with tender abscesses and draining fistulas will also respond within the first few weeks of treatment. However, therapy cannot be judged to have failed until 6 to 8 weeks into therapy. Some patients will show a very gradual yet progressive response with maximum benefit at 3 to 4 months. Patients should be encouraged to stay on full dosage, if tolerated for at least 3 months.

3. Can the Dose of Metronidazole Be Stopped Without Disease Exacerbation?

Our attempts to reduce the dose or discontinue metronidazole altogether were associated with worsening of disease activity in two-thirds of the patients. Discontinuation of therapy was attempted either because of complete healing or persistent paresthesia. Reactivation of perineal disease activity occurred at various intervals from 2 weeks to 3 months. In less than one-third of these patients could the metronidazole therapy be discontinued without exacerbation. In all those in whom metronidazole therapy was later reinstituted in full dosage, the perineal disease responded as it had originally.

Thus, our experience indicates that although it is safe to reduce or discontinue metronidazole therapy, in only a minority of patients will such an attempt be successful. Exacerbation of disease, while expected, should respond to reinstitution of therapy.

4. Does Crohn's Disease Become Resistant to Metronidazole Therapy?

The necessity of long-term continuing therapy with metronidazole raises the question of the likelihood of the disease becoming resistant to the drug's effect. Ours and other studies suggest that metronidazole continues to be an effective agent in the treatment of perineal and bowel disease for periods as long as six years. Only 2 of the more than 40 patients whom we have treated suffered exacerbation of the perineal disease while on full dosage; one after 8 months and one after 12 months of therapy.

IV. MECHANISM OF ACTION

The mechanism of action of metronidazole remains unknown. While immunosuppression has been shown in animals and improved leukocyte chemotaxis in human subjects, improvement in patients with intestinal Crohn's disease has only been correlated with the drug's antimicrobial effect. Thus, there is a rough correlation between symptomatic improvement and diminution of fecal colony counts for bacteroides by 3 log powers; that is, 99.9% reduction in colon counts. Normal controls show no reduction in the fecal population of bacteroides. While data on the absorption of metronidazole in Crohn's disease are conflicting, in general, patients with Crohn's disease excrete more metronidazole and its metabolites in the feces than do normal controls in whom fecal levels of the drug are extremely low. Moreover, patients with active disease or those with Crohn's colitis and ileocolitis, excrete more of the compound into the feces than do those subjects with quiescent disease or only small-bowel involvement. Metronidazole-induced healing of perineal disease, with the exception of abscesses and obvious infections, is not easily explained by the drug's antimicrobial properties.

V. ADVERSE REACTIONS

A. Reported Side Effects

Metronidazole is generally well tolerated by patients, although adverse reactions associated with short-term therapy are many. These include metallic taste, dark urine, nausea, diminished appetite, headache, urticaria, vaginal and urethral burning, and reversible neutropenia; most are dose related and easily handled by reducing the dosage by as little as 250 mg daily. A disulfiram-like effect has been reported in patients on metronidazole who drink alcoholic beverages, but we have yet to observe this reaction in any of our patients. Central nervous system side effects have been reported, although the more serious ones have been associated with doses of metronidazole (750 mg q6h) far exceeding those we have used.

The most significant side effect we have encountered with metronidazole therapy is paresthesia, which occurs in 50% of the patients and typically develops approximately 6 months after the initiation of drug therapy (11). Sensory peripheral nerves are affected, especially those innervating the lower limbs. Careful neurologic and laboratory testing in children has revealed an even higher incidence of sensory neural dysfunction and nerve conduction abnormalities (13). In contrast, in two separate studies in Sweden, not yet published but referred to by Ursing (16), 59 patients with Crohn's disease were investigated with electrophysiological measurements including motor and sensory nerve action potentials. Three groups of patients were examined. Eighteen were on metronidazole and had taken the drug for at least 12 months. Twenty patients had previously been treated with metronidazole for at least 12 months but treatment had been completed months or years before the examination. Twenty subjects who had never been on metronidazole acted as controls. No clinical or electrophysiological symptoms or signs of neuropathy attributable to the treatment with metronidazole were found and none of the groups differed from the other in respect to the neurophysiological findings.

Paresthesias in our patients appear to be dose related and, in some cases, gradually disappear after reducing the dosage by as little as 250 mg daily. Paresthesias were not progressive, but in some patients were quite prolonged if dosage was not decreased at their onset. In many patients, however, even after discontinuing therapy, paresthesia may persist for months to years before abating.

Metronidazole-induced peripheral neuropathy is believed to be due to axonal degeneration. In rodent experiments, metronidazole was found to bind selectively to neuronal RNA (21); this is in contrast to it antibacterial effect, which involves binding to the organism's DNA. In binding to neuronal RNA, metronidazole or its metabolites inhibit protein synthesis, resulting in axonal degeneration. Electron microscopic studies of human sural nerve biopsy specimens in two patients have shown loss of myelinated fibers, with additional fibers undergoing Wallerian degeneration. These changes reverted to normal with either discontinuation of the drug or reduction in the dosage (22).

Isolated instances of pancreatitis, liver abscess, fixed drug eruption, and probably unrelated leukemia and carcinomas have been reported.

B. Questions of Mutagenicity, Teratogenicity, and Carcinogenicity (23)

Metronidazole, its hepatic oxidative metabolites, and the reductive metabolites formed by bacteria are all mutagenic in the Ames test. In this test, the spontaneous mutation rate of certain histidine-dependent *Salmonella* is determined. Histidine is then removed from the growth medium and the test substance, for example, metronidazole is added. An increase in bacterial growth implies reversion to a wild nonhistidine-dependent mutant strain and shows good correlation with mutagenicity, teratogenic potential, and carcinogenicity in higher species. Despite the positive Ames test seen with metronidazole and its metabolites, a variety of mammalian test systems, including the dominant lethal test and micronucleus test, have not shown any mutagenic effects of the drug. In humans, no evidence of chromosomal damage was detected in 22 patients with Crohn's disease treated with sulfasalazine or metronidazole (800 mg daily) during repeated karyotyping over a 4-month period (24).

Neither embryotoxicity nor teratogenicity has been shown for mammalian species. In one study by Beard and colleagues, 771 woman were given metronidazole for the treatment of vaginal trichomoniasis. Use of metronidazole was documented during 57 of 698 pregnancies in this group, and in 23 instances this agent was administered during the first trimester without a significant increase in spontaneous abortion or congenital abnormalities (25). Nonetheless, the drug remains to be proven harmless during pregnancy, and in today's litigious climate, the drug should be avoided if possible until after delivery. However, since it is excreted in breast milk, it is contraindicated in the nursing mother.

The drug shows no oncogenicity in hamsters but the incidence of liver, mammary, and other carcinomas is increased in rats. However, this increase is considered questionable because the drug prolongs the life span of treated animals, and these tumors occur normally in aged rats. In mice, an increased number of pulmonary tumors and lymphomas was noted when 3 to 30 times the usual dosage employed for Crohn's disease was used. No statistical increase in tumor risk was demonstrated in the combined results of two studies performed over a 3 to 10-year follow-up period and including 3,231 subjects treated for *Trichomonas* infection (25,26). It should be remembered, however, that dosage was low, courses were short, and two decades may be an inadequate follow-up to detect drug-induced carcinoma. It is also prudent to remember that the drug is not yet approved by the Food and Drug Administration for the treatment of Crohn's disease, despite the many reports attesting to its effectiveness.

A study using the well-established 1,2-dimethylhydrazine model for colon neoplasia in rates (27), showed that a diet low in fiber enhanced colonic carcinogenesis and one high in fiber was protective. Much to the investigators' surprise, however, addition of metronidazole to the rat chow was associated with an increased incidence of colon cancer. Stool bacterioides counts were not depressed in the metronidazole-fed animals, nor was metronidazole detectable in the feces; both observations are in contrast to the patient with Crohn's disease in whom bacteroides counts are often depressed and metronidazole is assayable in stool. Metabolism of metronidazle in the rat is therefore different from that in patients with Crohn's disease, and these results, which show a cocarcinogenic effect of metonidazole, should not be translated into the clinical arena. However, while the evidence in mammalian systems for a carcinogenic effect of metronidazole is scanty, use of the drug over long periods in patients with premalignant disorders such as inflammatory bowel disease warrants concern.

VI. SUMMARY

Metronidazole at a dosage of 20 mg/kg is a useful agent for the treatment of Crohn's disease and especially for the perineal complications of the disease. It appears to be more useful in Crohn's colitis and ileocolitis than when disease is confined solely to the small intestine, and has an effect equal to that of sulfasalazine. Exacerbation of perineal disease is to be expected upon discontinuation of therapy. Although there are many minor side effects observed with metronidazole, the only troublesome side effect is paresthesia. Paresthesia appears to be dose related and not progressive, although it may persist for long periods after therapy has been discontinued.

Although no studies exist showing the drug to be mutagenic, teratogenic, or carcinogenic in humans, studies using the Ames test and tests in certain laboratory rodents raise concern about this possibility. The drug, therefore, should be stopped in three months if ineffective and repeated attempts should be made after six months to one year to discontinue therapy if disease activity is controlled. It is not a substitute for conservative perineal surgery, which may be utilized when the disease has stabilized and complete healing has not occurred.

REFERENCES

1. Shinn, D. L., Vincent's disease and its treatment, Excerpta Medica, 334-340 (1977).
2. Ursing, B., C. Kamme, Metronidazole for Crohn's disease, Lancet, 1:775 (1975).
3. Ursing, B., Metronidazole in Crohn's disease. In: Excerpta Medical Congress Series #386, The Management of Crohn's Disease, Amsterdam, Excerpta Medica Foundation, p. 189 (1975).
4. Ammann, R. W., J. Muller-Schoop, M. Knoblauch, Therapie des morbus Crohn in akuten schub mit ornidazol, Schweiz. Med. Wochenschr., 108: 1075 (1978).
5. Blichfeldt, P., J. P. Blonhoff, E. Myhre, et al., Metronidazole in Crohn's disease; a double-blind cross-over clinical trial, Scand. J. Gastroenterol., 13: 123 (1978).
6. Allan, R., W. T. Cook, Evaluation of metronidazole in the management of Crohn's disease, Gut, 18:A422 (1977).
7. Bardet, J. C., F. Besangon, J. P. Bourdias, Le traitment de la maladie de Crohn par le metronidazole. Resultats preliminaires d'un essai collectif, Gastroenterol., Clin. Biol., 2:342 (1978).
8. Kasper, H., H. Sommer, H. A. Hugn, Therapy of Crohn's disease with metronidazole–an uncontrolled trial, Acta HepatoGastroenterol., 26:217-221 (1979).
9. Ursing, B., Metronidazole in the treatment of Crohn's disease, Scand. J. Gastroenterol., 15:117 (1980).
10. Bernstein, L. H., M. S. Frank, L. J. Brandt, et al., Healing of perineal Crohn's disease with metronidazole, Gastroenterology, 79:357-365 (1980).
11. Brandt, L. J., L. H. Bernstein, S. J. Boley, et al., Metronidazole therapy for perineal Crohn's disease: a follow-up study, Gastroenterology, 83:383-387 (1982).
12. Ursing, B., T. Alm, F. Barany, et al., A comparative study of metronidazole and sulfasalazine for active Crohn's disease: The cooperative Crohn's disease study in Sweden, Gastroenterology, 83:550-562 (1982).

13. Duffy, L. F., F. Daum, S. E. Fisher, et al., Peripheral neuropathy in Crohn's disease patients treated with metronidazole, Gastroenterology, 88:681–684 (1985).
14. Demling, L., M. U. Schneider, S. Strobel, et al., Metronidazole in der behaandlung des morbus Crohn. Dtsch. Med. Wschr., 106:1126–1129 (1981).
15. Gabriel, R., C. M. Page, I. V. D. Weller et al., The pharmacokinetics of metronidazole in patients with chronic renal failure. In: Metronidazole. (Phillips, I., Collier, J., eds.), London, Academic Press, pp. 49–54 (1979). (Royal Society of Medicine International Congress and Symposium series no. 18.)
16. Ursing, B., Metronidazole therapy. In: Current Management of Inflammatory Bowel Disease. (Bayless, T., ed.), Toronto, Canada and Philadelphia, B. C. Decker (1988).
17. Onderdonk, A. B., J. A. Hermos, J. L. Dzink, J. G. Barlett, Protective effect of metronidazole in experimental ulcerative colitis, Gastroenterology, 74: 521–526 (1978).
18. Davies, P. S., J. Rhodes, R. V. Heatley, et al., Metronidazole in the treatment of chronic proctitis: a controlled study, Gut, 680–681 (1977).
19. Gilat, T., A. Suissa, G. Leichtman, G. Delere, M. Pavlotzky, A. Grossman, G. Fireman, A comparative study of metronidazole and sulfasalazine in active, not severe, ulcerative colitis, An Israeli multicenter trial, J. Clin. Gastroenterol., 9:415–417 (1987).
20. Chapman, R. W., W. S. Selby, D. P. Jewell, Controlled trial of intravenous metronidazole as adjunct to corticosteroids in severe ulcerative colitis, Gut, 27:1210–1212 (1986).
21. Schaffer, J. L., A. Kershaw, J. B. Houston, Disposition of metronidazole and its effect on sulphasalazine metabolism in patients with inflammatory bowel disease, Br. J. Clin. Pharmacol., 21:431–435 (1986).
22. Bradley, W. G., I. J. Karlsson, C. G. Rassol, Metronidazole neuropathy, Br. Med. J., 3:610–611 (1977).
23. Roe, F. J. C., Toxicologic evaluation of metronidazole with particular reference to carcinogenic, mutagenic, and teratogenic potential, Surgery, 93:158–164 (1983).
24. Mitelman, F., B. Strombeck, B. Ursing, No cytogenic effect of metronidazole, Lancet, 1:1249–1250 (1980).
25. Beard, C. M., K. L. Noller, W. M. O'Fallon, et al., Lack of evidence of cancer due to use of metronidazole, N. Engl. J. Med., 301-519 (1979).
26. Friedman, G. D., Cancer after metronidazole (letter), N. Engl. J. Med., 302: 519 (1979).
27. Sloan, D. A., D. M. Fleiszer, G. K. Richards, D. Murray, R. A. Brown, Increased incidence of experimental colon cancer associated with long-term metronidazole therapy, Am. J. Surg., 145:66–70 (1983).

6

Immunosuppressives

Burton I. Korelitz

Lenox Hill Hospital, New York, New York

The number of drugs effective against Crohn's disease and ulcerative colitis is small and in none is the mechanism of action thoroughly understood. While the dramatic effect of ACTH and corticosteroids is considered anti-inflammatory, their immunosuppressive action is commonly acknowledged. Sulfasalazine, 5-ASA, and metronidazole, too, are classified as anti-inflammatory, but their favorable actions might also be immunosuppressive. In common usage, however, the drugs which are thought to have their primary impact on cellular and humoral immunity are those for which the terminology immunosuppressive agents has been reserved. These in order of reported success in inflammatory bowel disease (IBD) include 6-mercaptopurine (6-MP), azathioprine, and cyclosporine.

Early enthusiasm for trials of 6-MP and azathioprine on the part of clinicians involved in management of IBD was influenced by the then new concept of autoimmune diseases, the possibility that Crohn's disease and ulcerative colitis belonged in this category, and the early success of immunosuppressive drugs in preventing the rejection of kidney transplants.

I. PHARMACOKINETICS OF 6-MP AND AZATHIOPRINE

6-MP and azathioprine are closely related, the latter being an S-substituted 6-mercaptopurine which is metabolized in vivo. Many or all of the pharmacological effects of azathioprine are actually due to the 6-MP degradation product.

6-MP was synthesized and developed by Hitchings, Elion, et al. at the Wellcome Research Laboratories (1,2). It is an analogue of the purine bases adenine and hypoxanthine and is converted by the enzyme HGPR Tase to the intracellular nucleotide thioinosinic acid which inhibits several reactions involving inosinic acid including an enzyme unique to the de novo pathway for purine ribonucleotide synthesis (2). Precisely which of the known biochemical effects of the drug are responsible for immunosuppression, or in fact whether it is immunosuppression that is responsible for its favorable effect on IBD, is not known. It has been demonstrated by Brogan et al. that the lymphoblastoid response to the tetanus toxoid in Crohn's disease patients is impaired when the disease is active, or improved on other drugs, but is normal when the disease is improved on 6-MP (3). They have also shown that both azathioprine and 6-MP selectively depress NK cell activity (3a). It is known that absorption in humans is incomplete and variable, but also that the biochemical effects of a single dose of 6-MP are evident long after the parent drug has disappeared from plasma.

Both 6-MP and azathioprine are manufactured in the form of 50 mg tablets by Burroughs-Wellcome, the 6-MP as Purinethol and the azathioprine as Imuran. Azathioprine has received the approval of the Food and Drug Administration for the treatment of rheumatoid arthritis and renal transplantation and 6-MP for the treatment of some leukemias, utilized mostly for those occurring in childhood. Burroughs-Wellcome has not applied for FDA approval for either drug for the treatment of IBD.

II. CLINICAL INVESTIGATION OF 6-MP AND AZATHIOPRINE

A. Historical Background

Historically, 6-MP was tried in IBD before azathioprine and its success was established in ulcerative colitis before Crohn's disease (4). Early enthusiasm was dampened by poor results and toxicity when the drug was initiated in the most severely ill ulcerative colitis patients (5). Nevertheless, many controlled and uncontrolled trials of azathioprine in the treatment of both ulcerative colitis and Crohn's disease of varying severity were undertaken in the 1960s and 1970s, encouraged by the favorable observations of Brooke et al. (6), who reported remarkable results with azathioprine in patients with extensive Crohn's disease including cases with fistulas. Uncontrolled trials showed favorable response (average 72%) in Crohn's disease (7,8) and a still more impressive result in ulcerative colitis (average 80%) (9–11) but controlled trials in both diseases showed no overall advantage of the drug over placebo (12–21). In some of these controlled trials it was noted that, in the patients receiving the azathioprine, steroids could be reduced to a greater extent than in those receiving the placebo.

In the mid-1960s studies were directed at children chronically ill with ulcerative colitis in whom corticosteroids could not be eliminated or required reintroduction soon after termination. The results were impressive. The choice of 6-MP over azathioprine in this study was fortuitous. It had been favored for three reasons: (a) A colleague in hematology, Dr. Nathaniel Wisch, who monitored the blood counts, had experience using 6-MP in the treatment of childhood leukemias but none with azathioprine; (b) no cases of cancer had been reported in which 6-MP had been implicated, and this was not the case with azathioprine; and (c) in ulcerative colitis, the immunosuppressive agent responsible for favorable responses had been 6-MP.

The enthusiasm engendered from the results of the uncontrolled trials in ulcerative colitis led to consideration of a controlled trial in Crohn's disease where, in contrast to ulcerative colitis, the incidence of complicating neoplasm was low, and where the chronicity of the disease without opportunity for cure by resection might warrant trial of a promising drug even if it carried a small risk of cancer.

A controlled double-blind cross-over study of 6-MP versus placebo in the treatment of patients with severe Crohn's disease who as yet had no absolute indication for surgical resection was initiated (22). Coincidentally, at approximately the same time, the National Cooperative Crohn's Disease Study (NCCDS) was launched as a collaboration of 14 centers (17). The choice of 6-MP in the one study was fortuitous since the outcome with this drug was favorable which was not the case with azathioprine. 6-MP is a metabolic byproduct of azathioprine and, therefore, the effective dose could be titrated more accurately. This was one of the distinctions from the NCCDS responsible for the failure of azathioprine in that study (23).

B. Controlled Trials in Crohn's Disease

1. *Overall Results*

In the double-blind controlled study, specific goals were defined for each patient, just as is done for Crohn's disease in its usual clinical management. The most common goals were the elimination of the primary bowel and systemic symptoms, the reduction and termination of corticosteroids, and the closing of fistulas. Other goals were the elimination of recurrent episodes of bowel obstruction, short bowel syndrome, and abdominal masses. These goals would pertain both to the primary involvement of the bowel with Crohn's disease or recurrent ileitis or colitis after resection. A later established goal was maintenance of remission once accomplished. Other drugs being taken by the patient at initiation of the study were not stopped. In the case of sulfasalazine, it was agreed the drug had failed overall, but its continuation would be less of a variable than its termination. In the case of corticosteroids, cessation of therapy would invite immediate exacerbation while the ability to reduce and eliminate could serve as a variable and a goal. In retrospect, this, too, was likely due to error in the design of the NCCDS where steroids had to be stopped in those randomized to another drug or to placebo (23).

In the course of the 6-MP study, patience was necessary for success since the worsening of symptoms, as defined in the protocol, warranted increase or reintroduction of steroids and this sequence might be indicated more than once. In retrospect, the mean time until response attributable to the 6-MP was 3.1 months. This signified that an immediate response was encountered rarely, consistent improvement without having to raise or reintroduce steroids occasionally, ups and downs over the first 3 months more commonly, and in some instances remission requiring close to a year to accomplish. Nevertheless the favorable results attributable to 6-MP were indisputable. This variable time for response, in retrospect, was another major difference from the protocol of the NCCDS which allowed for a trial limited to 17 weeks, thereby excluding many patients who might have been late responders (23).

The overall results of the double-blind 6-MP versus placebo trial can be summarized as follows. Of 83 patients, 39 received both placebo and 6-MP for one year each; 26 (67%) improved while receiving 6-MP; and only 3(8%) with placebo. This difference was highly significant ($p < 0.001$). In this group of 83 patients, 33 received only one drug, 6-MP or placebo; of the 19 receiving 6-MP the rate of improvement was 70% compared to the 29% improvement in the 14 treated with placebo ($p < 0.05$). To determine whether the outcome of the first year of trial had any influence on the outcome of the second year, a separate analysis of the first year data for 72 patients showed a highly significant difference favoring 6-MP; 26 of 36 (72%) versus 5 of 36 (14%) ($p < 0.001$).

2. Management of Steroids

In the 6-MP controlled study, 44 patients were receiving steroids at the outset; in 24 (55%) the steroids could be discontinued; and in another 9 (20%) reduced. Many patients with chronic disease entered into the study did not require steroids to control the disease while awaiting a response to 6-MP. Unpublished data show that the favorable outcome was the same whether patients had been on steroids or not. This was true also of sulfasalazine.

The favorable response of Crohn's disease to 6-MP occurs independent of the influence of steroids. Nevertheless, if the patient extremely ill with Crohn's disease is not treated with steroids, indications for surgery might arise before there has been an opportunity to respond to 6-MP. Therefore, steroids often should be introduced or reintroduced to "buy time" to realize the effectiveness of 6-MP. There is no apparent contraindication to using both drugs together. If anything, the leukocytosis caused by steroids counteracts the leukopenia accompanying 6-MP therapy, thereby permitting a larger dose if clinically warranted. Whether steroids and 6-MP have any direct synergistic therapeutic action has not been studied.

3. Effect on Fistulas

Fistulas, whether through compromise of quality of life by purulent discharge or by the pain of associated abscess formation, are distressing chronic complications of Crohn's disease. They rarely close spontaneously or in response to treatment with corticosteroids or sulfasalazine. Metronidazle has served to favorably influence the course of perirectal fistulas in some cases but has not been observed to help fistulas at other sites. Enteric fistulas have served as the most common complication of ileocolitis (24). Since ileocolitis is the most common distribution of Crohn's disease the enteric fistulas has been the most common indication for resective surgery. Less often perirectal abscesses and fistulas have led to diversionary surgery, usually with a colostomy. The results often have been disastrous with the risk of combinations of recurrent Crohn's colitis in the stoma, diversion colitis in the rectum, and persistence of perineal sepsis being realized.

6-MP is the first drug demonstrated to close internal fistulas in Crohn's disease (22,25) Abdominal wall fistulas improved or closed in 10 of 12 (83%), rectovaginal fistulas in 4 of 6 (67%), enteroenteric in 5 of 7 (71%), and vulval in 1 of 2 patients (50%); even perirectal fistulas, the least likely to respond to 6-MP without concomitant local anorectal surgery, closed or improved in 9 of 18 (50%). Recent experience with 6-MP in enterovesical fistulas has been reported (26). Overall the favorable response rate of fistulas to 6-MP has been 65% (Fig. 1).

4. Site of Involvement with Crohn's Disease

Analysis of data has consistently shown that moderate to excellent responses to 6-MP occur most often when the colon is involved with Crohn's disease. Crohn's disease of the colon, ileocolitis, and ileitis, in that order, have the best chance of improving on this agent. This is correlated with the relatively narrow lumen of small bowel compared to large and to obstruction being the most common complication of ileitis. Despite this, ileitis has improved on 6-MP in approximately 60% of cases.

5. Maintenance of Remission

In a controlled trial, O'Donoghue et al. (27) have demonstrated that remission in Crohn's disease once established was maintained by azathioprine in 70% at one year but not by placebo. Presumably, this success pertains to 6-MP as well.

Follow-up of 20 patients who participated in the controlled trial of 6-MP versus placebo and who continued to receive 6-MP for 18-72 months (mean 37 months) revealed that improvement was at least maintained in 16 and even bolstered in another 3 (95%), with only one patient suffering a relapse. Follow-up of 32 patients who stopped 6-MP after earlier favorable response showed that 26 (81%) relapsed while 6 (19%) did not. The time to recurrence of symptoms varied from 3 weeks to more than a year, so that at the end of one year 23 (72%) had relapsed and 9 (28%) had not. Nyman et al. (28) found that the

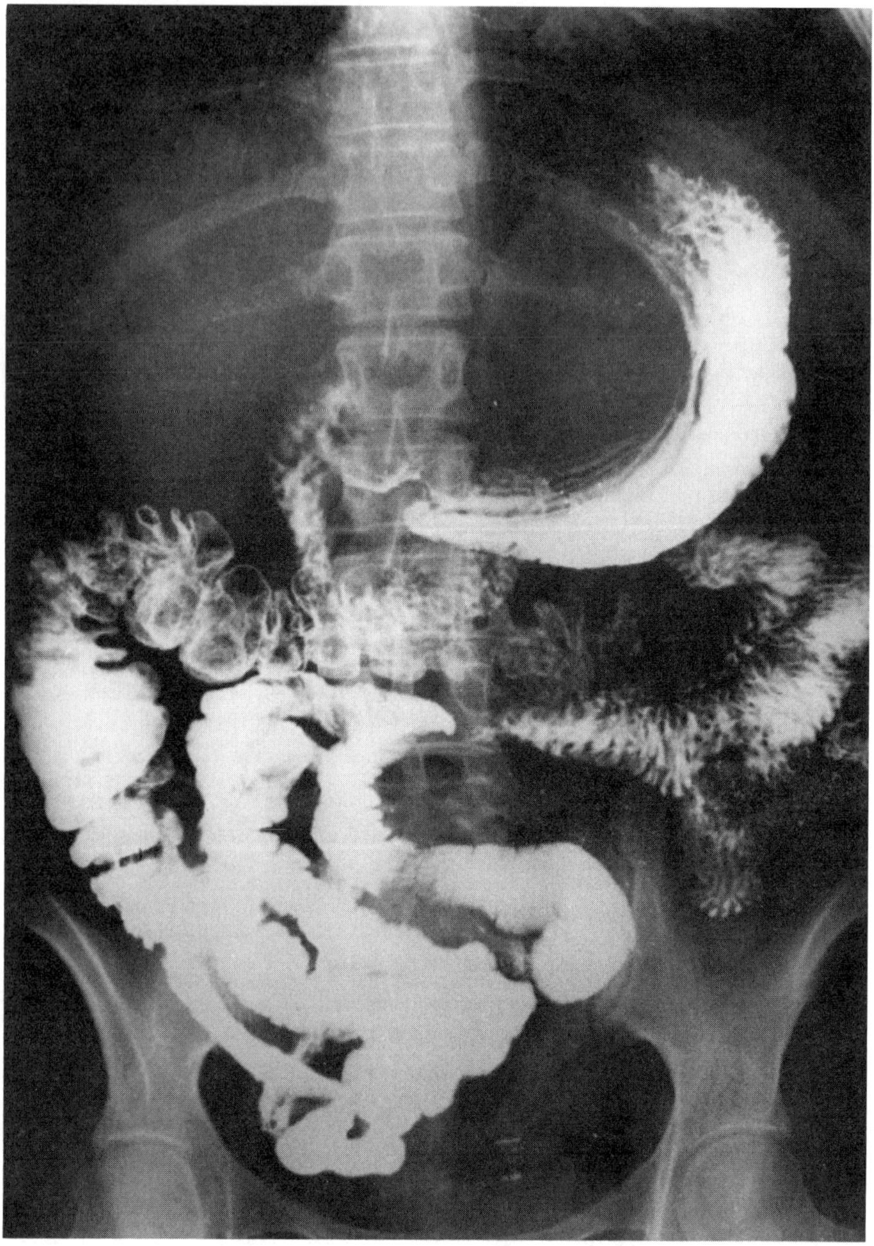

(a)

Figure 1 A 40-year-old woman with diarrhea and a rectovaginal fistula. (a) The upper GI and small bowel x-ray series showed nonstrictured ileitis. (b) After one year on 6-MP the rectovaginal fistula had closed and a repeat x-ray study showed a normal appearing terminal ileum.

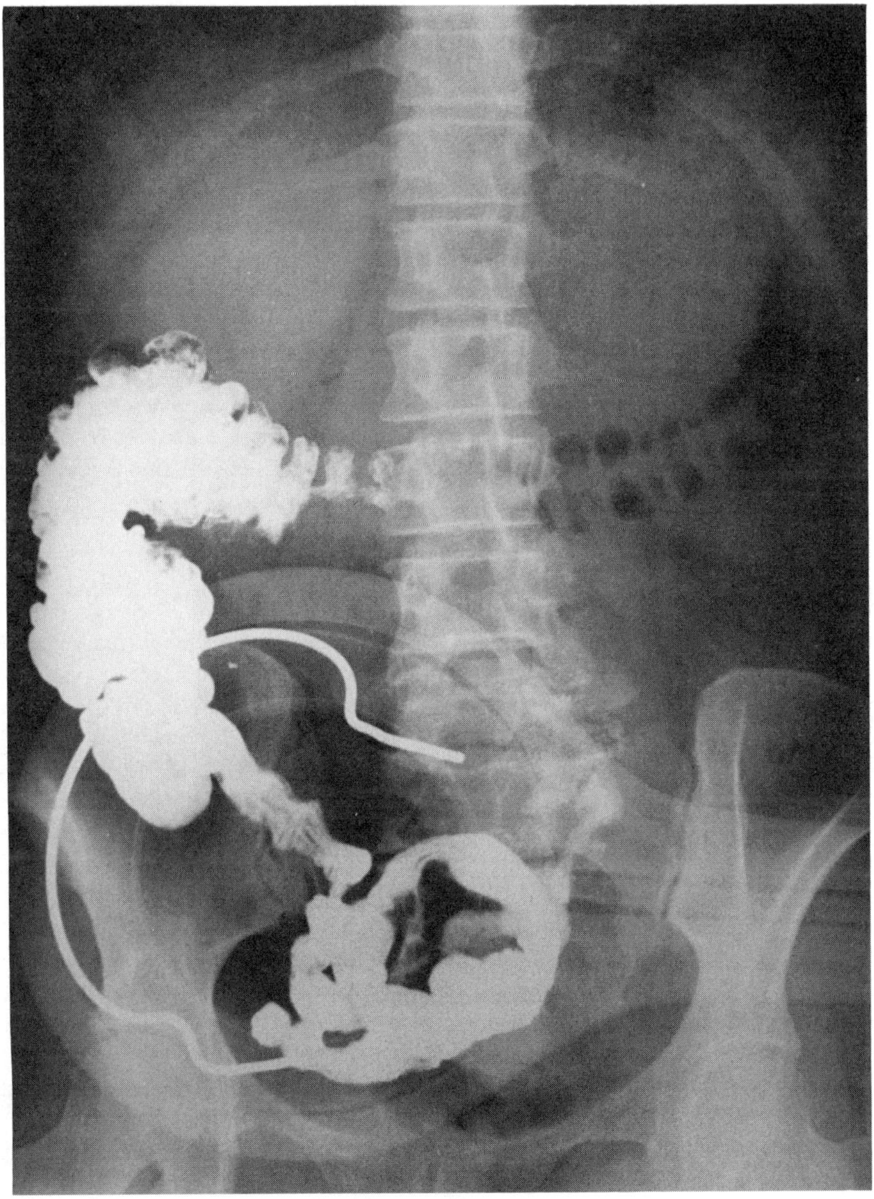

(b)

average time for maintaining remission after withdrawal of all drugs, including 6-MP or azathioprine in 10 patients, was 10 months. Our own experience with 6-MP has shown that the average time until relapse upon terminating the drug is 6 months, and our long-term follow-up data show that 90% of patients who stay on 6-MP will remain well.

6. Response to Second Course of 6-MP

Following completion of the controlled trial, 6-MP was reintroduced in 16 patients at some time after symptoms recurred with resulting improvement once again in all cases. This second course of 6-MP therapy was initiated from 5 to months (average 12 months) after termination of the first course. The mean response time for the second course of 6-MP was 1.5 months, considerably more rapid than the first course. Subsequent experience has not supported such confidence in the success of a second course. The failures, however, have been mostly patients with ileitis complicated by small bowel obstruction prior to the initial course of therapy.

C. Other Experience in Crohn's Disease

No other controlled trial has as yet been reported evaluating 6-MP or azathioprine in Crohn's disease. Nevertheless, since the completion of the Lenox Hill-Mt. Sinai and the NCCDS studies, others have recorded their observations: Goldstein has shared his experience over 18 years with 27 of 38 (70%) Crohn's disease patients treated successfully with azathioprine (29). Nyman et al. used either 6-MP or azathioprine in 42 patients with severe Crohn's disease and extensive colonic involvement, and all but one improved (28). Prednisolone could be withdrawn in 25 patients and reduced to less than 7.5 mg every other day in the others. Verhave et al. treated 15 pediatric Crohn's disease patients (mean age 13.4 years) with azathioprine starting at 2 mg/kg per day; after a mean follow-up of 1.25 years 6 of 12 had completely responded and another 3 showed partial improvement (30). The mean time until response was 4 months. Barreiro brought all 6 patients with Crohn's disease into remission for an average of 11 months on 50 mg of 6-MP daily (31).

Recently I have summarized my own experience over 16 years at Lenox Hill Hospital with 6-MP in the treatment of Crohn's disease (32). Adequate data could be collected in 124 patients, 73 without any prior bowel resection and 51 with an anastomosis or an ostomy. Goals were established for each case, just as in the original controlled study. This time, additionally an index of Crohn's Disease Activity was calculated prior to and following initiation of 6-MP therapy. Table 1 summarizes the goals, number of patients studied and rates of success.

All of the goals in Table 1 may serve as indications for 6-MP therapy in Crohn's disease. Other indications with substantial but less frequent success

Table 1 6-MP in the Treatment of Crohn's Disease

Goals	No. patients	No. achieved	Success
Eliminate steroids	105	75	71.4
Heal perianal abscesses and fistulas	28	18	64.4
Heal ileo- or colocutaneous fistulas	10	6	60
Heal enteroenteric fistulas	15	11	73.3
Heal recurrent ileitis or stomal abscess in an ileostomy	8	6	75
Prevent recurrent colonic obstruction due to strictures	6	5	83.3
Heal Crohn's disease of the stomach and duodenum	3	3	100
Heal Crohn's disease in a Kock pouch	1	1	100
Restore normal growth when retarded	4	3	75
Eliminate erythema nodosum	5	5	100
Heal pyoderma gangrenosum	1	1	100
Eliminate arthritis	8	7	87.5
Eliminate narcotics and other dependent drugs	3	2	66.6

include prevention of recurrent obstruction in ileitis and elimination of an abdominal mass where 45% and 50% success rates, respectively, were achieved with 6-MP. In many instances, the defined goal was one of multiple purposes to be accomplished.

One goal not addressed previously has now come into better focus, the opportunity to perform an elective resection. In many instances the bowel involvement with Crohn's disease appears so extensive, either in continuity or with skip areas, that resection seems contraindicated and the one remaining option is palliative drug therapy. Coincident with successful 6-MP treatment in these cases the zones of lesser involvement heal, and the remaining segments of most marked disease usually polypoid and strictured become better defined. This success then permits elective resection. This proved to be the case in 5 out of 5 cases in this most recent review. Usually prophylactic therapy with 6-MP is warranted thereafter.

The immunosuppressive drugs are the only ones demonstrated to affect maintenance of remission in Crohn's disease. Low-dose maintenance 6-MP following two resections should be considered. In some cases, because of the extensiveness or virulence of the disease, 6-MP should be used after even one resection. In the recently completed review there has been no sign of recurrence in 7 of 8 cases where the goal was prophylaxis after resection. The mean follow-up, however, has been only 40 months.

The overall success rate for all goals has been 69.8% for 6-MP in Crohn's disease. 6-MP was also responsible for reducing the numerical index of Crohn's disease activity in 79.8%. A greater than 35% reduction, signifying an obvious improvement in quality of life, was achieved in 65% of all cases. Therefore, once again 6-MP has served to achieve major therapeutic goals in 2 out of 3 patients with severe Crohn's disease so that surgical resection and subsequent extension is often postponed or eliminated.

D. Ulcerative Colitis

As mentioned earlier, initial successes with 6-MP in inflammatory bowel disease resulted from the treatment of ulcerative colitis rather than Crohn's disease. Uncontrolled trials showed response rates of 70–80%, but there was less enthusiasm for initiating controlled trials. One reason was fear of 6-MP or azathioprine accentuating the tendency toward the development of carcinoma of the colon. Another reason was that ulcerative colitis could be "cured" by resection of the colon, and therefore, any risk of an irreversible drug complication did not seem advisable. Finally, those pioneers who did undertake controlled trials in treating ulcerative colitis reported disappointing overall results (18,19,20,21). Nevertheless, Rosenberg et al. (20) noted that azathioprine permitted a significant reduction in steroid dosage and Carpilli et al. (21) found it was at least as effective as sulfasalazine.

Details of an initial 10-year favorable experience with 6-MP in the therapy of ulcerative colitis have been reported (10,33). More recently, Present (34a) gathered as yet unpublished information on 34 ulcerative colitis patients in the 14–70 age range whom he treated with 6-MP. These included 14 in whom the distribution was universal, 14 with left-sided disease and 6 with proctosigmoiditis, all resistant to steroids and sulfasalazine. There was a good to excellent response in 25 (73%) with discontinuation of steroids in 22. The mean time until response was 2.3 months considerably shorter than in Crohn's disease. In 22 of the 25 patients, the disease remained in remission during the period of follow-up, whether the patient remained on 6-MP or discontinued it.

A similar experience at Lenox Hill now under review suggests long-term favorable results of 6-MP therapy in patients with ulcerative colitis who otherwise would be committed to maintenance therapy with steroids and its complications or colectomy (34b). While some patients begin to show signs of recurrent activity, brief courses of steroids again lead to loss of symptoms and a normal sigmoidoscopic appearance of the mucosa. Remission for up to 11 months a year seems a desirable result. The frequency of exacerbations is clearly lessened by any increase in dose of 6-MP, a tact usually utilized when the blood count permits.

Most patients prefer a trial of therapy with 6-MP to total colectomy. This preference seems true despite the option of a sphincter saving ileopouch anal anastomosis which experience has shown is not consistently successful.

E. Recommendations for Therapy

1. Crohn's Disease

Even for purposes of the double-blind controlled trial only 14% of outpatients with Crohn's disease were entered. Patients who could be weaned from steroids, who had no complications such as fistulas serving to compromise the quality of life, and who could be maintained in remission by sulfasalazine (or a 5-ASA preparation), or metronidazole, even if requiring brief courses of prednisone intermittently, were not and are not started on 6-MP. The proportion of Crohn's disease patients now being treated with 6-MP has been increased, nevertheless. This likely can be attributed to caring for patients with a level of illness more severe than before, in whom all other available drugs have failed and in whom steroid toxicity is superimposed on the Crohn's disease. It must be kept in mind that the natural history of Crohn's disease is one of proximal extension after transection of the bowel. Many of the Crohn's disease patients seen for consideration of 6-MP therapy have already had one, two, or even three resections with varying degrees of malabsorption or short bowel syndrome. Others have extensive disease and chronic obstruction without any surgery. Despite any conservation in the choice of cases for 6-MP, seeing pateints with advanced incapacitating Crohn's disease cannot help but lead to reflection on initiating treatment much earlier, when proportionately there is more inflammation than fibrosis and greater expectation that the drug can be effective.

In all instances, consideration of treatment with 6-MP warrants careful clinical judgment, with special reference to the natural course of Crohn's disease, the specific manifestations and complications with which the patient presents and the assessment of the total patient and the patient's family. The virulence of the disease in a specific patient is usually established within the early years and the rate of progression and development of complications become apparent. At that point, a decision favoring 6-MP should be favorably influenced by the high rate of success when the extent of involvement is primarily colonic, when fistulas arising from the bowel are major manifestations, when the disease has had an early recurrence after surgery or when the disease is extensive with or without surgery. Additional clinical judgment is necessary in the decision to temporarily introduce steroids or to once again raise the dose of steroids, remembering that the mean time until there is an evident response to 6-MP is 3.1 months. The steroids buy time while waiting for 6-MP to take effect. Should the symptoms of Crohn's disease warranting the 6-MP be chronic but reasonably stable, the initial treatment with corticosteroids might not be necessary.

There are situations in Crohn's disease where the hope for success with 6-MP is not as great. The outstanding example is recurrent small bowel obstruction due to ileitis or recurrent ileitis after resection. If, however, it is clinically suspected that the segment of small bowel is narrowed due more to Crohn's disease inflammation than to fibrosis, then a trial of 6-MP might be warranted. Thc closest formula that serves as a guide to these circumstances suggests that a symptom-free interval of 8 months after establishing therapy with 6-MP indicates prolonged success thereafter (35). Another situation in Crohn's disease where at least initial success has not been great is that dominated by perirectal and perineal abscesses and fistulas. In some of these instances, a trial of metronidazole is warranted and in others it has already failed. Assuming the primary bowel disease does not dominate the picture, it is often appropriate to attempt eradication of the abscesses and fistulas with a modified Park's operation and multiple skip fistulotomies (36,37). Local anorectal surgery does not, as once thought, seem to provoke the primary bowel manifestations. Once this has been accomplished, 6-MP has been successful in bringing the primary bowel disease into remission and preventing recurrence of perineal sepsis.

Regardless of the indications for using 6-MP in Crohn's disease, considerations must be given to the intelligence, sophistication, character, and personality of the patient before the decision is made. No matter how ideal the candidate might seem to be on the grounds or duration, distribution, and complications of the organic disease, if the managing physician suspects on the basis of any of the above that compliance will be poor, the drug should not be used. The patient must understand the need to accurately participate in the monitoring and to contact the physician as directed. Once 6-MP has been started and it becomes evident that the patient is not compliant, termination of the drug should be considered.

2. *Ulcerative Colitis*

Those patients in whom corticosteroids cannot be eliminated and in whom sulfasalazine or 5-ASA products have failed, even with the support of brief intermittent courses of steroid therapy, might be candidates for 6-MP. The indication will rarely arise for ulcerative proctitis but consideration often occurs for universal and left-sided disease and sometimes for resistant cases of proctosigmoiditis.

It is frequently mentioned that treatment with 6-MP is not applicable to patients with ulcerative colitis, a disease that can be cured by total colectomy. This rationale has been considered to be supported by the advent of the ileo-pouch anal anastomosis. This stand, however, has been compromised by the lack of universal success with this sphincter-saving procedure and the inability as yet to predict who will do well with it and who will then have a new malady to contend with as a replacement for the old. Furthermore, most patients do not want to lose their colons, certainly as long as there is one other potentially successful nonoperative modality to try. Historically in the case of inflammatory bowel disease, postponement of surgery buys time for discovery of the etiology of the disease or at least of another potentially successful drug.

The above considerations do not markedly change the indications for surgery in ulcerative colitis. The surgical management of perforation, massive hemorrhage, carcinoma, and persistent dysplasia remain the same. In patients with toxic megacolon, the process may be reversed by nonoperative measures when recognized early, thus affording an opportunity to try 6-MP at a later stage. The main dilemma arises in those patients with universal disease of 10 years or greater duration who are theoretically at risk for developing carcinoma. There is no evidence that 6-MP increases this risk. However, this consideration must be shared with the patient before the decision is made. In some instances, chronic incapacity of 10 years or more should favor colectomy while less prolonged periods of debility might not. In those with universal or left-sided disease who do choose to try 6-MP, a conscientious surveillance program is encouraged. In all instances, the same considerations as to intelligence, sophistication, character, and personality with regard to potential compliance must prevail.

3. Dose and Monitoring

For the purpose of the controlled trial the initial dose of 6-MP, used in most of the earlier studies, was 1½ mg/kg. Since completion of the trial, further experience and concerns over leukopenia and even frank bone marrow suppression, have led to the use of an initial dose of 50 mg/day regardless of body weight. A blood count is scheduled weekly for the first 3 weeks until it is determined that the starting dose is safe. Following that, either the time between blood counts is extended or the dose is increased, depending on the needs of the individual patient. In general, when the patient is clearly doing well on the initial dose, it is not increased. If the clinical situation warrants trial of a larger dose, 6-MP is increased to 50 mg on one day alternating with 50 mg twice a day on the next day. The next increase would be 50 mg twice a day. The highest dose which has been used is 150 mg/day. At all times when the dose is raised a complete blood count is performed at least weekly for the next 3 weeks.

Monitoring always requires awareness of concomitant steroid therapy which serves to raise the white blood count while 6-MP lowers it. The timing between blood counts may be extended when steroids are reintroduced and decreased when the steroids are being lowered.

The managing physician must remain on constant alert to the patient's usual compliance habits. If the blood count is not done at the specified time and the patient does not heed additional warnings, a new prescription for the drug need not be given. Concern about this issue also is handled by limiting the size of the prescription and providing no refills.

The platelet count is monitored along with the white blood count. Only one case of possible 6-MP-related thrombocytopenia has been documented. Hemoglobin and hematocrit also are monitored. In no instance could anemia be attributed to 6-MP, but these tests helped the managing physician to recognize changes in the overall condtion–whether improving or worsening.

The patient is encouraged to have the clinical laboratory telephone the results of the white blood count, platelet count, hemoglobin, and hematocrit on the same day the tests are performed. This information is entered on the monitor form (Appendix III), which is checked to provide new directions in anticipation of the phone call from the patient. A judgment as to continuation or change of dosage and time until the next blood count is made by reviewing the last few white counts, the time that has passed between them, and the clinical goal in the particular case.

The above pertains in entirety to azathioprine as well as 6-MP. Although 6-MP is favored, should the patient develop an allergic reaction such as fever, joint pain, hepatitis, or pancreatitis, azathioprine is tried after the reaction has subsided. This has been successful in all types of allergic reactions except pancreatitis.

4. *Duration of Therapy*

On the basis of the results of the Crohn's disease controlled trial which showed that a convincing response to 6-MP might take up to 10 months with occasional further subsequent improvement, it is arbitrarily recommended that the 6-MP be continued for 2 years when it has been successful. The patient is not committed to 2 years of therapy and may stop the drug at any time. Most patients, once in remission on 6-MP, continue the drug for the minimal 2-year period. At that time, some patients continued fear of the drug leads them to discontinue it. By far, the majority of patients express their acknowledgment that their good health is attributable to the 6-MP and they prefer to continue on it. At that point, one other choice is offered. If during the period on 6-MP the disease has not been kept entirely in remission and one or more brief courses of steroids have been required, continuing the current 6-MP dose is recommended. If, however, the remission has been absolute for at least a year, the patient is offered the option of maintaining 6-MP therapy at a reduced dosage.

In those who have stopped the 6-MP treatment, the most common time lapse to recurrence has been 6 months, and three-quarters recur within a year. The recurrence is usually milder than the original disease and might then respond to other drugs. If it is decided to reintroduce the 6-MP it is usually once again effective. Once a second course of therapy has been chosen and has been successful, the patient then usually prefers to continue the 6-MP indefinitely. There are today many patients on 6-MP in whom the drug was first introduced 15–20 years ago during the controlled trial in the early 1970s. This has been the experience of Present (34a) and Goldstein (29) as well.

The most common reason for stopping 6-MP while it is successful is the desire for pregnancy. If the remission has been prolonged the decision to stop 6-MP is appropriate. If the remission has been brief, postponement of discontinuing the drug should be negotiated with the patient.

When it is clear that the goal to be achieved with 6-MP has not been accomplished, the drug should be stopped. Usually this decision can be made after 6 months of treatment. In some cases a longer trial is warranted.

III. ADVERSE EFFECTS

A. Historical Perspective

Experience with 6-MP in the treatment of leukemias and with azathioprine in rheumatoid arthritis and prevention of rejection of organ transplants disclosed that bone marrow suppression occurred and was dose related. Both leukopenia and thrombocytopenia have been reported. Hepatotoxicity has been observed in animals and humans. In humans it seems to have occurred when a dose of 2.5 mg/kg per day is exceeded and may occur early or late. The histopathology includes features of both intrahepatic cholestasis and parenchymal cell necrosis. The toxicity may in part or totally be a hypersensitivity reaction, and in some, jaundice has cleared on withdrawal of the 6-MP and reappeared with its reintroduction. Any kind of superinfection is theoretically possible and induction of immunity to vaccines might be compromised. The incidence of infections has been markedly greater in transplant cases than in rheumatoid arthritis patients treated with azathioprine.

Azathioprine and 6-MP cause chromosomal aberrations in animals and humans, but they are reversible in humans. They are carcinogenic in animals at the doses used and therefore may increase the risk of neoplasia in humans. This risk has been greater in transplant cases than in arthritis patients.

Women receiving 6-MP or azathioprine in the first trimester of pregnancy have an increased risk of abortion, but no malformation of the fetus has been observed.

Allopurinol, used to lower blood uric acid, may delay the catabolism of 6-MP resulting in accentuation of its usual toxicity. Therefore, when the two drugs are used concomitantly, the 6-MP should be reduced at least to one-third.

B. Toxicity Clearly Related to 6-MP

In a review of all possible complications occurring during or after treatment of IBD with 6-MP in 396 patients from the combined office-hospital services of Present and Korelitz, four types of toxicity were clearly related to the drug (38):

Pancreatitis was observed in 3.3% of patients; 12 with Crohn's disease and 1 with ulcerative colitis (39). All except one occurred within 32 days of starting 6-MP. The symptoms disappeared quickly on discontinuing the 6-MP; in all 7 rechallenged with 6-MP or azathioprine the symptoms recurred rapidly. Clinically the pancreatitis behaves like a hypersensitivity reaction, but attempts at desensitization were not successful.

Bone marrow depression requiring hospitalization occurred in 2%, all during the early years before accumulated experience with monitoring of blood counts and when the initial dose was based on weight (1.5 mg/kg). In these 8 patients, the white blood count ranged from 300 to 2500, fever occurred in 7, and blood cultures were positive in 3. There was accompanying anemia in 2 patients. There was no mortality. Characteristically the bone marrow depression was followed by a prolonged remission of the Crohn's disease or ulcerative colitis.

Leukopenia was noted at some time in most patients. White blood counts above 3500 were rarely associated with clinical problems and were managed by temporarily stopping the 6-MP or lowering its dose.

Allergic reactions occurred within the first three weeks of 6-MP treatment in 2%. These included fever in 8, rash in 2, joint pain in 1 and abdominal pain in 1 patient. Rechallenge with 6-MP or azathioprine produced similar reactions. None was associated with leukopenia.

Hepatitis occurred in 11 patients but in only one could it be attributed to the drug. In this patient, whose severe ulcerative colitis had gone into remission, liver function tests became normal on cessation of 6-MP and again became abnormal at a later date when he was rechallenged. In this case the hepatitis occurred after 4 months of therapy.

Overall toxicity clearly related to 6-MP occurred in 7.6%, was reversed in all upon stopping the drug, and no mortality resulted.

C. Infections Possibly Related to 6-MP

Almost every type of infection occurring during the course of treatment with 6-MP has also been reported in IBD patients not treated with immunosuppressive drugs. This pertains particularly to Crohn's disease.

The sickest patient in this category was a young woman who developed a fever, possibly related to her underlying ileocolitis, but did not stop 6-MP as all patients are directed to do under these circumstances. She developed a perforation and required a resection with anastomosis. This was followed by peritonitis, reexploration, drainage, and ileostomy. Thereafter, a series of intra-abdominal complications occurred including a pyrogenic liver abscess. Cytomegalovirus (CMV) and other organisms were cultured from different areas of the peritoneal cavity including the site of perforation. She recovered, and like other patients with severe infectious complications in the course of 6-MP therapy, there has been no sign of recurrence of Crohn's disease activity in 8 years.

One other patient developed a liver abscess which required drainage; there had been no bone marrow suppression in this case.

Five patients developed pneumonia; all responded to antibiotic therapy and stopping 6-MP. Subsequently, two additional cases of pneumonia were successfully treated on an ambulatory basis. Some patients have complained of frequent colds and upper respiratory infections but it is difficult to document an incidence greater than in the general population.

Herpes zoster occurred in 8 patients while they were taking 6-MP. In all, the "shingles" took its usual course despite the fact that 6-MP was continued in half of the patients. Many years later, one patient had a recurrence of herpes zoster on his trunk when he was again taking 6-MP and suffered a three-day syndrome consistent with encephalitis. There has been no residual defect during a 9-year follow-up and the ulcerative colitis has remained in remission.

A septic phlebitis occurred in one young woman with Crohn's disease while she was on steroid therapy and 6-MP; this was followed by bilateral necrosis of the hip joints which eventually required bilateral hip replacement. Her Crohn's disease remained in remission for many years thereafter.

A spiking fever and leukopenia occurred in one young woman with Crohn's disease and no source of infection was found. The fever resolved after 25 days and Crohn's disease remained quiescent for the following year.

Heptatitis not definitely due to 6-MP has occurred in 12 patients. In all instances except one with persistent enzyme elevations, the patient recovered, and in 7 6-MP was restarted without recurrence of liver abnormalities.

One patient developed Q-fever upon returning from a visit to Australia. Infectious mononucleosis was seen once. Warts were noted in 6 cases.

D. Neoplasms

Similar to the situation with infections, many neoplasms occur in patients with IBD who are not receiving immunosuppressive drugs. In Crohn's disease, particularly, an increased risk of extraintestinal neoplasms has been suggested (40). Nevertheless, influenced by the risk in transplant patients, an accurate appraisal was made of any neoplasms occurring in the 396 patients with IBD either during or after 6-MP therapy (38).

In one instance the neoplasm was considered to be probably related to 6-MP therapy. This was diffuse histiocytic lymphoma of the brain in a man with Crohn's disease who had taken 6-MP for approximately 9 months. He had stopped the drug 11 months prior to the onset of headaches, the evaluation of which led to the diagnosis. He did not respond to therapy.

One man with ulcerative colitis on 6-MP developed a malignant melanoma; the excision and axillary node dissection was curative.

Other malignant neoplasms occurring in patients who had earlier received 6-MP included an islet cell carcinoma, a carcinoma of the lung, a carcinoma of the breast, and basal cell carcinomas, none of which was felt to be related to the 6-MP.

Two carcinomas of the colon occurred in one patient with long-standing ulcerative colitis who had refused the recommendation of colectomy. In this case, the carcinomas clearly anteceded the initiation of 6-MP. Subsequently, one additional patient with long-standing left-sided ulcerative colitis who had been on 6-MP for one year developed a carcinoma of the rectum. Benign adenomatous polyps have been encountered on sigmoidoscopy or colonoscopy in patients on 6-MP; they have been removed endoscopically and no recurrence has been encountered despite continuation of 6-MP.

Benign tumors disclosed at follow-up of patients previously on 6-MP included one prolactinoma, a papilloma of the bladder, and several follicular adenomas of the thyroid.

E. Nausea

Nausea is a fairly common complaint during the first month of 6-MP therapy. Occasionally the dose of 6-MP has to be reduced temporarily. Rarely has the drug had to be terminated on this bases.

F. Considerations of Pregnancy

On theoretical grounds, conception has been contraindicated in patients on 6-MP, whether female or male. When pregnancy becomes the priority in women on 6-MP, it is recommended the drug be stopped for 3 months before eliminating contraceptives. In the toxicity study, 16 pregnancies occurred. In 10 cases, 6-MP had been terminated before conception as advised but in 6 cases the 6-MP had been continued for 3–4 weeks before the pregnancy was realized. In 3 of the 6, as well as the 10 who had stopped the 6-MP earlier, the patient continued the pregnancy, and all 13 delivered at full term. No abnormalities have been found in any of the 13 children. Goldstein (29) also described 4 women who became pregnant while taking azathioprine, chose to continue the pregnancy, then carried to term without appreciable ill effects on mother or child. Three of 6 who became pregnant while taking 6-MP and one reported by Goldstein proceeded with elective abortion as advised.

G. Mortality

In no patient with the exception of the one with a cerebral lymphoma could a death be attributed to 6-MP. Since there is a predilection for the brain in lymphomas developing in transplant patients (41) and in other patients receiving immunosuppressive drugs (42), it must be assumed that this tumor was caused by 6-MP. There are, however, reports of increasing numbers of lymphomas in patients with Crohn's disease (43,44) not receiving immunosuppressive drugs. In another study of 327 IBD patients treated with immunosuppressive drugs, no cases of lymphoma were seen (45).

IV. SUGGESTIONS FOR OBTAINING PERMISSION

Once 6-MP has been recommended, it is wise to have written as well as oral permission from the patient confirming that he or she understands its purpose, its potential risks, and the rationale for its use. This attitude is justified by the litigious society in which practice takes place and the lack of FDA approval for use of either 6-MP or azathioprine in either Crohn's disease or ulcerative colitis.

A signature is not enough. It is important to have a conversation with the patient and, if possible, the family, concerning the treatment with the drug and to record in the progress notes that this has been done. The conversation should include purpose, risks, benefits, and any alternatives. Notes should also be made documenting the patient's questions or concerns and that they were addressed. Subsequent questions and their answers, whether made by telephone or in person, should also be recorded.

Consider obtaining the signed permission on a different day then that on which the drug is recommended. After projecting a plan for further management and answering the questions necessary for orientation, it has been useful to provide the patient with an information form (Appendix I) along with a copy of the permission form (Appendix II), and the monitor form for recording blood counts and dose directions (Appendix III). The information form contains an introductory paragraph for orientation, background information on immunosuppressive drugs and specifically 6-MP, a summary of the outcomes of the controlled double-blind trial in Crohn's disease and the uncontrolled experience in ulcerative colitis, and information on experience with how long it takes the drug to be effective, side effects, and complications. The most space is devoted to leukopenia, monitoring, and the requirement to stop the drug on the occurrence of fever of any cause. Special mention is made of malignancies and pregnancy, the importance of the physician-patient partnership and quarterly clinical visits even when the patient is doing well. Finally, clarification is made of any charges to be rendered for the physician's time and that of his staff involved in monitoring.

After reading this material, another meeting between the physician and the patient is scheduled, whether in hospital or office; discussion is encouraged, and questions are answered. When the patient is satisfied and wants to proceed with the drug, the permission form is signed and witnessed. As an outcome of this exercise approximately 5-10% of patients decide not to use 6-MP; in some cases this decision is reversible. These few days taken between recommendation for using 6-MP and writing the prescription provide an opportunity to eliminate misunderstanding, reduce risk, and emphasize the partnership agreement.

V. CYCLOSPORIN

Cyclosporin, the immunosuppressive agent of choice for treatment to prevent rejection in transplant surgery has been tried in the treatment of IBD patients. It is a fungal metabolite representing a new generation of drugs which, more selectively and reversibly than 6-MP and azathioprine, has successfully suppressed cell-mediated immunity. It has been used with success for renal transplants, liver transplants, and bone marrow transplants (46).

A large variety of diseases, many considered "autoimmune," have been successfully treated with cyclosporin (47). These include uveitis, dermatomyositis, systemic lupus erythematosis, polymyalgia rheumatica, relapsing polychondritis, primary biliary cirrhosis, Graves' ophthalmopathy, thrombocytopenic purpura, rheumatoid arthritis, sarcoidosis, psoriasis, Type 1 diabetes mellitus, multiple sclerosis, and myasthenia gravis.

Success with cyclosporin has not been achieved without a price. A variety of side effects and toxic manifestations have been reported. They include hypertension, hepatic and renal dysfunction, gingival hypertrophy, dyspepsia, anorexia, vomiting, hyperkalemia, hyperuricemia, parasthesias, hirsutism, tremor, anemia, leukocytosis and lymphoma. Non-Hodgkin's lymphoma is the most common type of lymphoma and has been reported to occur earlier, more often and be more widespread in transplant cases treated with cyclosporin than with azathioprine. Cerebral lymphoma appears less often and in general the lymphoma is more likely to regress when cyclosporin is stopped as opposed to other immunosuppressive regimens. In contrast to 6-MP and azathioprine, cyclosporin has not been directly responsible for bone marrow depression, superinfection or pancreatitis.

Despite the complications attributable to cyclosporin, there is reason to consider a role for this drug in the treatment of IBD. Its action takes place within one to two weeks. Therefore, it is slower than corticosteroids but faster than 6-MP and azathioprine. Hopefully it would be effective for the sickest patients with Crohn's disease and ulcerative colitis, the subgroup where 6-MP azathioprine would be contraindicated. If the drug could be stopped before the patient is at risk for lymphoma and other complications, consideration of its use in IBD would be more attractive. Early experience has shown, however, that it is effective in patients with chronically active IBD where prolonged therapy might be required.

Experience with cyclosporin in the treatment of inflammatory bowel disease has been limited. Two out of 3 patients with Crohn's disease responded, while one had irreversible bowel obstruction (48,49). A 6-week report on a pilot study noted partial response in 2 of 5 cases (50). One patient with ulcerative colitis went into remission on cyclosporin (51). In the Canadian open study of 15 patients with Crohn's disease, 10 improved in 4 weeks, and in 7 of the 10 the improvement was maintained 952). In another open study, cyclosporin has been successful in treating severe ulcerative colitis as well as Crohn's disease (34a). A controlled study of cyclosporin in Crohn's disease has been initiated in Copenhagen after encouraging results in 8 of 11 patients with Crohn's disease in an open trial (53). In at least 3 reported cases the data suggest a diminished effect when cyclosporin is administered orally as opposed to intravenously, perhaps due to a shortened or diseased small bowel.

APPENDIX I

Information for Patients on 6-Mercaptopurine

Burton I. Korelitz, M.D.

Introduction

Your physician has recommended the use of 6-mercaptopurine, known as 6-MP for short, for the treatment of your Crohn's disease or ulcerative colitis. The purpose of this leaflet is to provide you with some background information on its use in treating these diseases, including its history, the way it is administered, and the methods used to follow its beneficial as well as its side effects. It is our opinion that the better informed you are, the better partner you can be in the project of treating your disease. It is also our hope that it will give you a framework on which you can build confidence in the treatment and to deal with your anxieties, which arise in all of us when we are ill. It is not meant to substitute for conversations between you and your gastroenterologist nor to try to answer every question you may have.

The nature of 6-MP

6-MP belongs to a class of drugs known as immunosuppressive agents. As suggested by that name, they theoretically could suppress the immune mechanism in our bodies; that is, they prevent or diminish our ability to respond to invasion by foreign elements, such as bacteria, for example. Originally, 6-MP was used to suppress certain kinds of childhood and adult leukemias. Furthermore, it was used to prevent rejection of a donor's transplanted organ, such as a kidney, by the recipient. Observations made during these phases of its history raised the possibility that the immunusuppressive qualities of 6-MP are the ones which work in Crohn's disease or ulcerative colitis. There is evidence that in the lower doses used in these diseases, it has, rather, an anti-inflammatory effect.

How long does it take to work?

Early experience with the drug showed that it is a slow-acting one. The average time it takes to begin to be effective is 3 months, though some patients react more rapidly and others more slowly. For this reason, it is important not to abandon existing therapy too soon after starting 6-MP. Though one of the goals in using 6-MP is to eliminate the use of steroids (prednisone, hydrocortisone, etc.), they should be reduced slowly rather than being discontinued abruptly. Ultimately, of course, it is intended that they will no longer be needed.

Side effects

There are side effects associated with the use of 6-MP as there are for most drugs, certainly all the other drugs used in treating inflammatory bowel disease. The commonest is leukopenia—the lowering of the white blood cell count. These cells are responsible, in part, for fighting infection so it is important to monitor this effect carefully. This is done with weekly blood counts until the dose is stabilized after which it is done less frequently. If the white count drops, the drug is discontinued until the count returns to normal. 6-MP is then resumed at lower doses. If the drop in white count is not as dramatic, the drug may be continued, rather than stopped, but at reduced dosage. If there is a fever suggesting an infection, 6-MP is stopped temporarily, regardless of the underlying cause. There have been instances in which the white count has fallen to low levels. Even in these few instances, it returned to normal after the drug was stopped.

The next most serious side effect is pancreatitis or inflammation of the pancreas. This occurs in 3-5% of patients and is often ushered in with abdominal pain, nausea, and vomiting. Though it, too, resolves on discontinuing 6-MP, this complication may suggest that further use of the drug is contraindicated.

Some patients report nausea, vomiting, or loss of appetite in the early stages of treatment but these symptoms usually disappear after a week or two. A still less common problem is fever due to the drug itself. This, too, subsides when the drug is stopped. Jaundice is a rare side effect of 6-MP in doses used in the treatment of inflammatory bowel disease.

Drug interaction

Allopurinol (Zyloprim), a drug often used in the treatment of gout, interferes with the breakdown of purines and, therefore, patients who take that drug must use much smaller doses of 6-MP.

Concern re: malignant disease and 6-MP

There has been some concern raised by the increased incidence of tumors in patients receiving kidney transplants who are treated with 6-MP. The doses used in those patients are much higher and multiple immunosuppressive drugs are used. Indeed, transplantation itself has been considered a predisposing factor to the development of malignancies. In over 700 patients treated with 6-MP, or the related drug azathioprine, one patient developed a lymphoma. More patients with Crohn's disease not treated with 6-MP have developed lymphomas. Nevertheless the small risk of tumor development must be weighed against the value of using 6-MP in chronic unrelenting diseases such as Crohn's disease and ulcerative colitis. There has been more than 18 years experience in hundreds of patients with Crohn's disease in very carefully conducted studies which show that 6-MP has been a very effective agent in its treatment. Clinical experience supports the view that it is similarly effective in ulcerative colitis.

The safety of 6-MP in pregnant women has never been established. It is recommended, therefore, that reliable methods of deferring pregnancy be used until the drug is stopped. If pregnancy does occur while a patient is on the drug, a therapeutic abortion is advised, though normal children have been born in several cases where this advice was not followed.

FDA status

Although we have now used 6-MP for 20 years in the treatment of Crohn's disease and ulcerative colitis, the drug company that manufactures it has never applied for FDA approval for this use of the drug. For that reason, use of the drug in inflammatory bowel disease patients warrants a signed permission even though it is no longer considered investigational. It should be made clear that 6-MP is a FDA-approved drug and is not an experimental agent. As pointed out before, it has had years of use in a very large number of patients and is quite well understood.

Physician–patient partnership

When inflammatory bowel disease is not responding adequately to other drugs, a trial of 6-MP should be considered and is relatively safe. A committed partnership between the patient and the physician is absolutely necessary to its successful use, however. That requires of the patient that the drug be taken exactly as specified and that any laboratory procedures be done promptly, as ordered. It also takes considerable patience because, as has already been pointed out, results may be slow in coming. It must also be remembered that no medication works in all patients with inflammatory bowel disease. It is important, for these reasons, that the patient have no reluctance in sharing his concerns and asking any questions that may come to his mind with his physician.

Costs of treatment

A final consideration is the cost of treatment. There will be laboratory fees, as is evident from the previous discussion. The physician must closely monitor the laboratory work, making the necessary adjustments in the dosage and time of the next blood test. For this time-consuming function, the physician's fee is $250.00 per year which can be billed monthly, quarterly, or yearly according to the patient's preference. Independent of this the patient must be seen at intervals not longer than 3 months, even when doing clinically well, to verify the drug used correctly and no complications have occurred.

After all issues have been considered and all questions answered, if the use of 6-MP seems advisable and agreeable to the patient, he/she should advise the physician of that decision, sign the permission form, and receive the prescription which can be filled in any drug store.

APPENDIX II

Authorization for Treatment with 6-Mercaptopurine

1. I authorize Dr. Burton I. Korelitz

   to treat ______________________________

   (State "myself" or name of patient.)

   with the drug presently identified as 6-Mercaptopurine (Purinethol)

   ______________________ for the following condition

   Crohn's disease/ulcerative colitis ______________________

   __________ (Describe symptoms or name of disease to be treated.)

   Inflammatory bowel disease ______________________

   ____

   ____

2. It has been explained to me that the safety and usefulness of the drug in the treatment of patients for the above condition has been and continues to be investigated.

3. I have read the material provided to me entitled *Information for Patients on 6-Mercaptopurine*. The following issues have been covered and my concerns and questions have been clarified or answered by Dr. Korelitz.

A. The nature and expected duration of the treatment:
Immunosuppressive drug-duration indefinite ______________________

____

B. The purpose of the treatment:
Bring Crohn's disease or ulcerative colitis or its complications under control or into remission ______________________________________

____

C. The method and means of the administration of the drug:
Orally dose monitored by blood counts ___________________________

____

D. The possible alternative methods of treatment:
Not using immunosuppressive drug; surgical resection _______________

____

E. The possible risk and attendant discomforts of the treatment:
Infections, pancreatitis, allergies, tumors, need for blood counts, inconvenience. Other less frequent complications may occur. _____________

____

F. The benefits reasonably to be expected of the treatment:
Controlling Crohn's disease or ulcerative colitis ____________________

____

G. I understand that I am free to ask any and all questions concerning this treatment and that any questions which I have chosen to ask have been answered to my satisfaction.

H. I understand that I am free to withdraw my consent at any time. I further understand that the withdrawal of my consent will not jeopardize my treatment in any way.

I have read this document in its entirety and I understand it fully.

______________________________________ __________

Signature of Patient Date

____________________________ ____________________

Witness Date

I have fully explained to the above-named patient the nature and purpose of this drug; the method and means of the adminstration of the drug; the possible alternative methods of treatment which might be advantageous; the benefits reasonably to be expected; the attendant discomforts and risks involved; the possibility that complications may arise from the use of this drug and the consequences and risks, if any, which might be involved if the patient decides to discontinue the prescribed drug regimen. I believe the patient fully understands the nature, purposes, benefits, risks and alternative methods of treatment associated with this drug. I have offered to answer any and all questions the patient has chosen to ask with respect to the use of this drug and I have completely and fully answered all such questions.

____________________________ ____________________

Signature of Physician Date

APPENDIX III

6-MP Record

Name: ________________ Date of Onset: ________________ Original Dose: ________

Date	WBC	HGB	HCT	Platelets	Last dose	Current directions/date	Next CBC to be done

REFERENCES

1. New York Academy of Sciences: 6-Mercaptopurine, Ann. N.Y. Acad. Sci., 60:359–507 (1954).
2. Elion, G. B., Biochemistry and pharmacology of purine analogues, Fed. Proc., 26:898–904 (1967).
3. Brogan, M., R. Stevens, J. Hiserodt, M. Oliver, B. I. Korelitz, S. Targan, Effects of 6-MP on the impaired in vivo humoral responsiveness in Crohn's disease (abstr.) Gastroenterology, 86(5):1035 (1984).

3a. Brogan, M., J. Hiserodt, M. Oliver, R. Stevens, B. I. Korelitz, S. Targan, The effect of 6-Mercaptopurine on natural killer cell activities in Crohn's disease, J. Clin. Immunol., 5(3):204 (1985).

4. Bean, R. H. P., The treatment of chronic ulcerative colitis with 6-Mercaptopurine, Med. J. Aust., 2:592–593 (1962).
5. Bowen, G. E., G. V. Jr. Irons, J. B. Rhodes, et al. Early experiences with azathioprine in ulcerative colitis, JAMA, 195:166–170 (1966).
6. Brooke, B. N., D. C. Hoffmann, E. T. Swarbuck, Azathioprine for Crohn's disease, Lancet, 2:612–614 (1969).
7. Drucker, W. R., K. N. Jeejeebhoy, Azathioprine: An adjunct to surgical therapy of granulomatous enteritis, Ann. Surg., 172:618–625 (1970).
8. Brooke, B. N., S. L. Javett, O. W. Davidson, Further experience with azathioprine for Crohn's disease, Lancet, 2:1050–1053 (1973).
9. Bean, R. H. D., Treatment of ulcerative colitis with antimetabolite, Br. Med. J., 1:1081:1084 (1966).
10. Korelitz, B. I., J. L. Glass, N. Wisch, Long-term immunosuppressive therapy of ulcerative colitis, Am. J. Dig. Dis., 18:317–322 (1973).
11. Theodor, E., Y. Niv, L. Bat, Imuran in the treatment of ulcerative colitis, Am. J. Gastroenterol., 76:262–266 (1981).
12. Willoughby, J. M. T., J. Beckett, P. J. Jumar, Controlled trial of azathioprine in Crohn's disease, Lancet, 2:944–947 (1971).
13. Rhodes, J., P. Beck, D. Bainton et al. Controlled trial of azathioprine in Crohn's disease, Lancet, 2:1273–1276 (1971).
14. Watson, W. C., M. Bukowsky, Azathioprine in management of Crohn's disease: A randomized cross-over study (Abstr), Gastroenterology, 66:796 (1974).
15. Klein, M., M. J. Binder, M. Mitchel et al., Treatment of Crohn's disease with azathioprine: A controlled evaluation, Gastroenterology, 66:916–922 (1974).
16. Rosenberg, J. L., B. Levin, A. J. Wall et al., A controlled trial of azathioprine in Crohn's disease, Dig. Dis., 20:721–726 (1975).
17. Summers, R. W., D. M. Switz, J. T. Sessions et al., National Cooperative Crohn's Disease Study: Results of drug treatment, Gastroenterology, 77: 847–869 (1979).
18. Kirk, A. P., J. E. Lennard-Jones, Controlled trial of azathioprine in chronic ulcerative colitis, Br. Med. J., 284:1291–1292 (1962).

19. Jewell, D. P., S. C. Truelove, Azathioprine in ulcerative colitis: An interim report on controlled therapeutic trial, Br. Med. J., 1:709–712 (1972).
20. Rosenberg, J. L., A. J. Wall, B. Levin et al., A controlled trial of azathioprine in the management of chronic ulcerative colitis, Dig. Dis., 20:721–726 (1975).
21. Caprilli, R. T., R. Carratu, M. Babbini, A double-blind comparison of the effectiveness of azathioprine and sulfasalazine in idiopathic proctocolitis. Preliminary report, Dig. Dis., 20:115–120 (1975).
22. Present, D. H., B. I. Korelitz, N. Wisch, J. L. Glass, D. B. Sachar, B. S. Pasternack, Treatment of Crohn's disease with 6-Mercaptopurine. A long term, randomized, double blind study, N. Engl. J. Med., 302:981–987 (1980).
23. Korelitz, B. I., D. H. Present, Shortcomings of the national Crohn's disease Study: The exclusion of Azathioprine without adequate trial, Gastroenterology, 80:193–196 (1981).
24. Farmer, R. G., G. Whelan, V. W. Fazio, Long-term follow-up of patients with Crohn's disease. Relationship between the clinical pattern and prognosis, Gastroenterology, 88:1818–1825 (1985).
25. Korelitz, B. I., D. H. Present, Favorable effect of 6-Mercaptopurine in fistulas of Crohn's disease, Dig. Dis. Sci., 30:58–64 (1985).
26. Margolin, M. L., B. I. Korelitz, Enterovesical fistulas in Crohn's disease (abstr.), Gastroenterology, 90:1534 (1986).
27. O'Donaghue, D. P., A. W. Dawson, J. Powell-Tuck, R. L. Brown, J. E. Lennard-Jones, Double-blind withdrawal trial of Azathioprine as maintenance treatment of Crohn's disease, Lancet, 2:955–957 (1978).
28. Nyman, M., I. Hansson, S. Eriksson, Long-term immunosuppressive treatment in Crohn's disease, Scand. J. Gastroenterol., 20:1197–1203 (1985).
29. Goldstein, F., Immunosuppressive therapy of inflammatory bowel disease, J. Clin. Gastroenterol., 9:654–658 (1987).
30. Verhave, M., H. S. Winter, R. J. Grand, Efficacy and safety of azathioprine in children with inflammatory bowel disease (abstr), Gastroenterology, 92: 1682 (1987).
31. Barreiro, M. A., 6-Mercaptopurine (6-MP) in the treatment of inflammatory disease of the bowel (abstr), Gastroenterology, 92(5), Part 2:1308 (1987).
32. Adler, D. J., B. I. Korelitz, Long term efficacy of 6-Mercaptopurine in the treatment of Crohn's disease (abstr), Gastroenterology, 92(5pt2):1288 (1987).
33. Korelitz, B. I., The treatment of ulcerative colitis with "immunosuppressive" drugs, Am. J. Gastroenterol., 76:297–298 (1981).
34a. Present, D. H., Personal communication.
34b. Adler, D. J., B. I. Korelitz, The therapeutic efficacy of 6-mercaptopurine in the treatment of ulcerative colitis, Am. J. Gastroenterol., 83(9):1042 (1988) (Abstr. 102).
35. Yaffe, B. H., B. I. Korelitz, Prognosis for non-operative management of small bowel obstruction in Crohn's disease, J. Clin. Gastroenterol., 5:211–215 (1983).

36. Sohn, N., B. I. Korelitz, M. A. Weinstein, Anorectal Crohn's disease: Definitive surgery for fistulas and recurrent abscesses, Am. J. Surg., 139:394–397 (1980).
37. Sohn, N., B. I. Korelitz, Local operative treatment of anorectal Crohn's Disease, J. Clin. Gastroenterol., 4(5):395–398 (1982).
38. Present, D. H., S. J. Meltzer, A. Wolke, B. I. Korelitz, Short and long term toxicity to 6-mercaptopurine in the treatment of inflammatory bowel disease (abstr), Gastroenterology, 88(5pt2):2:1545 (1985).
39. Haber, D. J., S. J. Meltzer, D. H. Present, B. I. Korelitz, Nature and course of pancreatitis caused by 6-mercaptopurine in the treatment of inflammatory bowel disease, Gastroenterology, 91:982–986 (1986).
40. Greenstein, A. J., R. Gennuso, D. B. Sachar et al., Extraintestinal cancers in inflammatory bowel disease, Cancer, 56:2914–2921 (1985).
41. Schneck, S. A., I. Penn, De-novo brain tumors in renal transplant recipients, Lancet, 1:983–986 (1971).
42. Penn, I., W. Hammond, L. Brettschneider, T. E. Starzl, Malignant lymphoma in the transplantation patients, Transplant. Proc., 1:106–112 (1969).
43. Glick, S. N., S. K. Teplick, L. R. Goodman, H. R. Clearfield, J. D. Shanser, The development of lymphoma in patients with Crohn's disease, Radiology, 153:337–339 (1984).
44. Greenstein, A. J., G. E. Mullin, J. A., Strauchen, T. Heiman, H. D. Janowitz, D. B. Sachar, Lymphoma in inflammatory bowel disease (abstr), Gastroenterology, 94(5):Part 2:A154 (1988).
45. Kinlen, L. J., Incidence of cancer in rheumatoid arthritis and other disorders after immunosuppressive treatment, Am. J. Med., 78(Suppl 1A): 44–49 (1985).
46. Weil, C., Cyclosporin A: Review of results in organ and bone marrow transplantation in man, Med. Res. Rev., 4:221–265 (1984).
47. Cyclosporin in autoimmune disease, Editorial, Lancet, 1:909–911 (1985).
48. Allison, M. C., R. E. Pounder, Cyclosporin for Crohn's disease, Lancet, 1: 902–903 (1984).
49. Bianchi, P. A., M. Modelli, F. Questo di Polo, T. Ranzi, Cyclosporin for Crohn's disease, Lancet, 2:1242 (1984).
50. Allison, M. C., R. E. Pounder, CyA and disease, a pilot study. Oral presentation at the International Workshop on Cyclosporin in Autoimmune Disease, Basel, March 18–20, Proceedings (in press).
51. Gupta, S., A. Keshavarzian, H. J. F. Hodgson, Cyclosporin in ulcerative colitis, Lancet, 2:1277–1278.
52. Peltekian, K. M., C. N. Williams, A. S. MacDonald, P. Roy, E. Czolpinska, Open study of Cyclosporin A (CyA) in Crohn's disease (CD) (abstr), Gastroenterology, 92(5pt 2):1571 (1987).
53. Brynskov, J., V. Binder, P. Riis, O. Schaffalitsky de Muckadell, K. Lauritsen, L. Freund, J. Fallingborg, S. Norby Rasmussen, P. Matzen, E. Krag, U. Tage-Jensen, Clinical experience with cyclosporin (Cyclosporin A) in chronically-active, therapy-resistant Crohn's disease (abstr), Gastroenterology, 92(5pt 2):1330 (1987).

7

Antidiarrheals, Antibiotics, Psychotropics, and Potential New Drug Therapies

Mark A. Peppercorn

Beth Israel Hospital, Harvard Medical School, Boston, Massachusetts

Previous chapters have dealt in depth with agents whose use is directed at the inflammatory process of patients with ulcerative colitis and Crohn's disease. These drugs have an accepted role in the therapy of inflammatory bowel disease (IBD) or have been well investigated and are likely to soon be of benefit. There are a number of drugs, however, which can be of great use in the individual patient with inflammatory bowel disease but whose action is not thought of as directed against the IBD itself. Moreover, there is emerging an increasing list of agents which on the basis of very preliminary reports appear to have some promise as first-line agents in IBD treatment. These drugs form the basis of this chapter.

I. ANTIDIARRHEALS

A. Opiates

For patients who have diarrhea related to intestinal resection but with minimal or no active disease and for patients with mild well-established chronic diarrhea despite specific therapy, the opiate drugs can be of welcomed benefit. Although both codeine and diphenoxylate hydrochloride (with atropine, as Lomotil) are frequently used in these settings, loperamide (Imodium) is the best studied and probably the safest and most effective of the opiate agents in IBD therapy (1).

Several controlled trials have investigated the utility of loperamide and Lomotil in patients with ulcerative colitis and Crohn's disease with ileostomies following colectomy or after intestinal resection and anastomosis. In general, patients from these studies had improved stool consistency and reduced stool frequency. Patients with some portion of the colon intact responded as favorably as did those with ileostomies (2–6).

Similar results have been reported for loperamide in outpatients with inflammatory bowel disease and chronic diarrhea not fully responsive to first-line drugs (7-10). As with patients who have undergone surgery, stool frequency can be reduced and stool weight decreased by as much as 40%.

Although not well studied in patients with acute, new-onset inflammatory bowel disease or in those with severe symptoms regardless of duration of the inflammatory bowel disease, opiate use should be discouraged in these settings because of their potential to produce ileus and precipitate toxic megacolon (11, 12).

Apart from the risk of toxic megacolon, opiate drugs in the IBD patient carry the same risks as those observed in normal subjects (1). Of the agents in common use, codeine is the most frequently associated with nausea, vomiting, drowsiness, and alterations of mood. Both codeine and Lomotil can produce physical dependence although this complication is rare with Lomotil when used at standard doses. The central nervous system side effects and addictive potential associated with loperamide are minimal probably because of exclusion of the drug by the blood-brain barrier.

B. Cholestyramine

Cholestyramine (Questran), an anionic resin that binds bile salts in the lumen of the gut, is the treatment of choice for bile salt diarrhea (13). Bile salt diarrhea which occurs most often after ileal resection for ileitis results from the impairment of colonic water absorption and promotion of colonic water secretion induced by the unabsorbed bile salts (14). On occasion, patients with unresected nonstenotic ileitis and mild diarrhea will benefit from cholestyramine therapy. Patients are instructed to begin treatment with one packet per day (4 g) in a glass of water and use up to 12 g/day in three divided doses. They must be warned about the potential for constipation. Moreover, the drug should be avoided in patients with strictures because concretions of cholestyramine at the site of narrowing can lead to clinical bowel obstruction. In patients with extensive ileal resections (>100 cm) and severe steatorrhea (>20 g/day), cholestyramine should be avoided as it will further deplete the bile salt pool making fatty acid-induced diarrhea worse. Such patients should be treated with a low-fat diet and medium-chain triglycerides.

Although cholestyramine is generally safe, it may aggravate heartburn and cause some patients to feel bloated. By depleting the bile salt pool, it may predispose to gallstone formation. An increased risk of colon cancer raised by certain animal studies (15) has not been seen in humans. Cholestyramine also is used to lower serum cholesterol levels and as an oxalate-binding agent in patients with oxalate renal stones (see Chap. 10).

C. Bulk Agents

Although most commonly used in patients with the irritable bowel syndrome, the hydrophilic mucilloids such as psyllium and methylcellulose can be of occasional use in the patient with IBD. Patients with proctitis or left-sided colitis may have frequent loose stools alternating with constipation, or constipation alone, patterns similar to that seen in functional bowel disorders. A trial of a bulk agent beginning with one teaspoon per day in a glass of water should be considered. The hydrophilic mucilloids also have a limited potential to bind bile salts and may be effective in bile salt diarrhea, especially when cholestyramine is not tolerated.

II. ANTIBIOTICS

A role for antimicrobial therapy in the treatment of inflammatory bowel disease led to the initial use of sulfasalazine which combines one of the first sulfonamides, sulfapyridine, with a salicylate analogue, 5-aminosalicylate (see Chap. 3). Although subsequent studies have established that the efficiency of sulfasalazine is related to the salicylate and not the sulfa moiety, speculations continue about a bacteria-mediated step in the initiation or perpetuation of the inflammatory process (16).

To date, the only antimicrobial which has been shown to be efficacious in inflammatory bowel disease in controlled trials in metronidazole, the nitroimidazole active against anaerobic bacteria. As discussed in detail in Chapter 5, metronidazole is as effective as sulfasalazine in Crohn's disease involving the colon (17). and appears to be of great benefit to certain patients with perianal complications of Crohn's disease (18). Since metronidazole has properties other than its antimicrobial ones, its mode of action in Crohn's disease has not been fully established.

Although not of proven benefit in controlled trials, a wide array of other antibiotics have been utilized in the therapy of IBD. In one series of 44 patients with Crohn's disease treated over a 5-year period with a variety of drugs including ampicillin, tetracycline, clindamycin, cephalothin, and erythromycin, a 93% success a rate in symptomatic improvement was reported. The authors observed clinical and radiologic resolution in the healing of fistulas, ulcerations, stenoses, and mass lesions (19). These results though intriguing suffer from their retrospective nature and lack of controls. Later in this chapter the possible role of antituberculous drugs in the treatment of Crohn's disease is reviewed.

Finally, antibiotics need to be considered as adjunctive therapy in the patient with severe colitis especially with signs of toxic megacolon and as primary treatment in the patient with Crohn's disease who presents acutely with localized peritonitis. Somewhat surprisingly, no controlled trials of antibiotics have been carried out in either of these two important clinical settings.

In the patient with severe colitis and a dilating colon on high-dose corticosteroids serosal seeding by bacteria undoubtedly often contributes to the pain and tenderness experienced by the patient. It is striking to see such patients suddenly improve with the addition of broad-spectrum antibiotics after failure to improve on steroids.

In the case of the patient with Crohn's disease and localized peritonitis, a local perforation of a stenotic area of diseased bowel has usually occurred. Treatment with antibiotics and bowel rest directed at the complication of contained bacterial infection almost always results in improvement. Clinicians vary in their choice of antibiotics. A regimen of parenteral amipicillin, an aminoglycoside, and metronidazole is often used, but the substitution of a cephalosporin for the penicillin and omission of the anaerobic agent is common and may be equally effective. Corticosteroids, if already begun, need to be continued and at times the dose raised depending on the stress to the patient. Whether steroids should be initiated in such patients acutely or are actually harmful because of their potential to mask inflammation is a matter of debate which awaits study (see Chap. 14).

III. PSYCHOTROPICS

A full discussion of the psychosocial issues confronting the patient with IBD is contained in Chapter 13, where the authors describe a therapetuic approach which takes into account the full complexity of the interactions of the diseases and the psyche. Although never a substitute for the concern and warm support of the physician and other caregivers, minor tranquilizers such as oxazepam, diazepam, and lorazepam (20) and, in selected cases, antidepressants such as amitriptyline doxepin and imipramine may prove useful. The anticholinergic properties of the latter agents have to be monitored in the IBD patient.

The clinician should be aware that the therapy itself may alter the psyche of the patient and produce changes in mental status. Although not widely reported, both sulfasalazine and metronidazole can cause excessive fatigue, mood swings, and even depression. If such symptoms occur coincident with their usage, the drugs should be stopped or doses lowered. Moreover, as noted in Chapter 1, corticosteroids, usually in high doses, frequently cause alterations in behavior including insomnia, restlessness, inability to concentrate, depression, and psychosis. These adverse effects will usually disappear as the dose of steroid is lowered. In the patient with severe IBD who requires high-dose steroids, the addition of lithium carbonate may prevent or modify the adverse psychic effects (21).

IV. POTENTIAL NEW DRUG THERAPIES

The promise of the new topical and oral aminosalicylates, the rapidly metabolized topical steroids, and cyclosporin has been described in previous chapters. This section discusses a number of other new agents which have shown potential efficacy in preliminary trials in patients with ulcerative colitis and Crohn's disease.

A. Sodium Cromoglycate

Sodium cromoglycate is used in the therapy of a variety of disorders such as asthma which are associated with hypersensitivity reactions mediated by IgE. Observations of an increased number of eosinophils and mast cells in rectal biopsies of patients with ulcerative colitis led to the use of oral sodium cromoglycate in such patients. No significant benefit of the drug was noted in either active colitis or disease in remission (22,23).

Recently patients with distal ulcerative colitis and proctitis showed improvement on cromoglycate enemas in a study which compared the drug with prednisolone enemas (24). Further studies of this agent in topical form in active and quiescent disease are anticipated.

B. Sucralfate

Sucralfate is a mucopolysaccharide used in the treatment of peptic disorders. Its mode of action likely includes cytoprotection through enhancement of local prostaglandin production. Colitis induced in rats by topical acetic acid responded to the installation of sucralfate directly into the colon (25). An open-label trial of sucralfate enemas in a small number of patients with distal ulcerative colitis suggested efficacy (26).

These findings led to a randomized prospective study comparing sucralfate enemas with prednisolone in active distal colitis. Although patients on sucralfate appeared to improve with regard to stool frequency, rectal bleeding, and sigmoidoscopic appearance, patients did significantly better on prednisolone, with 71% showing complete resolution of bleeding compared with 28% taking sucralfate (27). When sucralfate enemas were compared with placebo and topical 5-aminosalicylate in another study of active distal colitis, sucralfate proved no better than placebo (28). The latter experience corresponds to additional unpublished results and casts doubt on the utility of topical sucralfate in distal colitis.

C. Chloroquine

In vitro studies described a defect in the ability of certain antigen-bearing epithelial cells in IBD patients to stimulate suppressor T cells (29). Further studies suggested that this defect might relate to abnormal processing of foreign proteins and could be reverted by chloroquine which can slow antigen processing.

Based on these observations, an open trial of 10 patients with active ulcerative colitis and 4 with Crohn's disease was initiated using chloroquine therapy. At the end of 8 weeks, 8 of the 10 patients with ulcerative colitis improved clinically and sigmoidoscopically. The results in Crohn's disease, however, were not impressive (29). Side effects were limited to transient blurred vision and nasal congestion. A placebo-controlled trial is in progress.

D. Methotrexate

The anti-inflammatory properties of methotrexate have led to its successful use in psoriasis and rheumatoid arthritis and to its preliminary application in asthma, sclerosing cholangitis, and primary biliary cirrhosis (30,31). These experiences led to an open trial in 14 patients with Crohn's disease and 7 with ulcerative colitis (32). Patients were symptomatic despite therapy with steroids and/or azathioprine. After 12 weeks, 11 of the Crohn's disease patients showed endoscopic and histologic improvement on the methotrexate. Five of the ulcerative colitis patients had some improvement. Diarrhea, nausea, and transient leukopenia were noted as side effects. As with chloroquine, these promising early results need to be confirmed in randomized controlled trials.

E. Antituberculous Agents

The similarities of Crohn's disease and intestinal tuberculosis have long led to speculation about a causative infectious agent in the former. In recent years, several laboratories have isolated an atypical mycobacterium from the tissues of patients with Crohn's disease (33,34).

On the basis of these findings, six patients with severe refractory Crohn's disease were treated with streptomycin and rifabutin. After 4 months, all of the patients had improved with withdrawal of steroids, healing of fistulas, and improvement in the Crohn's Disease Activity Index (35). Similarly, 12 of 17 patients with active Crohn's disease improved after 6 months of treatment on a four-drug regimen (36). In a study of different design, combined rifabutin and ethambutol therapy did not affect the endoscopic appearance of recurrent ileitis following resection and anastomosis. Moreover, a high incidence of a flulike syndrome was noted (37). Randomized controlled trials of antituberculous agents in Crohn's disease are needed before the routine use of such drugs can be recommended.

F. Lipoxygenase Inhibitors: Eicosapentaeonic Acid (EPA)

In Chapter 3 it was noted that 5-aminosalicylate may be working via inhibition of the lipoxygenase pathway of arachidonic acid metabolism with a decreased production of leukotriene B_4 (LB_4), a potent chemotactic agent recruiting polys to sites of inflammation. EPA affects neutrophil function by competitively inhibiting the formation of LB_4.

While on EPA, the clinical response and neutrophil function in 6 patients with active ulcerative colitis were measured and compared to control patients (38). After 8 weeks of EPA therapy, the ulcerative colitis patients improved clinically and histologically and neutrophil function was altered. Further studies with EPA or similar specific arachidonic acid metabolism inhibitors may not only provide new drugs for treatment but offer further insights into the pathogenesis of IBD.

G. Immune Adjuvents

Agents which enhance cell-mediated immunity have been studied in Crohn's disease stimulated by evidence of possible transmissable viral agents in the disorder. A 6-month placebo-controlled trial of transfer factor revealed no clinical response in 33 patients with active Crohn's disease (39). Similarly, no benefit of BGG or coherin was found in active Crohn's disease (40). In contrast, a small number of patients with Crohn's disease appeared to benefit from 6 weeks of treatment with interferon although the trial was not controlled (41). Levamisole, an agent which enhances neutrophilic activity and has been utilized in rheumatologic disorders may be of benefit as maintenance therapy for Crohn's disease in remission (42). Finally, a different approach to manipulation of the immune system, T-lymphocyte apheresis has shown some success in Crohn's disease in preliminary trials (43).

REFERENCES

1. Barrett, K. E., K. Dharmathaption, Pharmacological aspects of therapy in inflammatory bowel diseases: Anti-diarrheal agents, J. Clin. Gastroenterol., 10:57–63 (1988).
2. Tytgut, G. N., K. Huibregtse, Loperamide and ileostomy output—placebo-controlled double-blind crossover study, Br. Med. J., 2:667 (1975).
3. Pelemans, W., G. Vantrappen, A double-blind crossover comparison of loperamide with diphenoxylate in the symptomatic treatment of chronic diarrhea, Gastroenterology, 70:1030–1034 (1976).
4. Tytgut, G. N., K. Huibregtse, J. Dageuos, A. van DenEude, Effect of loperamide on fecal output and composition in well-established ileostomy and ileorectal anastomosis, Am. J. Dig. Dis., 22:669–676 (1977).

5. Mainguet, P., K. Fiasse, Double-blind placebo-controlled study of loperamide (imodium) in chronic diarrhea caused by ileocolic disease or resection, Gut, 18:575–579 (1977).
6. Bergman, L., L. A. Djars, A comparative study of loperamide and diphenoxylate in the treatment of chronic diarrhea caused by intestinal resection, Ann. Clin. Res., 13:402–405 (1981).
7. Verhaegen, H., J. DeCree, V. Scheurmans, Loperamide a novel type of antidiarrheal agent. Arzneim. Forsch., 24:1654–1659 (1974).
8. Glambud, J. T., T. Hersch, S. Schroder, J. Wenger, Loperamide: A new antidiarrheal agent in the treatment of chronic diarrhea, Gastroenterology, 70:1026–1029 (1976).
9. Tytgut, G. N., K. Huibregtse, S. G. M. Meunissen, Loperamide in chronic diarrhea and ileostomy: A placebo-controlled double-blind crossover study, Arch. Chir. Neerlandicuin, 28:13–20 (1986).
10. Demeulenacre, L., S. Verbeke, M. Muls, A. Regutjcus, Loperamide: An open multicentre trial and a double-blind crossover comparison with placebo in patients with chronic diarrhea, Com. Ther. Res., 16:32–39 (1974).
11. Brown, J. W., Toxic megacolon associated with loperamide therapy, JAMA, 241:501–502 (1979).
12. Pittman, F. E., Adverse effects of lomotil, Gastroenterology, 67:408–410 (1974).
13. Hoffman, A. F., J. R. Poley, Cholestyramine treatment of diarrhea associated with ileal resection, N. Engl. J. Med., 281:379–402 (1969).
14. Mekhjian, H. S., S. F. Phillips, A. F. Hoffman, Colonic secretion of water and electrolytes induced by bile acids: Perfusion studies in man, J. Clin. Invest., 50:1509–1577 (1971).
15. Sachatello, C. T., H. Hedjecock, A. Armstrong, What can experimental colorectal cancer tell us about colorectal cancer in man, Dis. Colon. Rectum, 23:80–85 (1980).
16. Sack, D. M., M. A. Peppercorn, Drug therapy of inflammatory bowel disease, Pharmacotherapy, 3:158–176 (1982).
17. Ursing, B., T. Alm, F. Barany, Comparative study of metronidazole and sulphasalazine for active Crohn's disease: The cooperative Crohn's disease study in Sweden, Gastroenterology, 83:541–549 (1982).
18. Bernstein, L. H., M. S. Frank, L. J. Brandt, Healing of perineal Crohn's disease with metronidazole, Gastroenterology, 79:357–365 (1980).
19. Muss, A. A., J. V. Carbone, H. Y. Kressel, Radiologic and clinical assessment of broad-spectrum antibiotic therapy in Crohn's disease, Am. J. Roentgenol., 131:787–790 (1978).
20. Stokes, D. K., Jr., Loperamide in anxiety associated with chronic enteritis and ulcerative colitis, J. Clin. Psych., 39:53–57 (1978).
21. Goggans, F. C., L. J. Weisberg, L. M. Koran, Lithium prophylaxis of prednisolone psychosis: A case report, J. Clin. Psych., 44:101–102 (1983).

22. Buchnell, N. A., S. R. Gould, D. W. Day, Controlled trial of disodium cromoglycate in chronic persistent ulcerative colitis, Gut, 19:1140–1143 (1978).
23. Dronfield, M. W., M. J. S. Langman, Comparative trial of sulphasalazine and oral sodium cromoglycate in the maintenance of remission in ulcerative colitis, Gut, 19:1136–1189 (1978).
24. Grace, R. H., A. E. Gent, M. D. Hellier, Comparative trial of sodium cromoglycate enemas with prednisolone enemas in the treatment of ulcerative colitis, Gut, 28:88–92 (1987).
25. Zahaui, J., I. Avidar, H. Marcus, Effects of sucralfate in experimental colitis in the rat, Gastroenterology, 92:1707 (1987).
26. Carling, L., I. Kager, E. Borvall, Sucralfate enema - effective in inflammatory bowel disease, Endoscopy, 18:115 (1986).
27. Riley, S. A., I. Gupta, V. Mani, A comparison of sucralfate and prednisolone enemas in the treatment of active distal ulcerative colitis, Gastroenterology, 94:A377 (1988).
28. Campieri, M., P. Gienchetti, A. Belluzzi, C. Grigmola, G. M. Tabanelli, M. Migaldi, M. Migbiol, L. Bardara, 5-aminosalicylic acid, sucralfate and placebo enemas in the treatment of distal ulcerative colitis, Gastroenterology, 94:A58 (1988).
29. Mayer, L., D. B. Sachar, Efficacy of chloroquine in the treatment of inflammatory bowel disease, Gastroenterology, 94:A293 (1988).
30. Kaplan, M. M., S. Arora, S. H. Pincus, Primary sclerosing cholangitis and low-dose oral pulse methotrexate therapy, Ann. Intern. Med., 106:231–235 (1987).
31. Kaplan, M. M., T. A. Knox, S. Arora, Primary biliary cirrhosis treated with low-dose oral pulse methotrexate, Ann. Intern. Med., 108:429–431 (1988).
32. Kozarek, R. A., D. J. Patterson, M. D. Gelfund, V. A. Botoman, T. J. Ball, K. R. Wilske, Methotrexate induces clinical and histologic remissions in refractory inflammatory bowel disease, Ann. Intern. Med., 110:353–356 (1989).
33. Chiodini, R. J., N. J. Van Kruiningen, W. R. Thayer, R. S. Markal, J. A. Couta, Possible role of mycobacterium in inflammatory bowel disease, Dig. Dis. Sci., 29:1073 (1984).
34. Chiodini, R. J.,H. J. Van Kruiningen, R. S. Merkal, W. R. Thager, J. A. Couta, Characteristics of an unclassified mycobacterium species isolated from patients with Crohn's disease, J. Clin. Microbiol., 20:966 (1984).
35. Thayer, W. R., J. A. Couta, R. J. Chiodini, H. J. Van Kruiningen, Use of rifabutin and streptomycin in the therapy of Crohn's disease, Gastroenterology, 94:A458 (1988).
36. Parker, M. C., S. H. Savegmutter, J. J. McFadden, J. Herman Taylor, Results of quadruple antimycobacterial chemotherapy in 17 Crohn's disease patients completing six months treatment, Gastroenterology, 94: A1770 (1988).

37. Rutgeerts, P., G. Vantrappen, J. Van Isreldy, K. Gebres, Rifabutin therapy in patients with recurrent Crohn's disease after ileocolonic resection, Gastroenterology, 94:A391 (1988).
38. McColl, T., J. O'Leary, J. Bloomfield, C. A. O'Morain, Eicosapentaenoic acid, Gastroenterology, 94:A294 (1988).
39. Vicary, F. R., J. D. Chanders, P. Dhillion, Double-blind trial of the use of transfer factor in the treatment of Crohn's disease, Gut, 20:408–413 (1979).
40. Rahban, S., J. H. Sherman, G. Opelz, BGG treatment of Crohn's disease, Am. J. Gastroenterol., 71:196–201 (1979).
41. Vantrappen, G., G. Caremans, A. Billian, Treatment of Crohn's disease with interferon: A preliminary clinical trial, Acta Clin. Belg., 35:4–10 (1980).
42. Segal, A. W., G. Lowei, Neutrophil disfunction in Crohn's disease, Lancet, 2:219–222 (1976).
43. Bichs, R. O., K. Groshart, R. Chandler, The treatment of severe chronically active Crohn's disease by T lymphocyte apheresis, Gastroenterology, 90: 1346 (1986).

8

Enteral and Parenteral Nutrition

C. Richard Fleming

Mayo Clinic, Jacksonville, Florida, and Mayo Medical School, Rochester, Minnesota

Malnutrition is a commonly recognized complication of inflammatory bowel disease (IBD) that usually correlates with the severity and duration of the disease. The diarrhea, maldigestion, and malabsorption that most patients with IBD experience often result in deficiencies of multiple nutrients (e.g., protein, folate, vitamin B_{12}) which may further impair the integrity of the gut epithelium.

Nutrition in patients with IBD has been examined from several perspectives, including: (1) manifestations and mechanisms of protein-calorie malnutrition, (2) nutritional requirements, (3) selective nutritional deficiencies, (4) preoperative nutritional status and its influence on surgical outcome, (5) dietary characteristics of patients with IBD, (6) roles of specialized enteral and parenteral nutrition in management of patients with IBD, and (7) growth failure in children and adolescents. In this chapter, each of these areas will be addressed.

I. MALNUTRITION IN IBD: MANIFESTATIONS AND MECHANISMS

Malnutrition in patients with inflammatory bowel disease (IBD) is usually manifested as hypoalbuminemia and weight loss (1). The mechanisms contributing to these deficiencies include decreased intake of nutrients, malabsorption from decreased small bowel absorptive surface due to resection or disease, maldigestion of fat and fat-soluble vitamins after ileal resection, drug–nutrient interactions, and protein-losing enteropathy. Examples of drugs contributing to

Table 1 Frequency of Nutritional Deficiencies Reported in Inflammatory Bowel Disease

	Crohn's disease (%)	Ulcerative colitis (%)
Weight loss	65–75	18–62
Hypoalbuminemia	25–80	25–50
Negative nitrogen balance	69	a
Anemia	60–80	66
Iron	39	81
Vitamin B_{12}	48	5
Folic acid	54	36
Calcium	13	a
Magnesium	14–33	a
Potassium	6–20	a

[a]Observed but frequency not reported.
Source: Modified from Ref. 1.

malnutrition are sulfasalazine, which interferes with folate absorption (2); corticosteroids, which suppress calcium absorption (3); and cholestyramine, which impairs the absorption of fat and fat-soluble vitamins. Gut losses of blood, water and electrolytes, trace elements, and protein are often underestimated. Intestinal protein losses measured by [^{51}CR] chloride were excessive in 21 of 30 patients with Crohn's disease with maximal values more than 15 times normal (4). Protein losses from the gut correlate well with the length of diseased bowel. Steinfield et al. used I^{131}-labeled albumin to measure albumin kinetics in patients with IBD (5). Whereas albumin synthesis was preserved when compared to controls, stool losses of albumin were significantly greater, resulting in a net decrease in exchangeable albumin.

It is often stated that patients with IBD have increased energy requirements due to their chronic inflammatory disease. This is misinterpreted by some to mean that the basal energy expenditure is increased when, in fact, patients with IBD who are not septic or febrile do not demonstrate increased basal energy expenditure (6,7). The resting energy expenditure measured by indirect calorimetry in patients with clinically active Crohn's disease was not significantly higher than the predicted energy expenditure estimated from the Harris-Benedict equation (Fig. 1a). Also, patients with Crohn's disease who were the most underweight demonstrated the highest caloric needs when expressed on a body weight basis (Fig. 1b).

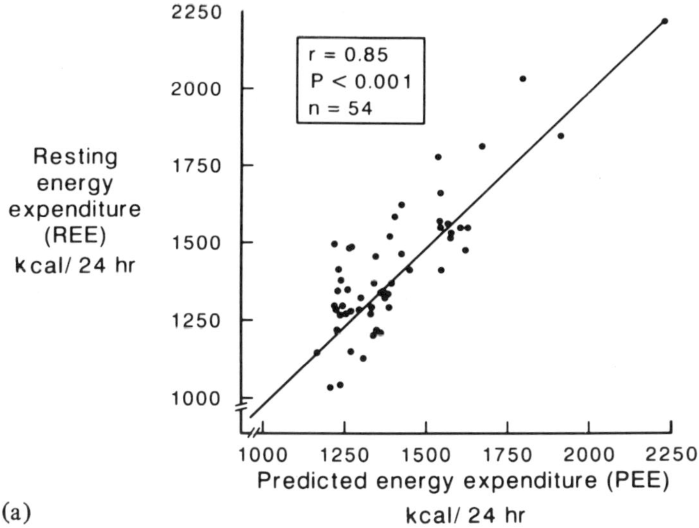

(a)

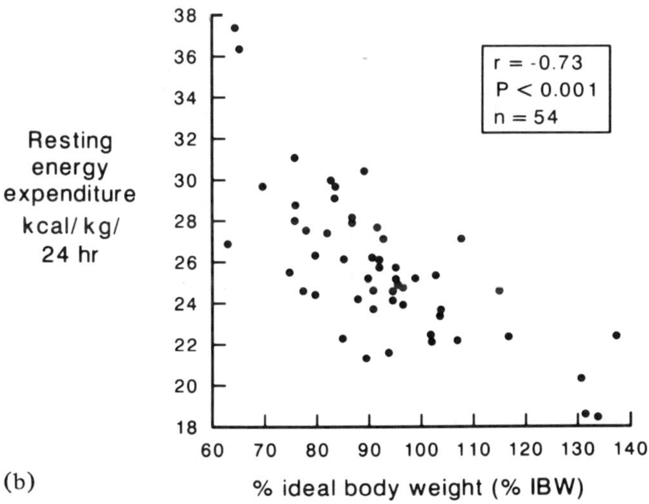

(b)

Figure 1 (a) Resting energy expenditure (REE) measured by indirect calorimetry in 54 patients with Crohn's disease correlated very well with the predicted energy expenditure (PEE) estimated by the Harris-Benedict equation. (b) Resting energy expenditure was the highest, when expressed on a body weight basis, in those patients who were the most underweight.

II. NUTRITIONAL REQUIREMENTS AND SELECTIVE NUTRITIONAL DEFICIENCIES

Basal energy expenditure (BEE) can be measured by indirect calorimetry or estimated by the Harris-Benedict equation. In general, malnourished patients with IBD will require approximately 35 kcal and 1.5 g of protein per kilogram body weight per day when fed by total parenteral nutrition (TPN) in order to gain weight at a rate of one-half pound per day and remain in positive nitrogen balance. The dual energy system (glucose and fat calories) rather than glucose alone for patients receiving TPN reduces fat and water retention while promoting increased nitrogen retention (8).

The delivery of adequate amounts of macroelements, trace elements, and vitamins is extremely important during nutritional restoration. Examples include data from Rudman and colleagues that demonstrated that omitting such elements as potassium and phosphorus resulted in a change in the quality of weight gain in that fat weight was increased and lean body mass was decreased (9).

With diarrhea and fistula drainage, there are increased losses of electrolytes and trace elements. There is usually a good correlation between stool weights and zinc losses; patients producing one liter of stool per day may lose 10 mg of zinc (10). Therefore, zinc deficiency may be common in patients with IBD. The serum zinc, however, is not a sensitive measure because hypoalbuminemia, which is frequently present in IBD, will result in a low serum zinc value since albumin binds at least 60% of circulating zinc. A combination of a low serum and urinary zinc is more suggestive of zinc deficiency (11).

Patients with IBD are susceptible to many additional trace nutrient deficiencies. Driscoll et al. reported that 25% of 82 patients with Crohn's disease had vitamin D deficiency as determined by very low 25-hydroxyvitamin D levels (12). Of 9 patients who had bone biopsies, 6 had osteomalacia and 3 had osteoporosis. Adequacy of replacement therapy, as proven by repeat biopsies, was assessed accurately by monitoring the serum 25-hydroxyvitamin D levels. Gerson and Fabry have reported low ascorbic acid levels in blood and intestine in Crohn's patients with fistulas (13). Vitamin A deficiency has been well described in 21% of patients with Crohn's disease, and those with plasma retinol < 0.8 μmol/l (<23 μg%) run a high risk of developing night blindness (14). Folate deficiency is of multiple origin: inadequate diet, malabsorption, and chronic (drug-induced?) low-grade hemolysis (15). An ileal resection of 60 cm or greater makes an abnormal Schilling test likely and should prompt vitamin B_{12} supplementation (16).

Magnesium depletion deserves special note, especially in Crohn's patients with a short bowel syndrome. It may be the cause of persistent hypocalcemia, despite adequate replacement of calcium and vitamin D. In one study of 17 patients with *severe* Crohn's disease, Mg^{2+} depletion was present in 15 (88%) and severe enough to cause symptoms in 2 patients (17). Twenty-four-hour urine levels of Mg^{2+} are more sensitive indicators of Mg^{2+} deficiency in humans than are serum levels. Hassov et al. found that urinary magnesium excretion decreased with increasing lengths of small bowel resected, as did the muscle concentration of magnesium (18).

III. PREOPERATIVE NUTRITIONAL STATUS AND ITS INFLUENCE ON SURGICAL OUTCOME

Lindor et al. determined that the risk of developing postoperative complications in Crohn's patients was inversely related to the concentrations of serum albumin and total iron-binding capacity (19). The rate of complications was 29% among patients with low (less than 3.1 g/dl) serum albumin levels but only 6% among patients with normal albumin levels. No correlations were noted between postoperative complications and preoperative weight loss or preponderance of Crohn's disease of the colon. The median duration of postoperative hospitalization was 24.5 days for the 16 patients with complications in comparison with only 10 days for patients without complications. Lehr and colleagues found significant depletion of intracellular potassium in Crohn's patients (20). Treatment before surgery to increase body potassium content resulted in a reduced surgical mortality and complications rate compared with a retrospective series of 56 patients in whom aggressive attempts to restore potassium losses were not made. Gerson noted that Crohn's patients with serum albumin levels less than 2.5 g/dl had longer hospital stays (21).

IV. DIETARY CHARACTERISTICS OF PATIENTS WITH INFLAMMATORY BOWEL DISEASE

Most observations on record regarding the diet of patients with IBD have emphasized low fiber and high sugar intakes. The preillness diets in 30 patients with Crohn's disease were approximately twofold greater in refined sugar and fourfold less in fruits and vegetables compared with diets of 30 healthy controls (22). Also, patients with Crohn's disease have been reported to add two- to threefold the amount of sugar to drinks both before and after symptoms compared with age- and sex-matched controls (23). No correlation has been found between the taste thresholds and the amount of the average daily sugar intake in patients with Crohn's disease (24).

These observations led to the use of a fiber-rich diet which showed that 32 patients with Crohn's disease taking the diet had a reduction in total hospital days and intestinal operations, when compared with historical controls treated with an ad lib diet (25). A more recent and prospectively controlled study argues against a high-fiber diet in patients with Crohn's disease (26). Twenty patients with Crohn's disease who had been brought into remission by TPN or an elemental diet were randomized to a diet which excluded specific foods to which the patient was intolerant or to a fiber-rich diet. At six months, 7 of the 10 on the exclusion diet were still in remission compared to 0 of 10 subjects on the high-fiber diet. However, significant differences in disease distribution and prior treatment with corticosteroids existed between the two groups. It should not be surprising that our heterogeneous population of Crohn's patients might respond similarly to more than one type of diet, and it is equally unlikely that all patients with Crohn's disease will benefit from the same dietary manipulations.

V. ROUTES OF NUTRITIONAL THERAPY

A. Enteral Nutrition

In general, dietary restrictions should be discouraged since caloric intake is often decreased in patients who need calories the most. Exceptions include low-residue diets for patients with strictures and partial bowel obstruction, low oxalate diets for those with hyperoxaluria and/or calcium oxalate renal stones, and lactose-free diets for the patient with IBD who is lactase deficient.

Superiority of elemental or defined formula diets over whole food has not been demonstrated for patients with IBD. However, these concentrated commercial diets (1-2 kcal/cc) have proved useful in some patients with IBD who cannot or will not eat enough. They can be used as supplements or as meal replacements.

Harris and colleagues demonstrated the usefulness of a supplemental defined formula in a crossover study involving 28 patients with Crohn's disease (27). Each patient received an ad lib select diet for two months and the same diet plus Ensure Plus designed to increase the daily intake to approximately 3000 calories for another two months. Ensure Plus contributed a mean of only ~500 kcals to the total 3000 kcal. Significant increases in the two months when Ensure Plus was added included anthropometrics such as arm muscle circumference and triceps skinfolds, serum proteins, 24-hr urinary creatinine-to-height index, and circulating T lymphocytes. Significant decreases included orosomucoid which is consistent with a decrease in inflammatory response. An earlier study illustrated that an elemental diet for 28 to 56 days in seven patients with extensive jejunoileal Crohn's disease decreased gut protein losses by 47% compared to an ad lib diet in the same patients (28).

O'Morain et al. conducted a controlled trial in which 21 patients acutely ill with exacerbations of Crohn's disease were randomized to either prednisone (0.75 mg/kg) or an elemental diet (Vivonex) for four weeks (29). Assessment at 4 and 12 weeks showed that patients treated with Vivonex (40-60 kcal/kg) improved clinically and biochemically as much as the steroid group and 80% of patients in both groups were in remission at four weeks. The patients on prednisone started to taper the drug at 4 weeks and were still on a large dose at 12 weeks, whereas patients on Vivonex stopped it and resumed whole food at the end of four weeks. Saverymuttu and colleagues also used an elemental diet as a meal replacement in a prospective trial (30). Thirty-seven patients with active Crohn's disease were randomized to either prednisolone and an ad lib diet or to an elemental diet and nonabsorbable antibiotics. The rationale for the latter regimen was to exclude both dietary and bacterial antigens from the gut lumen. Five patients could not tolerate the elemental diet and antibiotics. Of the 32 patients who completed the study, no differences in the two groups were detected with respect to changes in sedimentation rate, the Crohn's Disease Activity Index and fecal granulocyte excretion. Between 10 and 20% of patients in the studies by Harris et al. (27) and Saverymuttu et al. (30) were not able to take the formulas and were excluded from their data analyses. A more recent and prospective randomized trial of 107 patients with an acute phase of Crohn's disease concluded that a combination of prednisone and sulfasalazine was significantly more effective than enteral nutrition (an oligopeptide diet) in inducing clinical remissions during six weeks of therapy (31).

If elemental or defined formula diets are helpful in controlling clinical activity in some patients with Crohn's disease, how might they be working? Speculations include a reduction in intraluminal antigenic stimulation, improved immune function, modification of gut bacterial flora and provision of nutrients (i.e., glutamine) that provide selective fuel to the gut epithelium.

Patient compliance in drinking elemental diets over long periods is poor and often negates the potential benefits. Consequently, one may "bypass" the appetite by administering the diets through a nasogastric, gastrostomy, or jejunostomy tube. The formulas can be infused at a constant rate, using enteral feeding pumps, or given as periodic bolus feedings. Rees and colleagues showed that the administration of undiluted hypertonic elemental diets (630 mOsm) by constant nasogastric infusion to patients with IBD was safe and usually effective (32). Avoiding "starter regimens" led to increased nutrient intake and improved nitrogen balance.

B. Parenteral Nutrition

Total parenteral nutrition (TPN) is often used in IBD:

As adjunctive treatment to conventional medical or surgical treatment
As primary therapy for patients with extensive Crohn's disease and gut failure

Most data suggest that patients with Crohn's disease respond better to TPN and bowel rest than do patients with ulcerative colitis and that patients with Crohn's enteritis respond better than patients with Crohn's colitis.

1. Ulcerative Colitis

Total parenteral nutrition, with or without bowel rest, has been used in hopes of achieving clinical remissions and to support malnourished patients before and after surgery.

Clinical Remissions Dickinson and colleagues conducted a randomized trial of TPN and bowel rest in patients with acute colitis, most of whom had CUC (33). Control patients were fed an ad lib oral diet and the treatment group received TPN and bowel rest. Controls and TPN treated patients were taking comparable amounts of prednisone. Half of each group required surgery during the same hospitalization. Of those not requiring surgery, the time required of medical treatment to induce clinical remissions was comparable in the two groups. Thus, there was no difference in the outcome in the control and TPN groups with regard to frequency of surgery or duration of medical treatment. The compiled retrospective reports and another similar controlled study (34) also suggested that the addition of TPN and bowel rest will not prompt clinical remissions more often than the use of corticosteroids and hospitalization alone. However, these reports should not discourage the use of TPN in malnourished CUC patients in whom enteral nutrition is impossible or inadequate.

Postoperative TPN Collins et al. performed a controlled clinical trial in patients undergoing proctocolectomy, half of whom had IBD (35). Postoperatively, patients received one of three intravenous nutritional formulas: balanced amino acids without another caloric source, an intravenous water-electrolyte solution alone or conventional TPN. Eight of 10 TPN-treated patients were home with complete perineal wound healing by 4 weeks compared to only four of 10 patients in the water-electrolyte group and 3 of 10 patients in the amino acid group who had healed their wounds during the same period.

2. *Crohn's Disease*

Clinical Remissions Allowing for differences in authors' definitions of clinical remission, uncontrolled data suggest that 60-70% of patients treated with TPN will undergo an initial, in-hospital remission, but only 40-50% of those followed for three months remain in remission.

To define the effect of bowel rest (total and partial) and nutritional support (enteral and parenteral) as independent variables, a controlled trial was prospectively undertaken in patients with active Crohn's disease unresponsive to other medical management (36). Nutritional support for 21 days was randomized in 51 hospitalized patients to one of the following treatment groups: central parenteral nutrition and NPO (TPN, $n = 17$), defined formula diet given through a nasogastric tube (DFD, $n = 19$) or partial parenteral nutrition and oral food (PPN, $n = 15$). Clinical remission, defined as a CDAI < 150 and ability to ingest food without medication adjustment occurred in 12 patients on TPN (71%), 11 on DFD (58%), and 9 on PPN (60%). The mean interval to relapse after successful therapy was 7 months on DFD (9 of 11 patients), 9 months on TPN (4 of 12 patients), and 8 months on PPN (5 of 9 patients). Thus although TPN is a useful adjunct in the management of Crohn's disease, it proved no better than DFD or PPN.

Lochs performed a randomized trial comparing TPN with bowel rest with TPN without bowel rest in 20 patients with Crohn's disease (37). There was no apparent advantage by clinical scores or nutritional indices in the patients who were placed on bowel rest while receiving TPN.

Muller et al. treated 30 consecutive patients with complicated Crohn's disease with 12 weeks of TPN and bowel rest (38). No medications were given. Although surgery was initially avoided in 25 of 30 patients, the cumulative relapse rate was 60% after two years and 85% after four years. This was compared with the results of bowel resection, obtained from a 10-year period before TPN was begun at the same hospital, showing the cumulative recurrence rates after TPN to be four times higher than after resection.

Fistulas The use of TPN and bowel rest to permanently close enterocutaneous fistulas from Crohn's disease has been disappointing and surgery should not be delayed unnecessarily in the hope that the fistulas will close. Many such patients require TPN and bowel rest for restoration of adequate nutrition during the perioperative period.

Gut Failure Patients with diffuse small bowel Crohn's disease or severe short bowel syndrome that does not respond to conventional treatment often require home parenteral nutrition (HPN). Nutrition repletion during HPN is excellent and 75% of patients on HPN are rehabilitated and return to gainful employment, school, or homemaker activities (39,40). In 1985, our 40 active patients received HPN for a total of 14,420 days, only 5% of which were spent in the hospital. Of our first 88 patients, 50 (56%) discontinued HPN for one of four reasons: 25% improved enough and were able to maintain good nutrition with oral intake alone, 20% died, 6% chose to discontinue, and 5% were noncompliant and removed from HPN. Of our 19 HPN patients who died while still receiving HPN, 5 died from a HPN-related complication. Overall, there was a 6% (5/88) mortality rate associated with HPN (41).

VI. GROWTH FAILURE IN IBD

Fifteen percent of children or adolescents with chronic ulcerative colitis (CUC) and 30% with Crohn's disease are less than the third percentile for height sometime during their illness. The growth retardation may precede the onset of gastrointestinal symptoms by several months.

Adequate nutritional supplementation alone, regardless of the form, should stimulate growth. The caloric and protein requirements revert to those of the newborn infant: 75–100 kcal/kg and 2–3 g of protein/kg per day. For significant growth velocity to occur, the supplementation must begin prior to epiphyseal closure. Chronic malnutrition decreases circulating somatomedin C levels and growth velocity; therefore, monitoring these measurements will help determine nutritional sufficiency (42).

Kirschner and colleagues reported 7 teenagers with Crohn's disease and severe growth failure whom they were able to manage by oral nutrition alone (43). Through frequent visits to the dietician, the mean caloric intake increased from 56% of needed to 91% and the growth velocity, expressed as centimeters/year, increased from 1.8 to 6.2. It took approximately three to four years of oral nutritional intervention in some patients before preillness height percentiles were achieved. Morin found that continuous infusion through a nasogastric tube of an elemental diet for 6 weeks resulted in prompt increases in height and weight (44). This relatively short course of elemental enteral nutrition led to temporary resumption of growth. Once the patient's disease activity recurred, however, the previously abnormal growth patterns returned.

Although it promptly stimulates vertical growth, TPN is not necessary in most cases. Kelts et al. studied seven youngsters with delayed growth (45). Eighty percent or more of calories were given through a central venous catheter for 8 weeks or longer. Patients were given 75 kcal/kg/day and 2 g of protein/kg/day. The growth velocity increased from approximately 2 cm to 6.4 cm per year and the average weight gain was 4.8 kg. Interestingly, the growth that was demonstrated during and shortly after the nutritional support continued for as long as one year after stopping intravenous therapy. Excessive weight gain as fat and water rather than lean body mass often occurs during the initiation of TPN, especially in children receiving corticosteroids.

Some children with the most severe Crohn's disease or other gut diseases require HPN. Strobel and colleagues used HPN in 17 patients with Crohn's disease and growth failure (46). Of the 17 patients, 12 underwent clinical remission but only four had remission sustained longer than three months. On a more positive side, all 17 patients showed a significant increase in weight and 14 of 17 demonstrated increased height. Of these 14 patients, 10 showed "catch-up growth" defined as growth velocity greater than expected for age. Amarnath et al. showed that the mean growth velocity (cm/yr) in Crohn's patients treated with HPN increased more than fivefold and that patients who were younger and had their disease for a shorter period (<3 years) grew better than older patients with Crohn's disease who had their disease for a mean of 8 years (47). (For further discussion of nutritional therapy in children see Chap. 12.)

REFERENCES

1. Driscoll, R. H., I. H. Rosenberg, Total parenteral nutrition in inflammatory bowel disease, Med. Clin. North Am., 62(1):185–201 (1978).
2. Franklin, J. L., I. H. Rosenberg, Impaired folic acid absorption in inflammatory bowel disease: Effects of salicylazosulfapyridine (Azulfidine), Gastroenterology, 64:517–525 (1973).
3. Shultz, T. D., S. Bollman, R. Kumar, Decreased intestinal calcium absorption in vivo and normal brush border membrane vesicle calcium uptake in

cortisol-treated chicken: Evidence for dissociation of calcium absorption from brush border vesicle uptake, Proc. Natl. Acad. Sci. USA, 79:3542-3546 (1982).

4. Beeken, W. L., H. J. Busch, D. L. Sylvester, Intestinal protein loss in Crohn's disease, Gastroenterology, 62(2):207-215 (1972).
5. Steinfeld, J. L., J. D. Davidson, R. S. Gordon, The mechanism of hypoproteinemia in patients with regional enteritis and ulcerative colitis, Am. J. Med., 29:405-415 (1960).
6. Barot, L. R., J. L. Rombeau, I. D. Feurer, J. L. Mullen, Caloric requirements in patients with inflammatory bowel disease, Ann. Surg., 195:214-218 (1982).
7. Chan, A. T. H., C. R. Fleming, W. M. O'Fallon, K. A. Huizenga, Estimated versus measured basal energy requirements in patients with Crohn's disease, Gastroenterology, 91:75-78 (1986).
8. Macfie, J., R. C. Smith, G. L. Hill, Glucose or fat as a nonprotein energy source? A controlled clinical trial in gastroenterological patients requiring intravenous nutrition, Gastroenterology, 80:103-107 (1981).
9. Rudman, D., W. J. Millikan, T. J., Richardson, Elemental balances during intravenous hyperalimentation of underweight adult subjects, J. Clin. Invest., 55:94-104 (1975).
10. Wolman, S. L., G. H. Anderson, E. B. Marliss, K. N. Jeejeebhoy, Zinc in total parenteral nutrition: Requirements and metabolic effects, Gastroenterology, 76:458-467 (1979).
11. Fleming, C. R., K. A. Huizenga, J. T. McCall, J. Gildea, R. Dennis, Zinc nutrition in Crohn's disease, Dig. Dis. Sci., 26(10):865-870 (1981).
12. Driscoll, R. H., S. C. Meredith, M. Sitrin, I. H. Rosenberg, Vitamin D deficiency and bone disease in patients with Crohn's disease, Gastroenterology, 83:1252-1258 (1982).
13. Gerson, C. D., E. M. Fabry, Ascorbic acid deficiency and fistula formation in regional enteritis, Gastroenterology, 67:428-433 (1974).
14. Main, A. N. H., P. R. Mills, R. I. Russell, J. Broute-Stewart, L. M. Nelson, A. McClelland, A. Shenkin, Vitamin A deficiency in Crohn's disease, Gut, 24:1169-1175 (1983).
15. Elsborg, L., L. Larsen, Folate deficiency in chronic inflammatory bowel diseases, Scand. J. Gastroenterol., 14:1019-1024 (1979).
16. Thompson, W. G., E. Wrathell, The relation between ileal resection and vitamin B12 absorption, Can. J. Surg., 20:461-464 (1977).
17. Main, A. N. H., R. J. Morgan, R. I. Russell, Magnesium deficiency in chronic inflammatory bowel disease and requirements during intravenous nutrition, J. Parent. Enteral. Nutr., 5(1):15-19 (1981).
18. Hessov, I., C. Hasselblad, S. Fasth, Magnesium deficiency after ileal resection for Crohn's disease, Scand. J. Gastroenterol., 18:643-649 (1983).
19. Lindor, K. D., C. R. Fleming, D. M. Ilstrup, Preoperative nutritional status and other factors that influence surgical outcome in patients with Crohn's disease, Mayo Clin. Proc., 60:393-396 (1985).

20. Lehr, L., O. Schober, H. Hundeshagen, R. Pichlmayer, Total body potassium depletion and the need for preoperative nutritional support in Crohn's disease, Ann. Surg., 196(6):709–714 (1982).
21. Gerson, C. D., Small bowel malfunction and malnutrition, Mt. Sinai J. Med., 50(2):119–125 (1983).
22. Thornton, J. R., P. M. Emmet, K. W. Heaton, Diet and Crohn's disease: Characteristics of the pre-illness diet, Br. Med. J., 2:762–764 (1979).
23. Mayberry, J. F., J. Rhodes, R. Allan, R. G. Newcombe, G. M., Rejan, L. M. Chamberlain, K. G. Wragg, Diet in Crohn's disease. Two studies of current and previous habits in newly diagnosed patients, Dig. Dis. Sci., 26:444–448 (1981).
24. Kasper, H., H. Sommer, Taste thresholds in patients with Crohn's disease, Letter to Editor, J. Hum. Nutr., 34:455–456 (1980).
25. Heaton, K. W., J. R. Thornton, P. M. Emmet, Treatment of Crohn's disease with an unrefined-carbohydrate, fibre-rich diet, Br. J. Med., 2:764–766 (1979).
26. Jones, V. A., E. Workman, A. H. Freeman, R. J. Dickinson, A. J. Wilson, J. O. Hunter, Crohn's disease maintenance of remission by diet, Lancet, 177–180 (1985).
27. Harris, A. D., V. Danis, R. V. Heatley, L. A. Jones, R. Fifield, R. G. Newcombe, J. Rhodes, Controlled trial of supplemental oral nutrition in Crohn's disease, Lancet, 1:887–890 (1983).
28. Logan, R. F. A., J. Gillon, C. Ferrington, C. A. Ferguson, Reduction of gastrointestinal protein loss by a elemental diet in Crohn's disease of the small bowel, Gut, 22:383–387 (1981).
29. O'Morain, C., A. W. Segal, A. J. Levi, Elemental diet as primary treatment of acute Crohn's disease: A controlled trial, Br. Med. J., 288:1859–1862 (1984).
30. Saverymuttu, S., H. J. F., Hodgson, V. S. Chadwick, Controlled trial comparing prednisolone with an elemental diet plus nonabsorbable antibiotics in active Crohn's disease, Gut, 26:994–998 (1985).
31. Lochs, H., H. J. Steinhardt, B. Klaus-Wenz, P. Bauer, H. Malehow, Enteral nutrition versus drug treatment for the acute phase of Crohn's disease, Gastroenterology, 94(5):A267 (1988).
32. Rees, R. G. P., P. P. Keohane, G. K. Grimbel, Elemental diet administered nasogastrically without starter regimens in patients with inflammatory bowel disease, J. Parent. Enteral. Nutr., 10(3): 258–262 (1986).
33. Dickinson, R. J., M. G. Ashton, A. T. R. Axon, R. C. Smith, C. K. Young, G. L. Hill, Controlled trial of intravenous hyperalimentation and total bowel rest as an adjunct to the routine therapy of acute colitis, Gastroenterology, 79:1199–1204 (1980).
34. McIntyre, P. B., J. Powell-Tuck, S. R. Wood, J. E. Lennard-Jones, E. P. Hecketsweiler, J. P. Galmiche, R. Colin, Controlled trial of bowel rest in the treatment of severe acute colitis, Gut, 27:481–485 (1986).
35. Collins, J. P., C. B. Oxby, G. L. Hill, Intravenous amino acids and intravenous hyperalimentation as protein-sparing therapy after major surgery. A controlled clinical trial, Lancet, 1:788-791 (1978).

36. Greenberg, G. R., C. R. Fleming, K. N. Jeejeebhoy, Controlled trial of bowel rest and nutritional support in the management of Crohn's disease, Gut, in press.
37. Lochs, H., Has total bowel rest a beneficial effect in the treatment of Crohn's disease, Clin. Nutr., 2:61–64 (1983).
38. Muller, J. M., H. W. Keller, H. Erasmi, Total parenteral nutrition as the sole therapy in Crohn's disease—a prospective study, Br. J. Surg., 70:40–43 (1983).
39. Fleming, C. R., D. B. McGill, S. Berkner, Home parenteral nutrition as primary therapy in patients with extensive Crohn's disease of the small bowel and malnutrition, Gastroenterology, 73:1077–1081 (1977).
40. Fleming, C. R., R. W. Beart, S. Berkner, D. B. McGill, R. Gaffran, Home parenteral nutrition for management of the severely malnourished adult patient, Gastroenterology, 79:11–18 (1980).
41. Fleming, C. R., Comprehensive care of the gut failure patient: Present and future, Trans. Am. Climat. Assoc., 98:197–207 (1986).
42. Kirshner, B. S., M. M. Sutton, Somatomedin-C levels in growth-impaired children and adolescents with chronic inflammatory bowel disease, Gastroenterology, 91:830–836 (1986).
43. Kirshner, B. S., J. R. Klich, S. S. Kalman, M. V. Defavano, I. H. Rosenberg, Reversal of growth retardation in Crohn's disease with therapy emphasizing oral nutrition restitution, Gastroenterology, 80:10–15 (1981).
44. Morin, C. L., Continuous elemental enteral alimentation in children with Crohn's disease and growth failure, Gastroenterology, 79:1205–1210 (1980).
45. Kelts, D. G., R. J. Grand, G. Shen, J. B. Watkins, S. L. Werlin, C. Boehme, Nutritional basis of growth failure in children and adolescents with Crohn's disease, Gastroenterology, 76:720–727 (1979).
46. Strobel, C. T., W. J. Byrne, M. E. Ament, Home parenteral nutrition in children with Crohn's disease: An effective management alternative, Gastroenterology, 77:272–279 (1979).
47. Amarnath, R. P., C. R. Fleming, J. Perrault, Home parenteral nutrition in chronic intestinal diseases: Its effect on growth and development, J. Pediatr. Gastroenterol., 6(1):89–95 (1987).

9
Ileostomy Alternatives

John H. Pemberton and Keith A. Kelly

Mayo Clinic and Mayo Medical School, Rochester, Minnesota

Although primarily a medical problem, inflammatory bowel disease (IBD) often becomes resistant to effective medical management and surgery is required. Experience with surgery, particularly as elective treatment of the disease, has broadened. Operations performed upon patients in extremis have gratifyingly decreased in frequency; indeed, classic full-blown toxic megacolon is rarely seen today. This is likely due to aggressive early medical care and the willingness to intervene early in evolving fulminant disease.

As prognosis after surgery has improved, more patients have been referred earlier in the course of their disease, before becoming debilitated, which in turn, has facilitated the improved surgical results. Therefore, because candidates for elective operation today are often in good general health, surgeons have been increasingly willing to embrace alternatives to the more classic operations described for patients with inflammatory bowel disease, particularly chronic ulcerative colitis (CUC). The rationale and aims of surgery for CUC and surgery for Crohn's disease differ; in one, surgery is "curative," while in the other, it is usually a form of ongoing adjunctive management of a disease for which the ultimate prognosis is always in doubt. In patients with pancolitis, caused by CUC or Crohn's disease, the *standard approach*, has been proctocolectomy with an abdominal ileostomy. The operation effectively eliminates the colonic disease, but results in an incontinent stoma. In contrast, the general goal of *alternative surgery* is to control enteric outflow.

This chapter describes various alternatives to an incontinent ileostomy, details the rationale and goals of the operations, outlines technique, reports on clinical and functional results, and assesses what role these alternatives have in the modern surgical management of patients with inflammatory bowel disease.

I. BACKGROUND

The goals of the earliest surgical maneuvers to manage inflammatory bowel disease were to divert the fecal stream and to gain access to the lumen of the colon for irrigation with medication. To these ends, venting colostomy and appendicostomy were practiced widely in the late 19th and early 20th centuries (1,2). Ileostomy was first used for the treatment of IBD by Brown in 1913 (3). His goals were to put the bowel to rest for a defined period of time and then to close the ileostomy later. Brown's technique of siting the ileostomy in the midline wound was widely adapted and used for decades. However, it became increasingly evident that such an ileostomy would be permanent and that patients could not be returned to full health unless the diseased bowel itself was removed. Surgeons then adopted ileostomy as the initial stage in a two-stage surgical approach to IBD, consisting of a primary ileostomy followed by excision of the diseased bowel. In the 1950s, the single-staged operation of proctocolectomy and ileostomy was demonstrated to be effective and safe by Counsell and Goligher (4), Crile et al. (5), and Miller et al. (6).

Construction of early ileostomies was almost always accompanied, however, by severe morbidity and high rates of mortality. For example, reports from the Mayo Clinic in 1931 and 1932 documented a 40% *four-month* mortality after diverting ileostomy alone (7,8). Part of this mortality was undoubtedly caused by failure to remove the diseased bowel. However, the ileostomy itself caused physiologic abnormalities which sometimes were devastating. The most difficult of these problems was serositis. Serositis occurred because the serosa of the ileum was exposed to the air and fecal content; the results were a high stomal output and severe volume depletion early after operation, followed by stomal stricture and obstruction later. These rather debilitating complications were eliminated effectively by the simple technique of mucosal eversion introduced by Brooke (9), in 1952 and later by Crile and Turnbull (10), who advocated mucosal grafting. The simplicity of the Brooke method, however, has facilitated its acceptance by almost all surgeons. This method gave such improved functional and clinical results that the eponym "Brooke" appended to the conventional ileostomy is justified. Indeed, no major improvements in technique of constructing an ileostomy have occurred since.

II. PROCTOCOLECTOMY WITH BROOKE ILEOSTOMY

A. Aim and Rationale

The *aim* of the operation is to extirpate all diseased and potentially diseased bowel and to establish a well-functioning stoma, the output of which can be managed effectively by an ileostomy appliance. The *rationale* for the operation is that proctocolectomy "cures" the disease, and the stoma is easy to construct and to manage, the rate of complication is low, and the long-term function results are satisfactory.

B. The Operation

After mobilizing the abdominal colon, the ileum is transected 3–4 cm proximal to the ileocecal valve, sacrificing the ileal branch of the ileocolic artery. Loss of 3–4 cm of distal ileum is physiologically unimportant, yet the ileum is much more mobile and easily pulled through the abdominal wall if the ileal branch is divided. Mobilization of the perirectal tissue is performed close to the rectum itself beginning above the sacral promontory, taking care to ensure that the sympathetic nerves are protected at the sacral promontory and the hypogastric and perirectal plexuses are protected in the pelvis. The perineal phase of the operation is performed using an *intersphincteric* approach which excises only the internal sphincter and leaves the external anal sphincter, puborectalis muscle, and levator plate intact. In this way, the parasympathetic supply of the bladder and genitalia are not disturbed and the surgical defect is small and closed securely.

The proposed site of the ileostomy in the right lower quadrant must be chosen preoperatively. It cannot be stressed too strongly that *intraoperative* sitting of the stoma invariably results in incorrect placement of the stoma which leads to long-term functional problems for the patient. After the incision is closed, the ileostomy is matured immediately and fashioned so that it protrudes 3–4 cm from the skin surface (Fig. 1). This ensures that output from the stoma will empty into the appliance without pooling.

Several points of technique should be re-emphasized: (1) the skin and fascial defects should be no larger than two fingerbreadths, thus preventing parastomal herniation; (2) the ileal mesentery should be secured to the perioneum or an extraperitoneal technique should be used, this prevents prolapse and torsion; (3) the ileum must be loose above the level of the skin, thus preventing tension, which causes retraction; (4) the ileum should be secured to the fascia with non-absorbable sutures. This helps to prevent hernia and prolapse; (5) the ileum must be everted immediately to prevent serositis, contracture, and stenosis; (6) the blood supply must be adequate to prevent necrosis and subsequent retraction

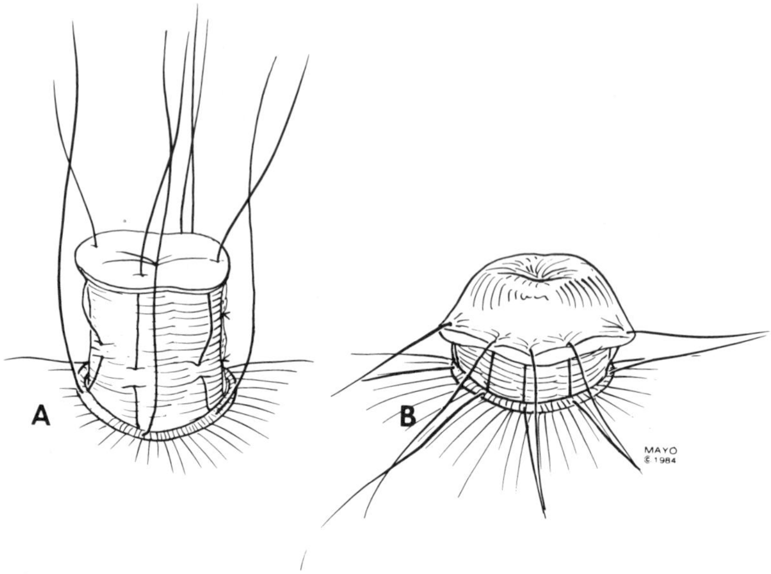

Figure 1 Brooke ileostomy. (A) Four sutures are placed, one in each quadrant, between the cut end of the ileum, the seromuscular layer of the ileum at skin level, and the subcuticular layer of the skin. (B) The ileum is everted immediately, using the four sutures as guides. Four additional simple sutures are placed between the cut ileal end and the subcuticular layer of the skin. No drains are placed. [From Pemberton JH, Beahrs OH: Brooke Ileostomy. In: Surgery of the Small Intestine. Nelson, R.L., Nyhus, L.M., eds.) Appleton-Century-Crofts, pp. 449–458 (1987)].

of the stoma; and (7) a protective appliance should be applied accurately in the operating room.

Adherence to these principles will help to avoid the major complications of hernia, retraction, erosion, prolapse, and serositis which have been historically associated with abdominal ileostomy. Using such techniques, a stomal reoperation rate of 10% or less should be achieved.

C. Complications

Overall, major and minor morbidity following proctolectomy and Brooke ileostomy has been reported to occur in between 19 and 70% of patients (11,12). Septic complications can occur in up to 30% (13,14), and about a third of patients experience breakdown of the perineal wound after primary closure of the perineum. Small bowel obstruction requiring laparotomy occurs in 5-16% of patients (11,15), which results in a late mortality of about 1% per year.

Bladder paresis and sexual dysfunction occur when the pelvic parasympathetic nerves are damaged; intersphincteric proctectomy has, however, rendered such devastating problems relatively rare (16,17). In the past, sexual dysfunction has been documented in 20-30% of men after proctectomy (18,19) and in 12% of women.

Complications related to the stoma itself have decreased in frequency since the mucosal eversion technique was widely adapted. However, problems still occur in 20-30% of patients (20). Gratifyingly, techniques of stomal management have advanced steadily over the past two decades with the introduction of intensive perioperative enterostomal therapy. Technical improvements in appliances have also rendered the quality of life of patients with ileostomies quite acceptable, although intermittent problems with skin irritation still occur.

D. Clinical, Functional, and Quality of Life Results

Rapid rehabilitation of patients with an ileostomy is the rule (21). As alluded to above, such rehabilitation has been facilitated by improvements in appliances and stomal care techniques such that most patients lead full active normal lives. Recently, the clinical and functional results of a large group of Brooke ileostomy patients were documented at our institution (22) in order to update a previous report by Roy et al. in 1970 (23). All patients who had a Brooke ileostomy constructed between 1966 and 1980 were sent a questionnaire. Of eligible patients, 81% responded: 53% of the patients were men and the median age was 35 years. The mean follow-up was 8 years. In all, 57% had the operation for ulcerative colitis while 35% had it for Crohn's disease.

Delayed healing of the perineal wound was experienced by 33% of patients while 18% required reoperation during the follow-up period. Stomal revision alone was performed in 11%.

The majority (99%) of the patients reported their diet to be satisfactory. Only 2% stated that they were unemployed, but 10% reported that their work was affected in some way by the stoma. Most patients (93%) had no problems managing the stomas, but 11% had to care for the stoma at night. Peristomal skin excoriation at some point after the operation was reported by 40% of the patients.

Patients were asked to judge the manner in which their ileostomy affected seven "activity status" categories (sexual function, sports, social activities, work at home, recreation, family relationships, and travel). More patients noted restriction and fewer noted improvements in the more physically demanding categories compared with more socially oriented activities. Fully 30% of patients indicated that their sexual activity had been restricted since their operation, whereas only 15% indicated it had improved. If the results in all categories are summed, 75% of patients indicated that, overall either the ileostomy had little effect or had affected an improvement in activity status.

Following the operation, 60% of patients indicated that their attitude toward the presence of an ileostomy had improved, 35% indicated their attitude had not been affected, and 5% indicated that it had deteriorated. We found no correlation between a change in attitude and the need for reoperation, sex of patient, or presence of prior disease.

Overall, 95% of patients were satisfied with their ileostomies. However, of patients who knew of alternatives to ileostomy, 40% desired a change. There was no correlation between a desire for change and sex of the patient or with the length of time after operation.

Furthermore, the functional and quality of life results of patients undergoing colectomy and Brooke ileostomy for Crohn's disease were compared to those who underwent the operation for chronic ulcerative colitis. The mean length of small bowel resected for chronic ulcerative colitis was 4 cm, but for Crohn's disease it was 25 cm. The perineal wound healing rate and the overall rate of reoperation did not differ between groups. Moreover, the daily stool output for patients with Crohn's and CUC did not differ. Patients with Crohn's disease, however, reported more restrictions in activity status compared to their ulcerative colitis counterparts. Finally, more CUC patients were satisfied with their Brooke ileostomies than were patients with Crohn's disease.

Although these results were quite acceptable, it was disturbing that in this latest group of Brooke ileostomy patients, the quality of life seemed to differ little from that reported previously by Roy et al. It appears, therefore, that the drawbacks and implications of Brooke ileostomy have remained almost unchanged since 1952. If so, the development of alternative procedures, at least for patients with chronic ulcerative colitis, seems justified.

E. Physiology

After surgery, ileostomy output decreases gradually and achieves a plateau at about 10 days (24). The total stool output range is 200–700 ml/day (25). There is little daily variation, but larger volumes are passed after meals. Gas and/or stool is ejected intermittently throughout the day and night. The influence of diet upon volume of ileal effluent is well known; large quantities of water result in no increase in effluent volume. A low-sodium diet, however, decreases ileostomy volume (26). Fasting also decreases the amount of ileostomy output dramatically to about 50–100 ml in 24 hours (27).

Malabsorption of fat is seen infrequently in ileostomy patients, but the amount of sodium lost in ileostomy effluent is about three times that lost in normal stool. The nature of the flora of the ileum after ileostomy has been described as partially colonic and partially small intestinal. The total number of organisms in ileostomy effluent is 80 times greater than in the normal terminal ileum while coliforms are 2500-fold more common (28). Transit time in ileostomy patients (mouth to stoma) has been studied (29), the time for 50% ($T_{1/2}$) of a labeled meal to transverse the small bowel is 317±40 min. The mean time to appearance of a marker at the stoma is 127±30 min. This time appears to be longer than in patients without an ileostomy (30), and may reflect the phenomenon of ileostomy adaptation.

Hill (31) has shown that despite adaptation, there is decreased total body water and exchangeable sodium in ileostomy patients compared with healthy persons. Ileostomy patients rarely, however, manifest symptoms of salt or water depletion. If high outputs occur for any reason, volume depletion develops rapidly.

Vitamin B_{12} malabsorption does not occur in ileostomy patients who have had a limited ileal resection (29,32). Whether or not ileostomy predisposes patients to cholelithiasis is controversial. However, patients with well-functioning ileostomies do have a slightly higher incidence of renal stones that the general population (7% vs. 3.8%) (33).

III. ILEOSTOMY ALTERNATIVES

Although patients with chronic ulcerative colitis are "cured" by proctocolectomy and Brooke ileostomy, by definition, they are incontinent of gas and stool and must wear a stool collecting appliance at all times. In the past, life with an ileostomy was thought by physicians and patients alike to sometimes be worse than the disease itself. Based on our review of performance status after ileostomy (22), and the observation that up to 45% of patients with stomas suffered depression, isolation, and difficulties with social interaction (34,35) it is apparent that ileostomies may indeed affect lifestyles adversely and therefore, remains a central issue in determining whether or even if patients are referred for surgery. Decisions to operate electively *should be* affected by these considerations if the choice of operation is limited to Brooke ileostomy.

The aim of alternative surgery is to provide continence for enteric contents and at the same time, eradicte the disease. The hypothesis is that if fecal discharge could be controlled, then the quality of life would be improved and the acceptance of the need for operation by the patient and physician would be faciliated.

A. Abdominal Colectomy and Ileal Rectal Anastomosis

1. *Aim and Rationale*

Ileal rectal anastomosis (ileorectostomy; IRA) was the first operation designed to eliminate the abdominal stoma in patients with inflammatory bowel disease to win wide acceptance. This operation was first performed in the 1940s (36). The *aim* of the procedure is to extirpate most of the diseased colonic mucosa in patients with CUC, thereby reducing the risks of hemorrhage, toxic dilation, perforation, and malignant degeneration, yet retain continence for stool and gas. In patients with Crohn's disease and minimal rectal involvement, ileorectostomy excises only the diseased colon, sparing the anorectal continence mechanisms.

The *rationale* for the operation for patients with chronic ulcerative colitis has been argued persuasively by Aylett (37), Grundfest et al. (38), and others (39-41). Ileorectal anastomosis avoids a permanent stoma, minimizes or eliminates injury to the pelvic nerves (thus sparing bladder and sexual function), is easy to perform, facilitates examination of the distal bowel, and other alternatives, should they be necessary, are not precluded. The rationale against the operation, however, is nearly as convincing (42,43), interval proctectomy is required in 6% to 37% of patients; poor results (>8 bowel movements per day, continuing need for steroids, incontinence, and poor general health) occur in 50% of patients (44), and finally the risk of developing carcinoma in the retained rectum approaches 17% after 27 years (45). There is little question, however, that the role of ileorectostomy in the management of Crohn's colitis with rectal sparing is secure (46,47), despite the observation that up to 70% will require proctectomy for recurrent disease (48).

2. *The Operation*

Before operation, the surgeon performs a proctoscopic examination to determine the distensibility of the rectum. If the rectum dilates easily, performing an ileorectal anastomosis is reasonable. If it does not, an anastomosis should not be performed because the rectum will act only as a nondistensible conduit for stool and incontinence would invariably result.

The abdominal colectomy is performed in standard fashion. The ileum is divided close to the cecum. If necessary, the rectum is partially mobilized gently, taking great care to spare the presacral nerve. Usually, the anastomosis can be constructed end to end, but need not be (Fig. 2). A diverting ileostomy is rarely performed at our institution, because if the surgeon judges that one is required, then the anastomosis probably should not be performed at all.

3. *Complications*

Operative mortality for elective ileal rectal anastomosis has been reported to vary between 2% and 8% (49). Nearly all deaths have been caused by anastomosis leakage (50,51), which occurred in between 3% and 15% of patients (46,52). Small bowel obstruction complicates the recovery of 14-20% of patients (53). Although, sexual function in men is usually preserved postoperatively, up to 50% of women have reported dyspareunia (19).

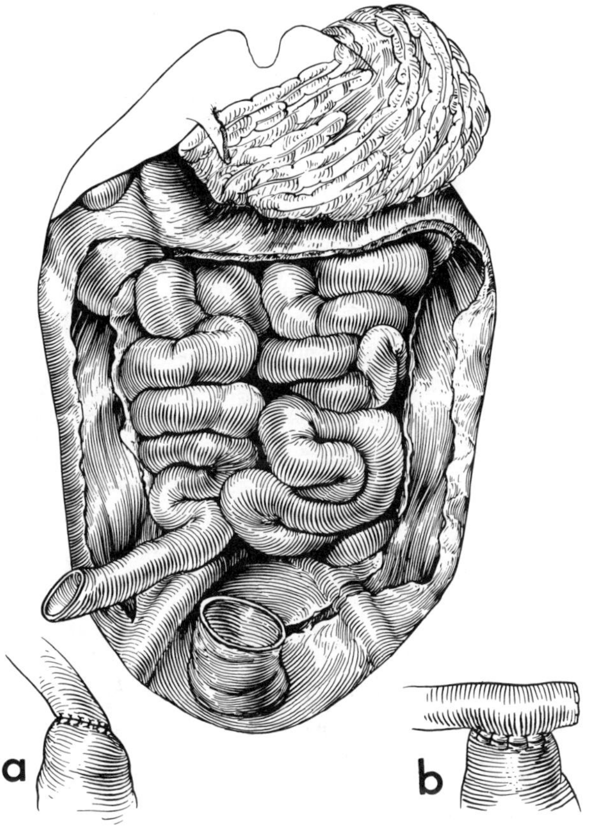

Figure 2 Ileorectostomy. The abdominal colectomy has been completed and the specimen removed. Intestinal continuity is restored with either an end to end (a) side to end (b) ileorectostomy. (From Ref. 47.)

4. Clinical, Functional, and Quality of Life Results After Ileorectal Anastomosis

Six months after ileorectal anastomosis, the mean stool frequency during 24 hours is about 4.5 (51). More than 80% of patients have fewer than six stools in 24 hours. Incontinence occurs in about 20% of patients (54), and about 50% of patients require bulking and constipating agents. Improvement of function occurs steadily over the first 12–18 months and plateaus thereafter.

Perhaps the best parameter with which to measure the successful clinical outcome of patients with ileorectal anastomosis is the interval proctectomy rate.

Late proctectomy is required for a variety of reasons including persistence or recurrence of disease (which is manifested by high stool frequency, incontinence, and bleeding), and the occurrence of rectal cancer. The late proctectomy rate for persistence or recurrence of disease varies between 5 (37) and 58% (55). At our institution, 24% of patients have required late proctectomy because of poor functional results (46). Importantly, the chance that a patient will have a good result after an ileorectal anastomosis, that is, have no requirement for steroids or other anti-inflammatory medication, be in good general health, have an acceptable stool frequency and a low incidence of incontinence, approaches 45% at our institution (46). This parallels the experience of others (19,55).

The risk of cancer developing in the retained rectum is an ever present, occurring in about 5% of patients at 15 years after operation and increasing to 15% at 30 years (49,55–57). Unfortunately, these cancers are usually of advanced grade and stage compared with type ordinaré colorectal cancer (49).

The quality of life after ileorectal anastomosis has been reported to be good (58); the satisfaction is high and an active, productive lifestyle can be preserved. Overall, satisfaction is tempered, however, by the fact that patients often feel they have not been cured because they must undergo frequent follow-up examinations.

5. *Physiology of Ileorectal Anastomosis*

The primary attraction of this operation is that most of the major anatomic mechanisms responsible for maintaining continence are retained; the rectal reservoir, the pelvic floor, the puborectalis muscle, and the internal and external anal sphincter together with their respective innervation and blood supply are preserved. However, the absorptive capacity of the proximal colon has been removed, and ileal content is continuously presented to the rectal remnant. Because this remnant is involved by inflammation in most patients, motor and absorptive functions are likely altered. It would be important to estimate how these alterations might affect the clinical and functional outcome of patients after ileorectal anastomosis.

6. *Maintaining Enteric Continence*

The three major factors which act together to maintain enteric continence are: (1) a reservoir which is capacious, which accommodates readily to increasing volume without concomitant increases in intraluminal pressure, and which evacuates completely; (2) an intact pelvic outlet which presents a mechanical impediment to aboral flow of content; and (3) content which is firm, easily recognized, and readily evacuated (59).

In order for the rectum to accommodate passively, it must be compliant and large; "compliance" is dependent on rectal wall elasticity. In active inflammatory disease of the rectum, compliant accommodation to content is impaired (60), and the elasticity coefficient is greater in patients with active inflammation than in those with quiescent disease. Moreover, the smaller the rectum, the greater the elasticicity coefficient; patients with active chronic ulcerative colitis have smaller rectums then controls (61). In patients *without* active colitis, rectal size, compliance, and elasticity did not differ from controls (58). Therefore, the lesser the mucosal inflammation and elasticity coefficient, the better the "compliance" and the fewer the stools per day.

Other investigators have observed that sphincteric function in patients with ileorectal anastomosis differs little from that in healthy people (62). Indeed, Mignon and Bonfils reported that patients with less than three stools per day after ileorectal anastomosis had "stronger" anal sphincters than patients with eight or more stools per day (58).

In summary, if the active inflammatory process in the rectum is minimal, the retained rectal reservoir will be compliant and will store content satisfactorily. If not, the rectum will not distend and will instead function merely as a rigid conduit for stool between the ileum and the anal sphincters.

7. *Absorption in the Rectal Remnant*

The abdominal colon is the primary site of water and salt conservation in humans; approximately 800-900 ml of the 1000 ml of ileal fluid presented to the colon each day is absorbed. In addition, the colon absorbs up to five liters of fluid upon demand (63). Little is know about the absorptive capacity of the rectum for water alone; the rectum, however, does have an absorptive capacity for sodium which is about a third of that of the entire colon and this may also be true of water absorption. To determine whether the rectum absorbed fluid and electrolytes after ileorectal anastomosis, Newton compared Brooke ileostomy and ileorectal anastomosis patients (64). He found that ileorectal anastomosis patients had a lower total stool output, lower stool sodium concentration, and higher potassium output than Brooke ileostomy patients. Therefore, it appeared that the rectal remnant *did* absorb sodium and water and excrete potassium, just as the colon. Importantly, however, the degree of mucosal inflammation in Newton's patients was not reported; such inflammation influences electrolyte and water movements in ulcerative colitis patients as shown by Edmonds and Pilcher (65). They also reported that in patients with *active* CUC, there was a loss of rectal mucosal absorption of sodium; indeed, a net absorption of salt occurred which reversed when the inflammation receded (65).

Therefore, in quiescent rectal disease, patients after IRA should be able to absorb water and sodium in the rectal remnant and the remnant will be capacious and distensible; a low stool frequency and little incontinence can be expected to occur. On the other hand, if the mucosa of the rectum is inflamed, little alteration of effluent volume will occur and patients will of necessity excrete between 500 and 1000 ml of stool per day. Moreover, the more inflamed the mucosa, the less capacious and distensible the rectal remnant; high stool frequency, urgency, and incontinence will follow.

B. Continent Ileostomy of Kock

In 1969, Nils Kock of Sweden published a report describing an intra-abdominal reservoir which provided continence of enteric content (66). He modified the procedure in 1973 by incorporating a "nipple-valve" in the outflow tract of the pouch; this one-way valve could be intubated to allow the reservoir to empty, but would not allow content to escape. Since that time, experience with more than 1600 continent ileostomy patients worldwide has been reported (67). Recently, use of the pouch as a reservoir for urine after cystectomy (which was, incidentally, one of the original uses devised for this procedure) has been advocated.

1. Aim and Rationale

The *aim* of the procedure is to extirpate the diseased colon and rectum entirely and to provide continence for feces and gas while maintaining a cosmetically acceptable stoma. The *rationale* for the procedure is that colectomy and proctectomy "cure" the disease, the ileal pouch functions as a storage reservoir for gas and stool, the nipple valve provides leak-proof continence, and the flush stoma is unobtrusive. By eliminating the necessity of wearing an external appliance, the quality of life of ileostomy patients would be improved.

2. The Operation

After completion of the colectomy and proctectomy, the distal-most 45 cm of ileum is used to construct the pouch, nipple valve, and outflow tract. Two 15 cm limbs of the bowel are sutured together and then opened (Fig. 3). The pouch is folded over, and one of the two anterior edges is closed. The nipple valve is fashioned by intussuscepting 10 cm of the distal ileum into the pouch after denuding its mesentery (Fig. 4). The 5-cm nipple valve is secured with staples. The remainder of the pouch is closed and checked (Fig. 5). The stoma is sited at the hairline in the right lower quadrant. The outflow tract is short, and the stoma is flush with the skin. A catheter is positioned in the pouch through the valve and drains the pouch continuously for 4 weeks postoperatively. At the end of 4 weeks, the patient removes that catheter and begins pouch intubation over gradually increasing intervals of time.

3. Complications

At Mayo, only one of 460 patients died after continent ileostomy (68). Summarizing the reported complications after continent ileostomy, Fazio and Church have reported that *early* complications included bowel obstruction (2-17%), hemorrhage (0.5-5%), sepsis (2-11%), and fistula (1-7%) (67). The primary late complications were valve extrusion, fistula, and nonspecific reservoir inflammation (pouchitis). In our series, valve extrusion usually occurred during the first year after operation (Fig. 6). Surgery to revise the valve was required in 43% of the patients early in our experience and in 22% later.

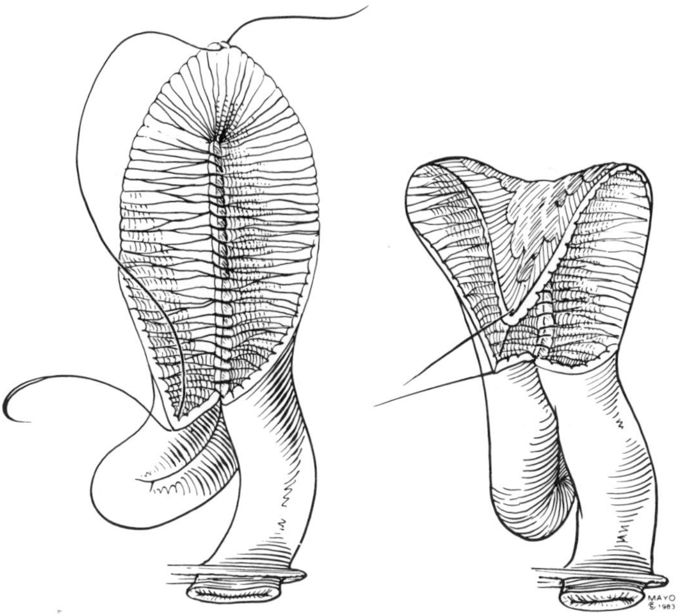

Figure 3 The continent ileostomy is constructed from the distal 45 cm of ileum. The reservoir is made from two 15-cm limbs of a single U-shaped loop which are incised on the antimesenteric border sutured together, and folded over to form the anterior and posterior walls. (From Ref. 68, pp. 180–191.)

"Pouchitis" occurs in between 7 and 30% of continent ileostomy patients (67). The etiology of pouchitis is not known, but treatment with metronidazole is usually effective. Interestingly, no continent ileostomy patients with familial polyposis in the Cleveland Clinic series experienced pouchitis (67).

Excision of the pouch was required in fewer than 5% of patients over the long term (68). The reasons for pouch excision were repeated valve malfunction, recurrent fistula, pouchitis unresponsive to medical management and unsuspected Crohn's disease.

4. Clinical, Functional, and Quality of Life Results

In the Mayo series (mean follow-up 3.5 years), only 3% of continent ileostomy patients wore an ileostomy bag (68). Of these patients, 75% were always continent of stool and gas while 23% had occasional leakage. In the Cleveland series, 91% of the patients were completely continent, and 5% occasionally leaked stool and gas (67). Kock's group reported that their success rate was 96% (69). Most patients more than 6 months after continent ileostomy intubated the pouch 3–6 times in 24 hours. McLeod and Fazio reported that 93% of continent ileostomy patients felt that their expectations had been fully met and that all of them

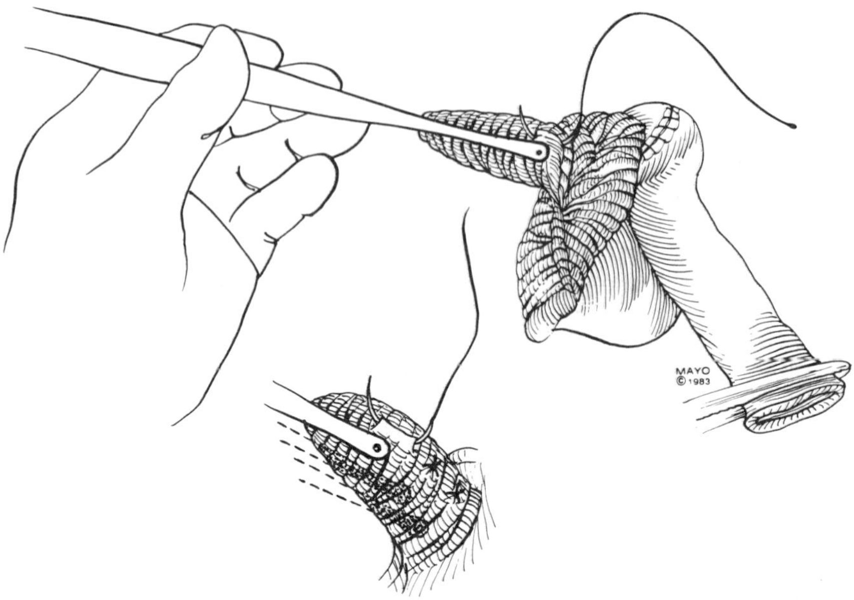

Figure 4 The 10-cm ileal segment immediately distal to the segment used to create the reservoir has been drawn back into the reservoir. The intussusceptum is held in its correct position with through-and-through sutures of 2-0 silk and staples. (From Ref. 68, pp. 180–191.)

would undergo the operation again (70). In contrast to these results, Valkamo has reported that only 37% continent ileostomy patients were satisfied after the initial operation, but this improved after revisional surgery (71).

In summary, although the complication rate and the rate of revisional surgery seems quite high after continent ileostomy, most patients appear to be satisfied and eventually achieve leak-proof stomal continence. Patients who fail do so during the first year after the operation. The rate of late failure (5–10 years) is unknown.

5. Physiology

The physiological consequences of constructing a continent ileostomy have been well studied. Many of the changes that occur in continent ileostomy patients also occur in ileoanal patients because in both operations, a pouch is constructed from the distal ileum.

At the time of construction, the volume of the ileal pouch is approximately 150 ml. This initial volume increases over 6 months to between 400 and 600 ml. Moreover, the pouch accommodates to increases in intraluminal volume passively.

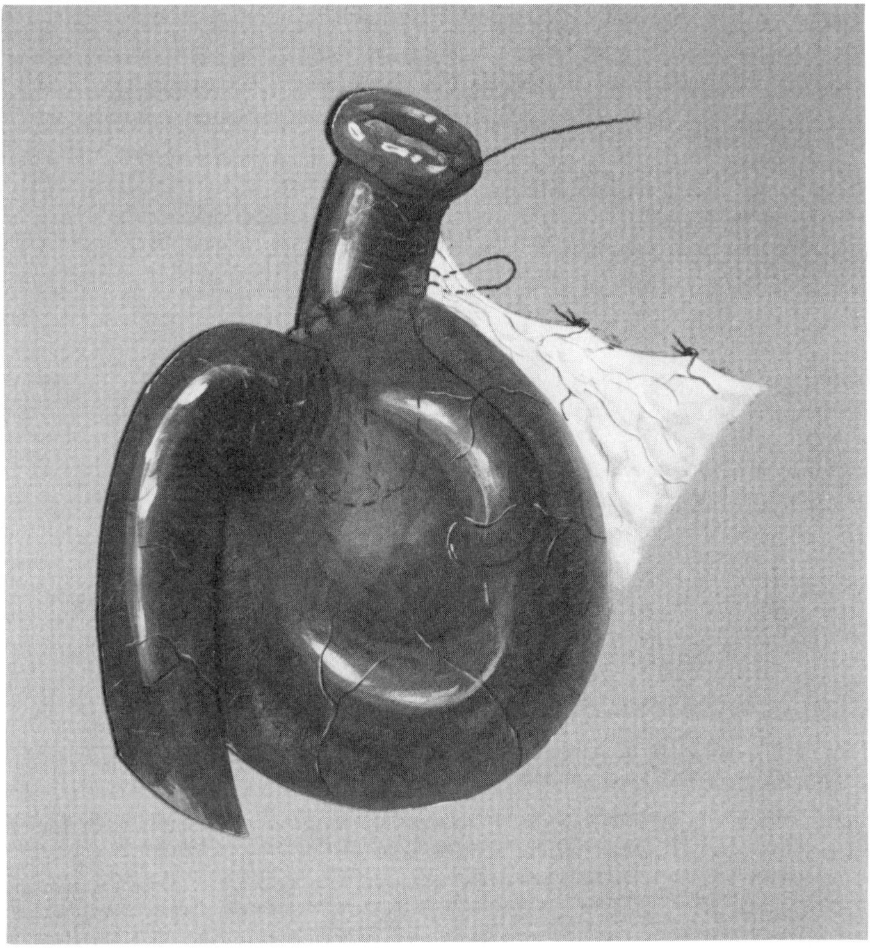

Figure 5 Appearance of continent Kock ileal stoma. Dotted lines represent position of nipple valve inside pouch. (From Ref. 118.)

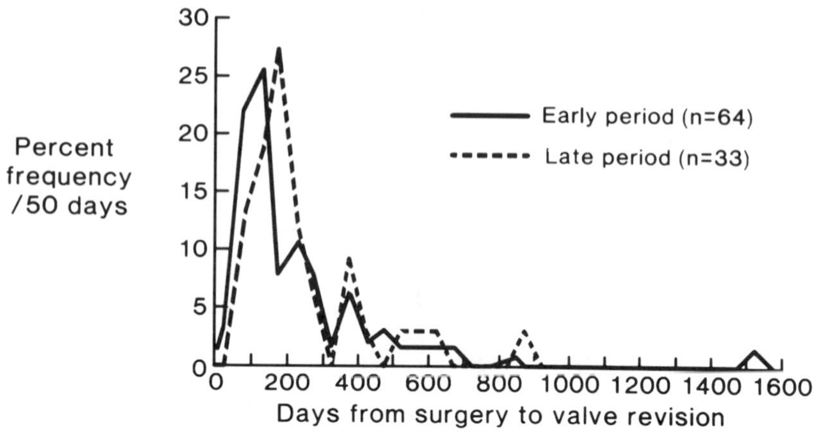

Figure 6 Interval between construction of continent ileostomy and first valve revision. Nearly all revisions were required within the first postoperative year. (From Ref. 68, pp. 180–191.)

Histologically, the villi of the pouch become blunted and take on a "coloniform" appearance (72), that is, in some areas of the pouch, the ileal mucosa resembles colonic mucosa. The long-term effects of this change are unknown; however, no patients have thus far developed an adenocarcinoma of the pouch.

Patterns of small bowel motility within the pouch also have been studied (73). Small intraluminal pressure waves (amplitude, <10 cm H_2O; frequency, 5–7 min) constituted the basal motor activity which was similar to the normal terminal ileal motor pattern. However, upon distension of the pouch to >60% of its maximum capacity, high-pressure waves (HPWs; amplitude >25 cm H_2O; frequency 1 every 3 min) were superimposed on this basal motor pattern (Fig. 7). These waves were associated with fullness and discomfort.

The bacteria present in a well-functioning continent ileostomy resembles colonic flora (74). The effect of such a colonic type of flora constantly bathing the ileal mucosa is unknown. The large numbers of anaerobic bacteria in the pouch have been implicated as the etiology of acute pouch inflammation (pouchitis) in continent ileostomy patients, but data from our institution do not support this (74). Finally, several studies have documented that ileal absorption of salt, vitamin B_{12}, and secretion of bicarbonate remains unchanged (75,76). This occurs despite the development of "abnormal" histology in the pouch. Moreover, the total fecal output is not different from that of a well-functioning Brooke ileostomy (77).

In summary, while the ileal pouch does act as a passive storage reservoir for enteric content, it is capable of generating high pressure waves. Such waves may cause leakage of content or promote valve slippage. Although the mucosa is

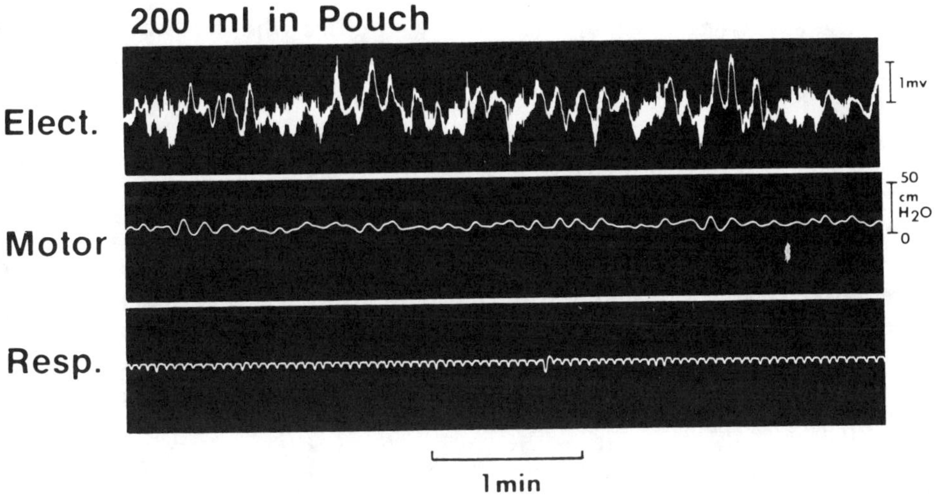

(a)

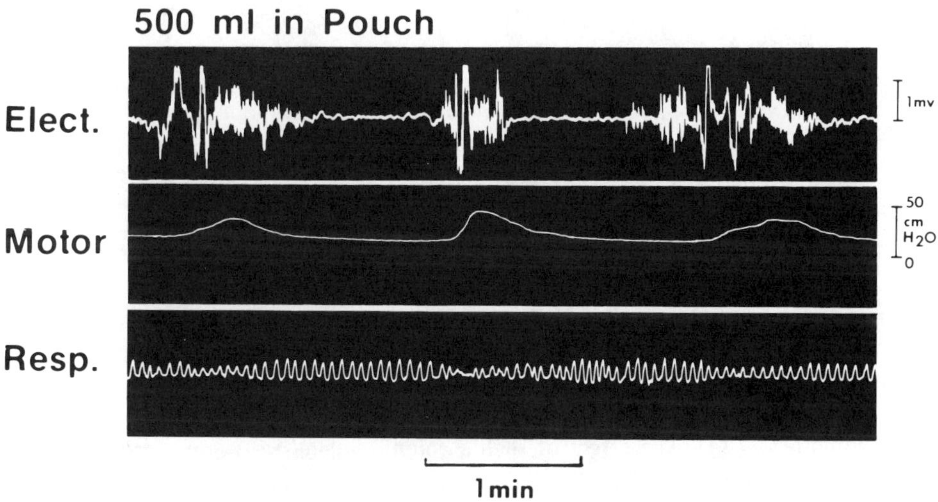

(b)

Figure 7 Effect of intrapouch distention on electrical ("Elect.") and motor activity of Kock pouch during fasting. (a) At 25% of maximal distention, action potentials occur randomly without associated high-pressure with high-pressure waves. (b) At 63% of maximum distension, action potentials are associated with high-pressure waves lasting up to 1 min. Resp. = respiratory pattern. (From Ref. 73.)

histologically changed, absorption of salt and vitamin B_{12} and secretion of bicarbonate is normal. Patients do not develop a "closed loop" syndrome despite stasis and bacterial proliferation, probably because the pouch is emptied regularly.

C. Ileal Pouch-Anal Anastomosis

The development of the ileal pouch-anal anastomosis operation has been described in detail by several authors (78-81). The resurgence in popularity of the operation can be credited to the report by Martin and colleagues in 1977 (82). The other significant development in the evolution of the procedure was the suggestion of Parks et al. (83), and Utsonomiya et al. (84) that constructing a pelvic pouch would improve results. Currently, at our institution, all patients undergoing ileoanal anastomosis in reality undergo ileal pouch-anal anastomosis, usually using a "J" pouch design (84).

1. *Aim and Rationale*

The *aim* of the operation is to extirpate all diseased and potentially diseased mucosa of the colon and rectum while concomitantly restoring fecal continence and allowing defecation to occur via the normal anatomic pathology. The *rationale* for the operation is that abdominal colectomy, proximal proctectomy, and distal mucosal rectal resection remove all potentially premalignant mucosa, but preserve the anal sphincter apparatus. The addition of an ileal pouch restores reservoir capacity. Moreover, because the distal rectal mucosal resection is performed endorectally, normal bladder and sexual function should be preserved. Finally, a perineal wound is avoided.

2. *The Operation*

The operation is performed in two stages. The abdominal colectomy, proximal proctectomy, distal rectal mucosal resection, and diverting ileostomy are performed as the first stage. At a second stage, 2 to 3 months later, the diverting ileostomy is closed.

The abdominal colectomy is performed and the ileum transected close to the cecum. The attachments of the ileal mesentery are divided to the level of the pancreas providing mesenteric mobility. When mobilizing the rectum, the nerves at the sacral promontory are swept away from the superior hemorrhoidal vessels. The dissection is carried down close to the rectal wall to the level of the coccyx posteriorly, to the midvagina or midprostate anteriorly, and to the levators laterally. The pouch is constructed from the distal 24-34 cm of ileum using either the GIA stapling device (85) or a handsewn technique (86).

At the dentate line, a submucosal plane is developed circumferentially for a distance of 3-5 cm. The specimen is removed and the apex of the pouch is delivered through the rectal muscular cuff to the dentate line. The pouch is anchored to the puborectalis muscle. The apex of the pouch is incised and the ileal pouch-anal anastomosis is constructed. Figure 8 depicts the construction and eventual anatomical location of the ileal pouch-anal anastomosis.

A loop ileostomy is placed in the right lower quadrant at a premarked site. The stoma is matured immediately.

Closure of the ileostomy takes place about 8 weeks following the operation. Patients undergo preclosure manometric and radiographic studies. A resting anal canal pressure of more than 40-50 mmHg and a voluntary squeeze pressure that is double the resting pressure is desirable. The capacity of the pouch is then measured with a balloon; a volume in excess of 120-140 ml is ideal. Finally, an ilial pouch radiograph is obtained to ensure that no sinuses, fistulas, or leaks are present.

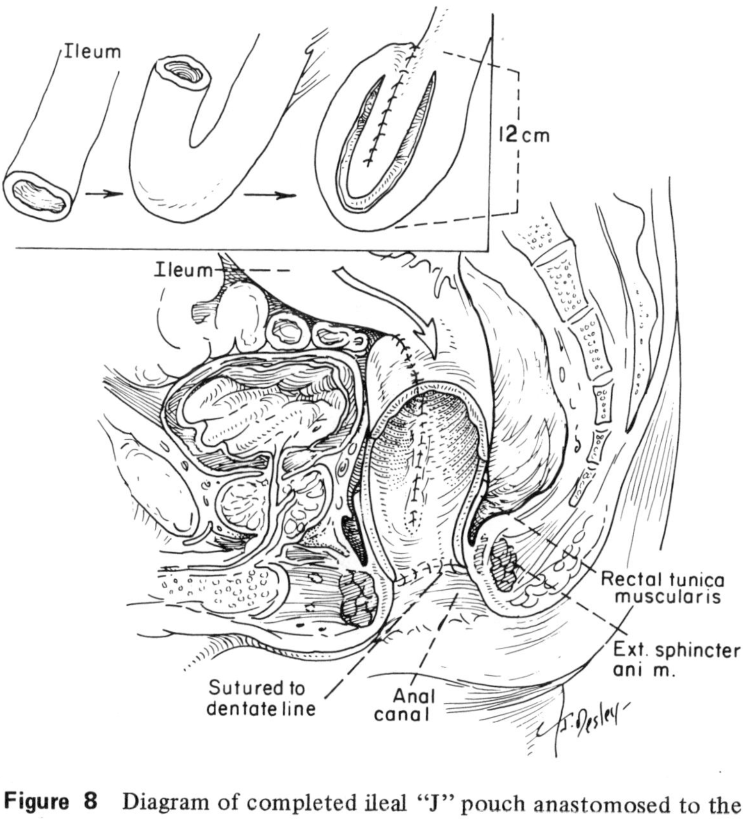

Figure 8 Diagram of completed ileal "J" pouch anastomosed to the internal sphincter and the anoderm. (From Ref. 119.)

In summary, the *technical* goals of the operation are to preserve the innervation of the bladder and genitalia, the anal sphincter and puborectalis muscles, and to construct a leak-proof pouch and tension-free anastomosis. If these goals are achieved, complications are minimized, and functional results will be predictably good.

3. Clinical Results

Recently, we reported the long-term results of the ileal pouch-anal anastomosis in 390 adults with chronic ulcerative colitis who had a "J" pouch constructed and who were followed a mean of 2.3 years (range 6 months to 5 years) (87).

4. Early Results

One of the 390 patients (0.2%) died of a pulmonary embolism two weeks after dismissal from the initial operation. Overall, 29% of patients had a postoperative complication (Table 1). After the first operation, the most frequent complication was small bowel obstruction, which occurred in 13%. Slightly less than half of these patients required reoperation, primarily to lyse adhesions, whereas the remainder resolved spontaneously. Pelvic sepsis, which occurred in 5% of the patients, was manifest clinically as fever, leukocytosis, and localized abdominal tenderness. One third of the patients with pelvic sepsis were treated successfully

Table 1 Postoperative Morbidity after Ileal Pouch-Anal Anastomosis and After Closure of the Ileostomy in 390 Patients

Complication	% of patients with complication
After ileal pouch-anal anastomosis	
Small bowel obstruction	13
Transient	8
Required reoperation	5
Pelvic sepsis	5
Antibiotics alone	3
Required reoperation	2
Wound infection	3
Urinary retention	7
Transient	5
Required catheterization	2
After closure of ileostomy	
Small bowel obstruction	9
Transient	4
Required reoperation	5
Anastomotic leakage	2

by antibiotic therapy alone, whereas the other two thirds required operative drainage. Abdominal wound infections occurred in 3%. Urinary retention occurred transiently in 7% but required intermittent catheterization in less than 2%

After closure of the ileostomy, 9% of patients had a small bowel obstruction for which operative correction was required in one half. Anastomotic leakage at the site of ileostomy closure occurred in 2%.

5. *Late Results*

The principal late complications were anastomotic stricture and "pouchitis." Many patients had weblike strictures at the anastomosis at the time of ileostomy closure; these were easily dilated and did not recur. Five percent of the patients, however, had persistent strictures that required dilation over time.

Pouchitis occurred at variable times throughout the postoperative period in 14% of patients. The mean (±SD) interval from operation to occurrence of pouchitis was 16 ± 14 months. Multiple episodes occurred in 4% of patients. Administration of metronidazle (250 mg q.i.d.) nearly always resulted in prompt subsidence of symptoms. Several patients, however, have required low-dose metronidazole therapy *continuously* to prevent recurrence of the syndrome.

Sexual dysfunction occurred in 11% of the men and 12% of the women overall. Of the men, 1.5% were impotent and 4% complained of retrograde ejaculation. Dyspareunia was the principle complaint in women and occurred in 7%.

Nearly all patients had a favorable outcome over the long term (Fig. 9); only 6% had a permanent ileostomy established and, therefore, failed the operation. The causes of failure, alone or in combination, were recurrent pouchitis, multiple stools, gross nighttime fecal incontinence, and granulomatous ileitis. Of the patients who failed, 75% did so within one year. No patient failed more than three years after the operation.

Table 2 and Figure 10 detail the stool frequency, pattern of continence, ability to discriminate gas from stool, and use of medication from 6 months to 5 years after ileal pouch-anal anastomosis. The daytime and nighttime stool frequency as well as the patern of daytime continence did not change over time. In contrast, the incidence of nocturnal incontinence and dependency on medication declined. Interestingly, whereas the mean ± SD stool frequency was 9 ± 5 stools/day *before* operation, it had decreased to 6 ± 2 stools/day after operation ($p<0.0001$).

6. *Predictors of Outcome*

We found that older patients had more stools during the day than did the younger patients (≤50 years; 6 ± 3 stools/day; >50 years; 8 ± 4 stool/day; $p=0.05$). Women and men had the same stool frequencies. Women, however, had more episodes of occasional incontinence than did men both during the day and at night. (Day: women 33% vs. men, 14% $p<0.001$; night: women 56% vs. men 44% $p<0.02$).

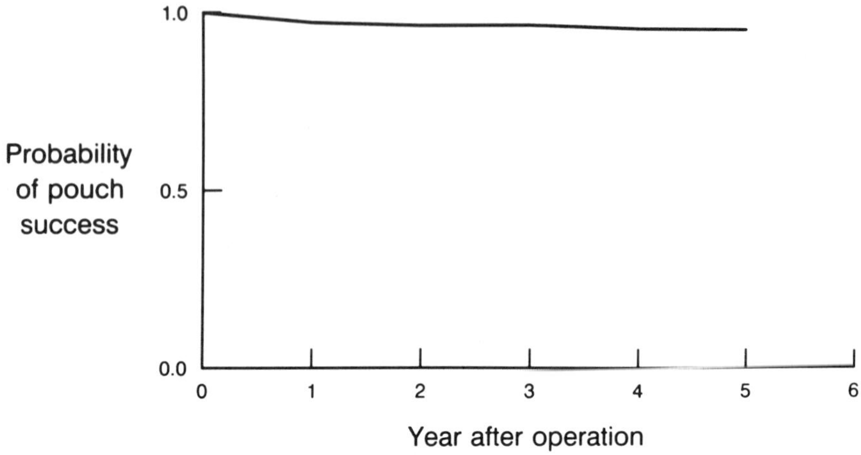

Figure 9 The probability of successful outcome with functioning pouch against year after operation. No patient failed after 3 years. (From Ref. 87.)

Patients who developed pelvic sepsis were no more likely to fail the operation than those who did not and they did not have more sexual or urinary problems. We did find that the incidence of incontinence during follow-up was significantly affected by the *preoperative* stool frequency; the more stools before the operation, the more likely patients were to be incontinent after the operation ($p<0.03$).

Table 2 Functional Results of Ileal Pouch-Anal Anstomosis from 6 Months to 6 Years Postoperatively in 389 Patients

	Follow-up					
Parameter	6 mo	1 yr	2 yr	3 yr	4 yr	5 yr
No. of stools (mean±SD)						
Day	5±2	5±3	6±3	6±2	6±3	6±2
Night	1±1	1±1	2±2	2±1	1±1	2±1
Able to discriminate gas from stool (% of pts)	69	77	73	84	77	86
Lomotil (% of pts)	26	19	17	25	6	4
Metamucil (% of pts)	43	36	40	38	30	27

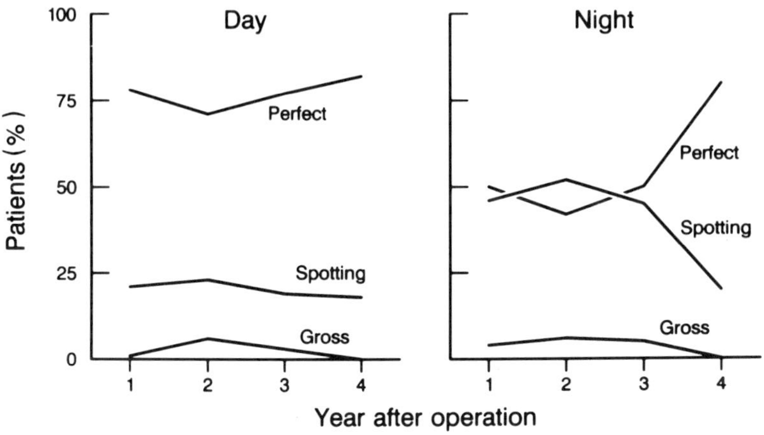

Figure 10 Daytime and nighttime continence after ileal pouch-anal operation against the years after operation. Perfect = no fecal leakage. Spotting - fecal spotting of underclothes, 3 cm or less in diameter, two times or less per week. Gross = gross fecal incontinence more than two times per week. Data points are connected for illustrative purposes. (From Ref. 82.)

7. *Quality of Life*

In order to determine whether there was any difference in the quality of life between patients with a ileal pouch-anal anstomosis (IPAA) and those with a Brooke ileostomy (BI), we surveyed 50 ileal pouch-anal anastomosis patients (mean follow-up 24 months) and compared results to the 675 Brooke ileostomy patients (mean follow-up 96 months) surveyed earlier (88). The mean ages of the patients were similar (IPAA = 31 years; BI = 35 years) as were the rates of reoperation. The great majority of both groups were satisfied with their operation (IPAA 95%; BI 93%). However, when asked to evaluate their ability to take part in certain activities, (sports, sexual activity, recreation, social relationships, work at home, and travel) more IPAA patients improved and fewer were restricted compared with patients with Brooke ileostomies. We concluded from this preliminary study that IPAA patients may experience an improved quality of life compared with patients with Brooke ileostomy.

8. *Physiologic Consequences of Ileal Pouch-Anal Anastomosis*

The ileal pouch-anal anastomosis operation is successful in most patients because the operation preserves and restores the mechanisms responsible for maintaining enteric continence and facilitating defecation.

Anal Canal High-Pressure Zone The anal canal high-pressure zone in healthy people is about 4 cm in length, being slightly longer in men than in women (4.6 cm vs. 3.7 cm) (89).

Resting Pressure The external anal sphincter (EAS) and internal anal sphincter (IAS) are responsible for maintaining resting pressure. The (IAS) contributes about 80% of total resting tone (90). the mean resting anal canal pressure in healthy adults is approximately 65 ± 5 mmHg (91,92).

After ileal pouch-anal anastomosis, the length of the anal canal did not differ from controls (92). However, resting pressures were lower than in corresponding healthy controls (patients, 56 ± 3 mmHg vs. controls, 65 ± 3 mmHg; $p<0.05$) (92). this decrease may be due to stretching of the anal canal intraoperatively.

Squeeze Pressures Voluntary contractions of the EAS and the puborectalis muscle generate squeeze pressures within the anal canal. With maximum effort, such pressures are twofold greater than resting pressures but last only 40-60 sec, because the EAS tires rapidly (93); the squeeze mechanism may, therefore, act simply as an emergency mechanism which prevents leakage of content at inopportune times.

After ileal pouch-anal anastomosis, squeeze pressures were maintained (patients, 126 ± 6 mmHg vs. controls, 131 ± 9 mmHg; $p>0.05$) (92). However, patients who had impaired continence postoperatively had lower maximum squeeze pressures than patients who did not (1004 ± 7 mmHg vs. 143 ± 7 mmHg; $p<0.05$) (92).

The technique of ileal pouch-anal anastomosis, therefore, preserves the integrity of anal canal high-pressure zone, although in slightly altered form; resting pressures were lower in patients after ileal pouch-anal anastomosis, but squeeze pressures were not. Patients who had problems with continence after the operation, however, had lower resting *and* squeeze pressure than those who did not.

The Anorectal Angle The anorectal angle is formed at the junction of the rectum and anal canal and is enveloped by the puborectal muscle. In health, at rest, this angle varies between 60° and 105° (94,95). The puborectal muscle pulls the anorectal junction anteriorly, thus accentuating the anorectal angle. Parks (96), ascribed a "flap valve" function to the anorectal angle, but Bartolo et al. (97), assert instead that the puborectal muscle acts as a *sphincter* at the anorectal junction. Whatever the mechanism, during times of rapidly increasing intra-abdominal pressure (cough, Valsalva, laughing) fecal content is kept from entering the anal canal by the action of the puborectal muscle.

The anorectal angle must open, however, in order to defecate. This is accomplished by squatting and flexing the hips to 90° (the angle opens to >100°) and by straining (the puborectal muscle often becomes electrically silent and relaxes).

Using a new low-dose radiation technique for imaging the anorectal angulation (98), we found that in 13 healthy controls, the mean (± SD) anorectal angle was 102 ± 18°. The angle did not change with standing but did increase to a mean (± SD) of 119 ± 17° upon sitting. Maneuvers which favored continence (squeezing) or stressed continence (Valsalva maneuver), made the angle more acute. In six patients after ileal pouch-anal anastomosis, an anopouch angle *was* present in each, and movements of the angle resembled movements of the anorectal angle in health (Fig. 11).

Ileal pouch-anal anastomosis, then, preserves the anatomic relationships of the pelvic floor such that an anorectal angle is reconstructed, which in general, functions as in health. Subtle differences from the situation in health do remain.

Anorectal Sensation and Reflex Mechanisms The anorectal sensory mechanisms facilitate discrimination of the character of the enteric content as well as its presence within the rectal lumen.

Rectum Balloon distension of the rectum produces a sensation of pelvic fullness and the desire to defecate. The site of the receptors for this sensation may lie in the rectal muscularis and/or in the pelvic floor musculature (99).

Anal Canal The cephalad half of the anal canal is lined by mucosa, the distal 1.5 to 2 cm of which contains sensory nerve endings (100). Roe et al. (101), have found this area to be sensitive to electrical stimulation. In health, this zone of mucosal sensitivity may supplement receptors present in the rectal and/or pelvic floor musculature at the anorectal junction and be responsible for "fine tuning" of the continence mechanism.

After ileal pouch-anal anastomosis, patients continue to detect the need for evacuation and can discriminate between gas and stool (87,102). These observations support previous suspicions that the rectal mucosa is not needed for rectal sensation. There is little question, however, that sensory mechanisms are not completely intact as some patients do leak small amounts of mucus and stool and sometimes mistake gas for stool.

An interesting argument has recently appeared in the literature concerning the necessity for sparing the mucosa of the transitional zone just proximal to the dentate line. Johnston et al. (103) found improved sensation and better rates of perfect continence in patients in whom the transitional zone was spared. Keighley et al. (104) agreed that sensation was diminished after excision of the transition zone, but found no demonstrable improvement in continence in patients in whom the zone was retained. We have no experience with leaving transitional zone mucosa intact but have found clinically that sensation does persist after ileal pouch-anal anastomosis and complete rectal mucosal resection, but in a somewhat blunted form.

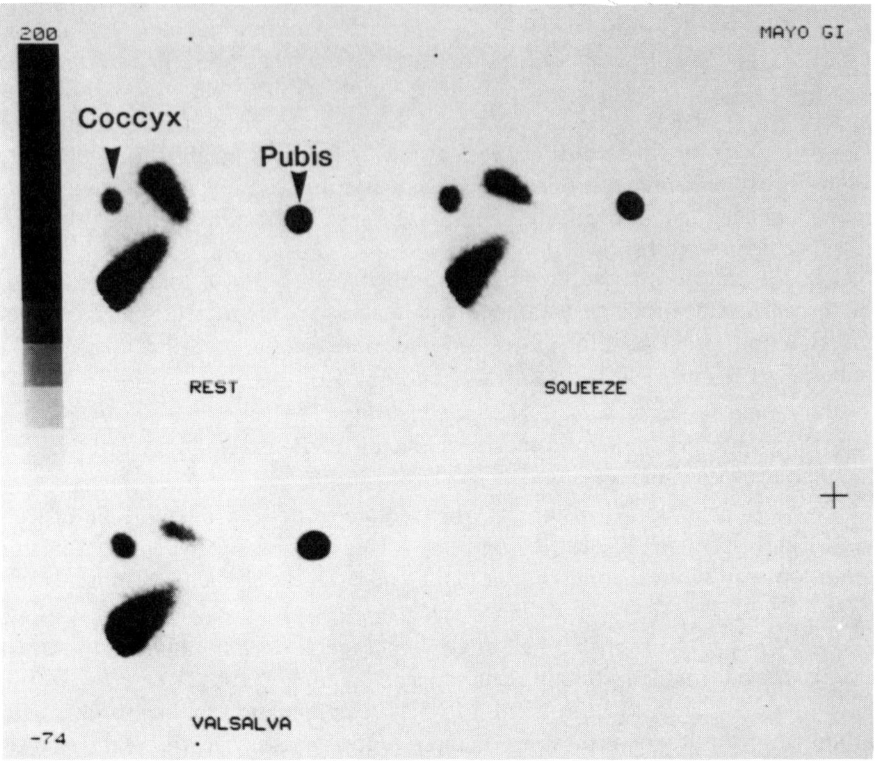

(a)

Figure 11 (a) Scintigraphic image of balloon device in place in a healthy volunteer. During maneuvers which facilitate continence (sphincter squeeze) or stress continence (Valsalva), the anorectal angle sharpens from its resting position. (b) Scintigraphic image of balloon device in place in a patient after ileal pouch-anal anastomosis. An angle is present between the pouch and the anal canal. As in health, this angle sharpens from its resting position during sphincter squeeze and the Valsalva maneuver. (From Ref. 95.)

Rectal Anal Sphincter Inhibitory Response Upon distending a balloon in the rectal amupulla acutely, the proximal portion of the anal canal (IAS) relaxes while the distal portion (EAS) contracts (105,106). This rectal-anal sphincter inhibitory response (RASIR) is present in all healthy adults, but is absent in patients with Hirschsprung's disease. The hypothesized role of the RASIR is that the relaxed IAS would allow rectal contents to come in contact with the sensitive transitional zone mucosa transiently while the contracted EAS would prevent leakage (106).

After ileal pouch-anal anastomosis, we have found that the response is abolished (91,107); discrimination and recognition of the urge to evacuate,

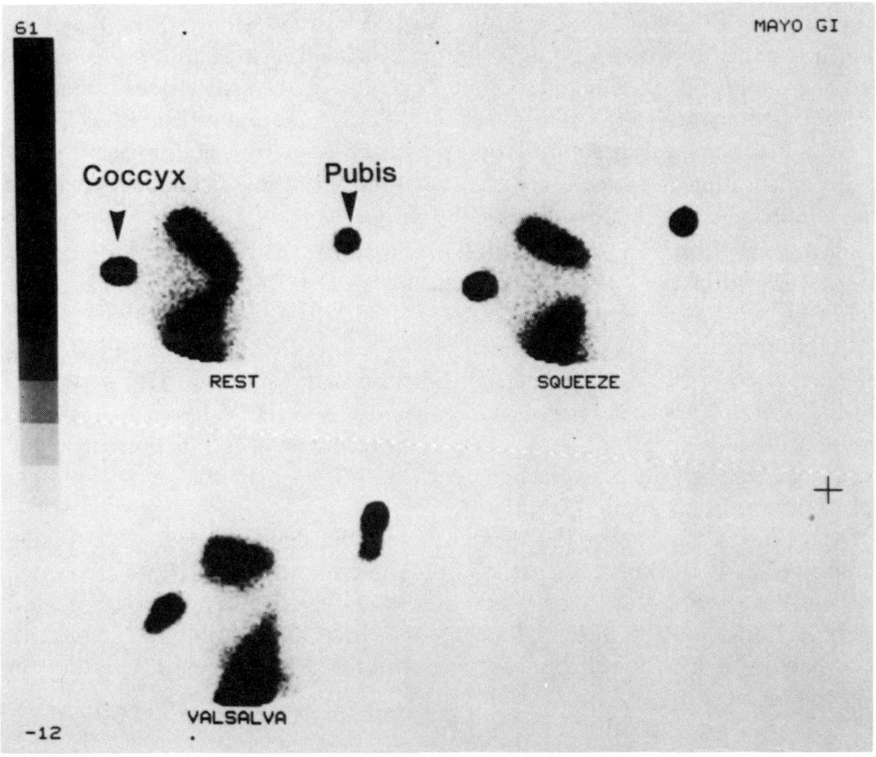

(b)

however, are retained (102). Because the response *has* been demonstrated in some patients after ileal pouch-anal anastomosis with a long rectal muscular cuff (10–12 cm) (108), it is likely mediated by receptors in the more proximal rectal muscular wall (above 4 cm) and carried intramurally or submucosally to the IAS (109).

In summary, the RASIR cannot be demonstrated in most patients after ileal pouch-anal anastomosis, yet discrimination and the urge to defecate remain intact. The traditional role of the reflex, therefore, may be in question.

Neorectal Capacity, Distensibility, and Motility In health, the rectum accommodates to distension; the maximum tolerable capacity is approximately 400 ml, yet even at this volume, intraluminal pressure rarely exceeds 15-20 mmHg. By plotting the slope of $\Delta P/\Delta V$ and taking its reciprocal, distensibility (or "compliance") of the rectum can be calculated. In health, the distensibility of the rectum is 16.8 ± 2 ml/ cm H_2O. By comparison, distensibility of the terminal ileum is 1.9 to 0.05 ml/cm H_2O (29).

The capacity of the J pouch 6 months or more after ileal pouch anastomosis is similar to the capacity of the healthy rectum (110). Likewise, the distensibility of a well-functioning J pouch is approximately 15 ml/cm H_2O, which is similar to the rectum. If an ileal pouch-anal anastomosis is *not* constructed and a segment of ileum anastomosed directly to the anus instead, capacities are tiny (less than 70 ml), and distensibility is only 1.3 ± 0.4 ml/cm H_2O (111).

Well-functioning ileal pouches are as distensible and capacious as healthy rectums. In addition, we have found that the more distensible the pouch, the lower the frequency of stooling postoperatively (111).

Neorectal Motility Rectal motility is characterized by infrequent small amplitude contractions which usually do not exceed 10 cm H_2O, no matter the volume to which the rectum is distended.

In contrast, there are two types of pelvic ileal pouch contractions (112,113); one is a wave of small amplitude and short duration (<10 mmHG; 3-6 s) (Fig. 12). These latter waves, termed high-pressure waves (HPWs) (which are analogous to the high-amplitude waves seen in the Kock pouches), are propulsive and are associated with the passage of content (113). The apparent stimulus for these waves is luminal distension (Fig. 13).

Neorectal filling triggers the HPWs when a "threshold volume" of distension is attained (45% maximum capacity) (114). Interestingly, the HPWs are associted with the *urge* to evacuate. Upon evacuation, the HPWs are abolished until the pouch fills and the threshold volume is reached once again (107) (Fig. 13). This pattern of motility clearly contrasts with the pattern of motility present in the normal rectum.

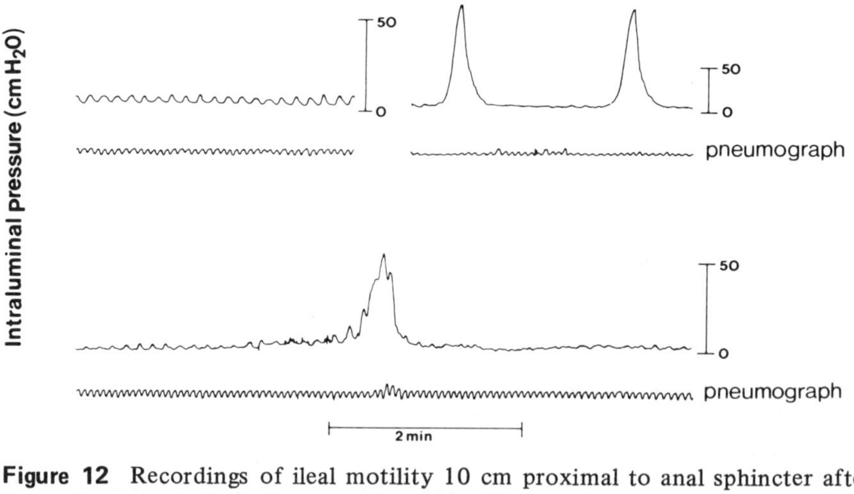

Figure 12 Recordings of ileal motility 10 cm proximal to anal sphincter after ileoanal anastomosis in humans. Top left: Changes in intraluminal pressure of small amplitude and duration. Top right: Changes in intraluminal pressure of large amplitude and duration. Bottom: Changes in intraluminal pressure of both small and large amplitude. (From Ref. 113.)

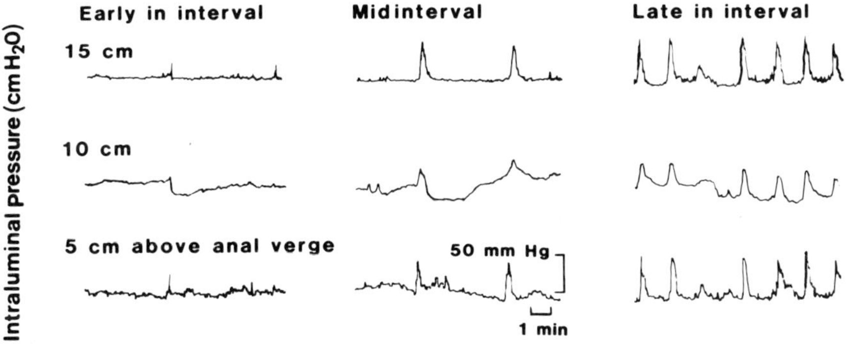

Figure 13 Recordings of high-pressure waves from ileal pouch after ileal pouch-anal anastomosis. As the pouch fills (late in interval), the frequency of these waves increases. (From Ref. 107.)

Neorectal Emptying The ileal pouch should not only store content effectively but should evacuate efficiently. J-shaped pouches do empty spontaneously and nearly completely; in health, about 73 ± 7% of instilled artificial stool is evacuated compared with 57 ± 3% in patients with J pouches (115). Because the rate of content evacuation is rapid and because defecation can be willed, raised intra-abdominal pressure and not pouch contractions is likely responsible for defecation after ileal pouch-anal anastomosis.

After ileal pouch-anal anastomosis, the volume excreted each day varies between 400 and 800 ml and is not different from the volume excreted by well-functioning Brooke ileostomies (114). The most important determinant of stool frequency after ileal pouch-anal anastomosis may be the total content output in 24 hours (110). Measures that would increase absorption and moderate net output would be welcome. Absorption and secretion studies analogous to those performed in continent ileostomy patients have not been performed in ileal pouch-anal anastomosis patients.

In summary, the ileal pouch-anal anastomosis operation achieves its goal of maintaining enteric continence and facilitating defecation because the anal sphincters and pelvic floor are preserved and because a capacious, readily distensible and completely evacuable reservoir is restored.

IV. BENEFIT/RISK ANALYSIS OF THE ALTERNATIVE PROCEDURES (TABLE 3)

Although Brooke ileostomy is a safe and reliable procedure which has broad applicability to patients with inflammatory bowel disease, it is not entirely free of complications; up to 30% of patients have a septic complication, 20-25%

Table 3 Comparison of Alternatives

	Applicability CD/CUC	Stoma	Continent	Mortality (%)	Overall morbidity (%)
Brooke ileostomy	Both	Yes	No	<1.0	19–70
Ileorectostomy	Both	No	Yes	2.5–8	16–20
Continent ileostomy	CUC	Yes	Yes	<1.0	15–60
Ileal pouch-anal anastomosis	CUC	No	Yes	<1.0	30–50

[a]Maximum follow-up, 8 years.
Abbreviations: CD = Crohn's disease; CUC = Chronic ulcerative colitis.

require stomal revision, 15% have recurrent small bowel obstruction, and stomal dysfunction can occur in up to 30%. These data should be kept in mind when reviewing the performance of the alternative procedures.

A. Ileal-Rectal Anastomosis

The primary benefit of ileorectostomy is that the rectum is undisturbed by the operative dissection; the normal pathway of defecation is left in situ and the incidence of bladder or sexual problems is very low. Moreover, there is no perineal wound. In many patients, the overall functional results are reasonably good. The major problem with this procedure is that diseased and potentially diseased mucosa is left in situ. In a few patients, inflammatory changes will resolve, but in most, the disease process continues unabated. The sequelae of leaving disease behind include (1) poor anastomotic healing which is responsible for the high mortality seen after ileal rectal anastomosis (in *distinct* contrast to the low mortality reported after continent ileostomy and ileal pouch anal anastomosis); (2) continued need for steroid medications; (3) continued bleeding and mucous discharge; (4) incontinence and high stool frequency if the disease flares and; (5) the possibility that cancer will occur. Between 20 and 40% of IRA patients require proctocolectomy for one or several of these complications.

Physiologically, if rectal inflammation is minimal, absorption of content can occur and the rectum will accommodate passively to distension and empty efficiently. If mucosal disease is active, however, the rectum cannot accommodate and acts merely as a rigid connection to the anal sphincters; incontinence and high stool frequency will result.

Obstruction (%)	Perineal wound compl. (%)	Stools/ 24 hr	Failure (%)	Disease removed?	Cancer risk (%)
12	33	N	–	Yes	0
15	N	4-6	24–40	No	15(30 yrs)
7	35	3–5	5	Yes	0
10	NA	5–7	6	Yes	0[a]

B. Continent Ileostomy

Although a stoma is constructed, the major benefit is that the stomal discharge can be controlled without using an external appliance. Moreover, in patients with chronic ulcerative colitis, all disease is removed. The principal problem with continent ileostomy is the impressively high complication rate. Most complications involve the nipple valve and invariably lead to incontinence or alternatively to complete outflow obstruction. These, in turn, almost always require an operation. Often the valve problems recur and some patients must undergo multiple reoperations. Nonspecific reservoir inflammation occurs in 10 to 20% of patients and can usually be controlled with metronidazole. A perineal wound, of course, accompanies this operation; the wound fails to heal in about a third of the patients. Encouragingly, whereas, the initial reoperation rate was more than 50%, it has now dropped into the 15–25% range.

In general, the physiological sequelae for patients with an ileal pouch are the same as for patients with brooke ileostomies. However, pouchitis can occur which leads to volume depletion and valve malfunction. Moreover, the bacteriology and histology of the pouch changes dramatically; these changes have not been associated with any long-term problem.

C. Ileal Pouch-Anal Anastomosis

The ileal pouch-anal anastomosis operation successfully restores enteric continence in the great majority of patients, but has a complication rate of about 30%. Occasional incontinence occurs in nearly all patients very early during the postoperative course, particularly at night. Major episodes of daytime incontinence occur in nearly 10% of patients but this incidence declines to nearly zero by four years. Other complications such as pelvic infection, stricture, fistula, sinus tracts, pouch leakage, small bowel obstruction, and pouchitis continue to occur. As experience with the operation has broadened, however, these complications have decreased in frequency.

Despite these problems, the benefits of ileal pouch-anal anastomosis are clearly profound; all disease is removed, the patients do not have a stoma, defecation is transanal, willful and controlled, and in the great majority of patients, continence is maintained and bladder and sexual function is normal.

Ileal pouch-anal anastomosis preserves continence because the physiologic mechanisms responsible are preserved or restored by the operation. The major challenge to homeostasis in ileal pouch-anal anastomosis patients is the occurrence of "pouchitis" which, if severe and recurrent can result in failure of the operation.

V. IMPLICATIONS OF ILEOSTOMY ALTERNATIVES FOR THE SURGICAL MANAGEMENT OF INFLAMMATORY DISEASE

A. Crohn's Disease

If a patient requires an operation for pancolitis caused by Crohn's disease, Brooke ileostomy is the treatment of choice. The failure rate of continent ileostomy and ileal pouch-anal anastomosis in this setting is so unacceptably high that these operations should not be considered in such patients. This statement is made with full knowledge that Bloom et al. (116), have suggested that some patients with Crohn's disease will do well with the Kock pouch.

In patients with Crohn's colitis in whom sparing of the rectum can be proven via endoscopy and in whom no anal disease is present, ileal rectal anastomosis is a reasonable alternative. Although late results of this operation in patients with Crohn's disease are somewhat disappointing (up to 70% proctectomy rate), IRA is the *only* operation which can provide a stoma-free life for patients with extensive colonic Crohn's disease and, therefore, is probably worthwhile. Even if proctectomy is required later, little small bowel length is sacrificed during conversion to a Brooke ileostomy.

B. Chronic Ulcerative Colitis

The criteria for an ideal alternative to proctocolectomy and Brooke ileostomy for patients which chronic ulcerative colitis are that all disease is excised, the transanal route for defecation is maintained, and the principal mechanisms for achieving and maintaining enteric continence are preserved. The *one* alternative that fulfills this criteria is ileal pouch-anal anastomosis. The ileal rectal anastomosis falls short principally because the disease process is left in situ, while the continent ileostomy operation necessitates an abdominal stoma.

This does not imply, however, that these latter procedures have no application to patients with chronic ulcerative colitis. There are several specific instances in which ileorectal anastomosis may be the procedure of choice. One indication might be when a young person requires an operation, but he or she has yet to start a family or, for that matter, finish school. In these patients, ileal rectal anastomosis may be considered a "bridging" operation; that is, an operation which will see them safely through adolescence without the problems of sexual or bladder dysfunction which might complicate ileal pouch-anal anastomosis. Moreover, patients of *any age* who are unwilling to accept *any* risk of sexual or bladder dysfunction should be offered ileal rectal anastomosis. Of course, the rectum must retain some degree of distensibility and not be strictured if the operation is to be successful.

Another application for ileal rectal anastomosis is in patients with indeterminate colitis (approximately 10% of all patients operated upon for colitis). Finally, ileal rectal anastomosis can be considered when a patient does not fit the criteria for the ileal pouch-anal anastomosis because of age (>50–55 years), or body habitus (obesity) but who wishes to avoid a permanent stoma. However, patients undergoing ileal rectal anastomosis must be fully informed that further surgery may be required for unrelenting disease, development of dysplasia, or for cancer. These patients must be willing, therefore, to undergo follow-up examinations at regular intervals and be amenable to proctectomy (and perhaps ileal pouch-anal anastomosis) when it is indicated.

Continent ileostomy also has a role, albeit a rather minor one, in the management of patients with chronic ulcerative colitis. Continent ileostomy remains an option for patients who have already had a proctocolectomy and who desire control of the stoma. In addition, in those few patients in whom an ileal pouch-anal anastomosis cannot be performed because of the presence of a short mesentery, continent ileostomy can be performed instead. Finally, continent ileostomy can be offered to patients who are unwilling to stool 4–8 times a day.

While no operation can restore a patient to "normality" after colectomy for chronic ulcerative colitis, the ileoanal anastomosis procedure appears to come closest *without leaving disease in place*. Ileal pouch-anal anastomosis is not a perfect operation, it is difficult to perform, not all patients are candidates, the complication rate is moderate, and not all patients have a successful outcome. However, a critical review of the published clinical experience suggests that in most patients, ileal pouch-anal anastomosis achieves its goals.

Selection of patients is critical to success of the operation. Patients who are compromised severely preoperatively or in whom an urgent or emergency operation is contemplated should undergo a simple and straightforward procedure. If the rectum can be left in place, however, this burns no bridges for future procedures and should be considered strongly. Moreover, patients less than 50 years of age and patients who are thin, have a better functional result than do older, obese patients. Steroids per se are not a contraindication to ileal pouch-anal anastomosis.

In conclusion, ileal pouch-anal anastomosis, which is as safe as Brooke ileostomy and continent ileostomy (and is safer the ileorectostomy) should be considered an important advance in the surgical management of chronic ulcerative colitis. Just as the spector of life with a Brooke ileostomy may have influenced the decision of when to intervene surgically in patients with chronic ulcerative colitis in the past, so should the availability of ileal pouch-anal anastomosis influence present-day decisions. Although not applicable to *all patients*, ileal pouch-anal anastomosis should be considered the alternative treatment of choice in most young patients with chronic ulcerative colitis.

REFERENCES

1. Makins, G. H., Ulcerative colitis, Proc. R. Soc. Med., 2:75–79 (1909).
2. Corbett, R. S., A review of the surgical treatment of chronic ulcerative colitis, Proc. R. Soc. Med., 38:277-290 (1945).
3. Brown, J. Y., The value of complete physiological rest of the large bowel in the treatment of certain ulcerative and obstructive lesions of this organ, Surg. Gynecol. Obstet., 16:610–613 (1913).
4. Counsell, J. C. Goligher, Surgical treatment of ulcerative colitis, Lancet, 2: 1045–1050 (1952).
5. Crile, G. Jr., C. Y. Thomas, The treatment of acute toxic ulcerative colitis by ileostomy and simultaneous colectomy, Gastroenterology, 19:58–68 (1951).
6. Miller, G. G., C. McG. Gardner, C. B. Ripstein, Primary resection of the colon in ulcerative colitis, Can. Med. Assoc. J., 60:584–585 (1949).
7. Rankin, F. W., Total colectomy: Its indication and technic. Trans. Am. Surg. Assoc., 49:263–285 (1931).
8. Bargen, J. A., P. W. Brown, F. W. Rankin, Indications for and technique of ileostomy in chronic ulcerative colitis, Surg. Gynecol. Obstet., 55:196–202 (1952).
9. Brooke, B. N., Management of ileostomy including its complications, Lancet, 2:102–104 (1952).
10. Crile G. Jr., R. B. Jr. Turnbull, The mechanism and prevention of ileostomy dysfunction, Ann. Surg., 140:459–465 (1954.
11. Ritchie, J. K., Ulcerative colitis treated by ileostomy and excisional surgery: Fifteen years' experience at St. Marks' Hospital, Br. J. Surg., 59:345–351 (1972).
12. Beauchamp, G., D. Beliveau, A. Archambault, Death and complications after total colectomy for inflammatory bowel disease, Can. J. Surg., 24: 463–466 (1981).

13. Binder, S. C., H. H. Miller, Deterling R. A. Jr., Emergency and urgent operation for ulcerative colitis: The procedure of choice, Arch. Surg., 110: 284-289 (1975).
14. Steinberg, D. M., R. N. Allan, B. N. Brooke, W. T. Cooke, J. Alexander-William, Sequelae of colectomy and ileostomy: Comparison between Crohn's colitis and ulcerative colitis, Gastroenterology, 68:33–39 (1975).
15. Sirinek, K. R., C. E. Tetirick, N. R. Thomford, W. G. Pace, Total procto-colectomy and ileostomy: Procedure of choice for acute toxic megacolon, Arch. Surg., 112:518–522 (1977).
16. Lee, E. C. G., B. L. Dowling, Perimuscular excision of the rectum for Crohn's disease and ulcerative colitis: A conservation technique, Br. J. Surg., 59:29–32 (1972).
17. Lyttle, J. A., A. G. Parks, Intersphincteric excision of the rectum, Br. J. Surg., 64:413–416 (1977).
18. Burnham, W. R., J. E. Lennard-Jones, B. N. Brooke, Sexual problems among married ileostomists: Survey conducted by the Ileostomy Association of Great Britain and Ireland, Gut, 18:673–677 (1977).
19. Gruner, O-P. N., R. Naas, B. Fretheim, E. Gjion, Marital status and sexual adjustment after colectomy: results in 178 patients operated on for ulcerative colitis, Scand. J. Gastroenterol., 12:193–197 (1977).
20. Ritchie, J. K., Ileostomy and excisional surgery for chronic inflammatory disease of the colon: A survey of one hospital region. I. Results and complication of surgery, Gut, 12:528–536 (1971).
21. Morowitz, D. A., J. B. Kirsner, Ileostomy in ulcerative colitis: A questionnaire study of 1803 patients, Am. J Surg., 141:370–375 (1981).
22. Pemberton, J. H., S. F. Phillips, R. R. Dozois, l. J. Wendorf, Conventional ileostomy: Current clinical results. In: Alternatives to Conventional Ileostomy. (Dozois R. R., ed.) Chicago, Yearbook Medical publishers, pp. 40–50 (1985).
23. Roy, P. H., W. G. Sauer, O. H. Beahrs, G. M. Farrow, Experience with ileostomies: Evaluation of long-term rehabilitation of 497 patients, Am. J. Surg., 119:77–86 (1970).
24. Hill, G. L., W. S. J. Mair, J. C. Goligher, Impairment of "ileostomy adaptation" in patients after ileal resection, Gut, 15:982–987 (1974).
25. Kramer, P: The effect of varying soidum loads on the ileal excreta of human ileostomized subjects, J. Clin. Invest., 45:1710–1718 (1966).
26. Kramer, P., M. M. Kearney, F. J. Ingelfinger, The effect of specific foods and water loading on the ileal excreta of ileostomized human subjects, Gastroenterology, 42:535–545 (1962).
27. Pemberton, J. H. (unpublished data).
28. Gorbach, S. L., L. Nahas, L. Weinstein, R. Levitan, J. F. Patterson: Studies of intestinal microflora. IV. The microflora of ileostomy effluent: A unique microbial ecology, Gastroenterology, 53:874–880 (1967).
29. Pemberton, J. H., J. A. Van Heerden, R. W. Jr. Beart, K. A. Kelly, S. F. Phillips, B. M. Taylor, A continent ileostomy device, Ann. Surg., 197:618–625 (1983).

30. Kerlin, P., A. Zinmeister, S. F. Phillips, Relationship of motility to flow of contents in the human small intestines, Gastroenterology, 82:701–706 (1982).
31. Hill, G. L., Ileostomy: Surgery, Physiology, and Management. New York, Grune & Stratton (1976).
32. Hulten, L., S. Kewenter, E. Persson, C. Ahren, Vitamin B_{12} absorption in ileostomy patients after operation for ulcerative colitis, Scand. J. Gatroenterol., 5:113–116 (1970).
33. Bambach, C. P., W. G. Robertson, M. Peacock, G. L. Hill, Effects of intestinal surgery on the risk of urinary stone formation, Gut, 22:257–263 (1981).
34. Druss, R. G., J. F. O'Connor, J. F. Prudden, L. O. Stern, Psychologic response to colectomy, Arch. Gen. Psychiatry, 18:53–59 (1968).
35. Failes, D., The Kock continent ileostomy: A preliminary report, Aust. N. Z. J. Surg., 45:125–130 (1976).
36. Devine, H., A method of colectomy for desperate cases of ulcerative colitis, Surg. Gynecol. Obstet. 76:136–138 (1943).
37. Aylett, S. O., Three hundred cases of diffuse ulcerative colitis treated by total colectomy and ileorectal anastomosis, Br. Med. J., 1:1001–1005 (1966).
38. Grundfest, S. F., V. Fazio, R. A. Weiss, D. Jagelman, I. Lavery, F. L. Weakley, R. B. Jr. Turnbull, The risk of cancer following colectomy and ileorectal anastomosis for extensive mucosal ulcerative colitis, Ann. Surg., 193:9–14 (1981).
39. Watts, J. M., E. S. R. Hughes, Ulcerative colitis and Crohn's disease: Results after colectomy and ileorectal anastomosis, Br. J. Surg., 64:77–83 (1977).
40. Khubchandani, I. T., H. D. Trimpi, J. A. Sheets, J. J. Jr. Stasik, F. S. Kleckner, Ileorectal anastomosis for ulcerative and Crohn's colitis, Am. J. Surg., 135:751–756 (1978).
41. Jones, P. F., Munro, A., S. W. B. Ewen, Colectomy and ileorectal anastomosis for colitis: Report on a personal series, with a critical review, Br. J. Surg., 64:615–623 (1977).
42. Vink, M., H. J. P. Beerstecher, A critical evaluation and analysis of total colectomy and ileorectal anastomosis for patients with ulcerative colitis, Arch. Chir. Neerl., 25:107–117 (1973).
43. Gruner, O. P. N., A. Flatmark, R. Naas, B. Fretheim, E. Gjone, Ileorectal anastomosis in ulcerative colitis, Scand. J. Gastroenterol., 10:641–646 (1975).
44. Adson, M. A., A. M. Cooperman, G. M. Farrow, Ileorectostomy for ulcerative disease of the colon, Arch. Surg., 104:424–428 (1972).
45. Johnson, W. R., F. T. McDermott, E. S. R. Hughes, E. A. Pihl, B. J. Milne, The risk of rectal carcinoma following colectomy in ulcerative colitis, Dis. Colon Rectum, 26:44–46 (1983).
46. Farnell, M. B., J. A. Van Heerden, R. W. Jr. Beart, L. H. Weiland, Rectal preservation in nonspecific inflammatory bowel disease of the colon, Ann. Surg., 192:249–253 (1980).

47. Farnell, M. B., M. A. Adson, Current results: The Mayo Clinic experience, In: Alternatives to Conventional Ileostomy. (Dozois R. R., ed.) Chicago, Year Book Medical Publishers, pp. 100–121 (1985).
48. Goligher, J. C., The long-term results of excisional surgery for primary and recurrent Crohn's disease of the large intestine, Dis. Colon. Rectum, 28:51–55 (1985).
49. Baker, W. N. W., R. E. Glass, J. K. Ritchie, S. O. Aylett, Cancer of the rectum following colectomy and ileorectal anastomosis for ulcerative colitis, Br. J. Surg., 65:862–868 (1978).
50. Aylett, S. O., Ulcerative colitis treated by total colectomy and ileorectal anastomosis: A ten year review, Proc. R. Soc. Med., 56:183–190 (1963).
51. Parc, R., E. Levy, P. Frileux, J. Loygue, Current results: Ileorectal anastomosis after total abdominal colectomy for ulcerative colitis. In: Alternatives to Continent Ileostomy. (Dozois R. R., ed.) Chicago, Year Book Medical Publishers, pp. 81–99 (1985).
52. Baker, W. N. W., The results of ileorectal anastomosis at St. Mark's Hospital from 1953 to 1968, Gut, 11:235–239 (1970).
53. Aylett, S. O., Diffuse ulcerative colitis and its treatment by ileorectal anastomosis, Ann. R. Coll. Surg. Engl., 27:260284 (1960).
54. Newton, C. R., W. N. W. Baker, Comparison of bowel function after ileorectal anastomosis for ulcerative colitis and colonic polyposis, Gut, 16:785–791 (1975).
55. Lindham, S., R. Langercrantz, Ulcerative colitis in childhood: Should the rectum be preserved at surgery? Long-term results in 50 patients, Scand. J. Gastroenterol., 15:123–127 (1980).
56. Grundfest, S. F., V. Fazio, R. A. Weiss, D. Jagelman, I. Lavery, F. L. Weakley, R. B. Jr. Turnbull, The risk of cancer following colectomy and ileorectal anastomosis for extensive mucosal ulcerative colitis, Ann. Surg., 193:9–14 (1981).
57. Devroede, G., W. F. Taylor, On calculating cancer risk and survival of ulcerative colitis patients with the life table method, Gastroenterology, 71:505–509 (1976).
58. Mignon, M., S. Bonfils, Altered physiology in ulcerative colitis patients with ileorectal anastomosis. In: Alternatives to Conventional Ileostomy. (Dozois R. R., ed.) Chicago, Year Book Medical Publishers, pp. 61–80 (1985).
59. Pemberton, J. H., K. A. Kelly, Achieving enteric continence: Principles and application, Mayo Clin. Proc., 61:586–599 (1986).
60. Denis, P. H., R. Colin, J. P. Galmiche, Y. Geffroy, P. H. Hecketsweiler, R. Lefrancois, P. Pasquis, Elastic properties of the rectal wall in normal adults and in patients with ulcerative colitis, Gastroenterology, 77:45–48 (1979).
61. Farthing, M. J. G., J. E. Lennard-Jones, Sensibility of the rectum to distension and the anorectal distension reflex in ulcerative colitis, Gut, 19:64–69 (1978).
62. Henriksen, F. W., B. Antonisen, Measurement of the anal sphincter strength by a simple method suitable for routine use, Scand. J. Gastroenterol., 7: 555–558 (1972).

63. Schultz, S. G., Ion transport by mammalian large intestine. In: Physiology of the Gastrointestinal Tract, Vol. 2. (Johnson L. R., ed.) New York, Raven Press, pp. 991–1002 (1981).
64. Newton, C. R., Comparison of the bowel function after colectomy and ileostomy or ileorectal anastomosis for inflammatory bowel disease (Abstr.). Gut, 13:855 (1972).
65. Edmonds, C. J., D. Pilcher, Electrical potential difference and sodium and potassium fluxes across rectal mucosa in ulcerative colitis, Gut, 14:784–789 (1973).
66. Kock, N. G., Intra-abdominal "reservoir" in patients with permanent ileostomy: Preliminary observations on a procedure resulting in fecal "continence" in five ileostomy patients, Arch. Surg., 99:223–230 (1969).
67. Fazio, V. W., J. M. Church, Complication and function of the continent ileostomy at the Cleveland Clinic, World J. Surg., 12:148–154 (1988).
68. Dozois, R. R., K. A. Kelly, R. W. Jr. Beart, O. H. Beahrs, Continent ileostomy: The Mayo Clinic experience. In: Alternatives to Conventional Ileostomy. Chicago, Yearbook Medical Publishers, pp. 163–175 (1985).
69. Kock, N. G., H. E. Myrvold, L. O. Nilsson, B. M. Phillips, Continent ileostomy: The Swedish experience. In: Alternatives to Conventional Ileostomy. (Dozois R. R. ed.) Chicago, Yearbook Medical Publishers, pp. 163–175 (1985).
70. McLeod, R. S., V. W. Fazio, Quality of life with the continent ileostomy, World J. Surg., 8:90–95 (1984).
71. Valkamo, E., Ileostomy in ulcerative colitis: Academic dissection (thesis). Second Department of Surgery. University Central Hospital Helsinki Fairbairn (1981).
72. Cameron, A., The continent ileostomy, Br. J. Surg., 60:785–790 (1973).
73. Akwari, O. E., K. A. Kelly, S. F. Phillips, Myoelectric and motor pattern of continent pouch and conventional ileostomy, Surg. Gynecol. Obstet., 150:363–371 (1980).
74. Kelly, D. G., S. F. Phillips, K. A. Kelly, W. M. Weinstein, M. J. R. Gilchrist, Dysfunction of the continent ileostomy: Clinical features and bacteriology, Gut, 24:193–201 (1983).
75. Gadacz. T. R., K. A. Kelly, S. F. Phillips, The continent ileal pouch: Absorptive and motor features, Gastroenterology, 72:1287–1291 (1977).
76. Jagenburg, R., N. G. Koch, B. Phillipson, Vitamin B_{12} absorption in patients with continent ileostomy, Scand. J. Gastroenterol., 10:141–144 (1975).
77. Jagenburg, R., G. Dotervall, J. Kewenter, N. G. Kock, B. Philipson, Absorption studies in patients with "intra-abdominal ileostomy reservoirs" and with patients with conventional ileostomies, Gut, 12:437–441 (1971).
78. Pemberton, J. H., J. Heppell, R. W. Jr. Beart, R. R. Dozois, R. L. Telander, Endorectal ileoanal anastomosis, Surg. Gynecol. Obstet., 155:417–424 (1982).

79. Stryker, S. J., R. R. Dozois, The ileoanal anastomosis: Historical perspectives. In: Alternatives for Conventional Ileostomy. (Dozois R. R., ed.) Chicago, Yearbook Medical Publishers, pp. 255–265 (1985).
80. Williams, N. S., D. Johnston, The current status of mucosal proctectomy and ileoanal anastomosis in the surgical treatment of ulcerative colitis and adenomatous polyposis, Br. J. Surg., 72:159–168 (1985).
81. Wong, W. D., D. A. Rothenberger, S. M. Goldberg, Ileoanal pouch procedure, Curr. Probl. Surg., 1–78 (1985).
82. Martin, L. W., C. LeCoultre, W. K. Schubert, Total colectomy and mucosal proctectomy with preservation of continence in ulcerative colitis, Ann. Surg., 186:477–479 (1977).
83. Parks, A. G., R. J. Nicholls, P. Belliveau, Proctolectomy with ileal reservoir and anal anastomosis, Br. J. Surg., 67:533–538 (1980).
84. Utsonomiya, J., T. Iwama, M. Imago, S. Matsuo, S. Sawai, K. Yaegashi, R. Kirayama, Total colectomy, mucosal proctectomy, and ileoanal anastomosis, Dis. Colon Rectum, 23:459–466 (1980).
85. Ballantyne, G. H., J. H. Pemberton, R. W. Jr. Beart, B. G. Wolff, R. R. Dozois, Ileal J pouch-anal anastomosis: Current technique, Dis. Colon. Rectum, 28:197–202 (1985).
86. Kelly, K. A., Ileal pouch-anal anastomosis after proctocolectomy, Surg. Rounds, 8:48–52 (1985).
87. Pemberton, J. H., K. A. Kelly, R. W. Jr. Beart, B. G. Wolff, D. M. Ilstrup, Ileal pouch-anal anastomosis for chronic ulcerative colitis: Long-term results, Ann. Surg., 206:504–511 (1987).
88. Pemberton, J. H., S. F. Phillips, R. L. Ready, A. Zinmeister, Comparing performance status after Brooke ileostomy and ileal pouch-anal anastomosis (abstr.), Gastroenterology, 88:1535 (1985).
89. Nivatvongs, S., H. S. Stern, D. S. Fryd, The length of the anal canal, Dis. Colon Rectum, 24:600–601 (1981).
90. Frenckner, B., C. V. Euler, Influence of pudendal block on the function of the anal sphincters, Gut, 16:482–489 (1975).
91. Heppell, J., K. A. Kelly, S. F. Phillips, R. W. Beart, R. L. Telander, J. Perrault, Physiology aspects of continence after colectomy, mucosal proctectomy and endorectal ileoanal anastomosis, Ann. Surg., 195:435–443 (1982).
92. O'Connell, P. R., S. J. Stryker, A. M. Metcalf, J. H. Pemberton, K. A. Kelly, Anal canal pressure and motility after ileoanal anastomosis, Surg. Gynecol. Obstet., 166:47–54 (1988).
93. Phillips, S. F., D. A. W. Edwards, Some aspects of anal continence and defecation, Gut, 6:396–406 (1965).
94. Hardcastle, J. D., A. G. Parks, A study of anal incontinence and some principles of surgical treatment, Proc. R. Soc. Med., 63(Supp):116–118 (1970).
95. Barkel, D. C., J. H. Pemberton, S. F. Phillips, K. A. Kelly, M. L. Brown, Scintigraphic assessment of the anorectal angle in health and following ileal pouch-anal anastomosis, Ann. Surg., 208:42–49 (1988).

96. Parks, A. G., Anorectal continence, Proc. R. Soc. Med., 68:681-690 (1975).
97. Bartolo, D. C. C., A. M. Roe, J. Locke-Edmunds, J. Virjee, N. J. McC. Mortenson, Flap-valve theroy of anorectal continence, Br. J. Surg., 73: 1012-1014 (1986).
98. Barkel, D. C., J. H. Pemberton, S. F., Phillips, K. A. Kelly, M. L. Brown, Scintigraphic assessment of the anorectal angle in health and after operation, Surg. Forum, 37:183-186 (1986).
99. Winckler, G., Remarques sur la morphologie et l'innervation du muscle releveur de l'anus, Arch. Anat. Histol. Embryol. (Strasb.), 41:77-95 (1958).
100. Duthie, H. L., F. W. Gairns, Sensory nerve endings and sensation in the anal region of man, Br. J. Surg., 47:585-595 (1960).
101. Roe, A. M., D. C. C. Bartolo, N. J. McC. Mortenson, New method for assessment of anal sensation in various anorectal disorders, Br. J. Surg., 73:310-312 (1986).
102. Beart, R. W. Jr., R. R. Dozois, B. G. Wolff, J. H. Pemberton, Mechanisms of rectal continence: lessons from the ileoanal procedure, Am. J. Surg., 149:31-33 (1985).
103. Johnston, D., P. J. Holdsworth, D. G. Nasmyth, D. E. Neal, J. N. Primrose, N. Womack, A. T. R. Axon, Preservation of the entire anal canal in conservative proctocolectomy for ulcerative colitis: A pilot study comparing end-to-end ileoanal anastomosis without mucosal resection with mucosal proctectomy and endoanal anastomosis, Br. J. Surg., 74:940-944 (1987)
104. Keighley, M. R. B., M. C. Winslet, K. Yoshioka, R. Lightwood, Discrimination is not impaired by excision of the anal transition zone after restorative proctocolectomy, Br. J. Surg., 74:1118-1121 (1987).
105. Gowers, W. R., The automatic action of the sphincter ani, Proc. R. Soc. Med., 26:77-84 (1877).
106. Duthie, H. L., R. C. Bennett, The relation of sensation in the anal canal to the functional anal sphincter: A possible factor in anal continence, Gut, 4: 179-182 (1963).
107. Stryker, S. J., K. A. Kelly, S. F. Phillips, R. R. Dozois, R. W. Jr., Beart, Anal and neorectal function after ileal pouch-anal anastomosis, Ann. Surg., 203:55-61 (1986).
108. Becker, J. M., J. L. Raymond, Ileal pouch-anal anastomosis: A single surgeon's experience with 100 consecutive cases, Ann. Surg., 204:375-381 (1986).
109. Pezim, M. E., J. H. Pemberton, R. R. Dozois, Enteric continence and the ileal pouch-anal procedure, Semin. Surg. Oncol., 3:92-98 (1987).
110. O'Connell, P. R., J. H. Pemberton, K. A. Kelly, Motor function of the ileal pouch and its relation to clinical outcome after ileal pouch anal anastomosis, World J. Surg., 11:735-741 (1987).
111. Heppell, J., B. M. Taylor, R. W. Jr. Beart, R. R. Dozois, K. A. Kelly, Predicting outcome after endorectal ileoanal anastomosis, Can J. Surg., 26: 132-134 (1983).

112. Code, C. F., A. G. Rogers, J. Schlegel, N. C. Jr. Hightower, J. A. Bargen, Motility patterns in the terminal ileum: Studies on two patients with ulcerative colitis and ileal stomas, Gastroenterology, 32:651–665 (1957).
113. Heppell, J., J. H. Pemberton, K. A. Kelly, S. F. Phillips, Ileal motility after endorectal ileoanal anastomosis, Surg. Gastroenterol., 1:124–127 (1982).
114. O'Connell, P. R., J.J. Pemberton, M. L. Brown, K. A. Kelly, Determinants of stool frequency after ileal pouch-anal anastomosis, Am. J. Surg., 153: 157–163 (1987).
115. O'Connell, P. R., J. H. Pemberton, M. L. Brown, K. A. Kelly, Neorectal emptying after "J" pouch-anal anastomosis (abstr.). Br. J. Surg., 72:1026 (1985).
116. Bloom, R. J., C. P. Lasen, R. Watt, H. A. Jr. Oberhelman, A reappraisal of the Kock continent ileostomy in patients with Crohn's disease, Surg. Gynecol. Obstet., 162:105–108 (1986).
117. Pemberton, J. H., O. H. Bealus, Brooke ileostomy. In: Surgery of the Small Intestine. (Nelson, R. L., L. M. Nyhus, eds.) Appleton-Century-Crofts, pp. 449–458 (1987).
118. Kelly, K. A., Advances in Surgical Management: Topics in Gastroenterology, vol 12 (Jewell, D. P., P. R. Gibson, eds.) London, Blackwell Scientific Publishers, pp. 163–177 (1985).
119. Taylor, B. M., R. W. Beart, Jr., R. R. Dozois, K. A. Kelly, S. F. Phillips, Straight ileoanal anastomosis vs ileal pouch-anal anastomosis, Arch. Surg., 118:696–701 (1983).

II
SPECIFIC MANAGEMENT PROBLEMS

10
Extraintestinal and Malignant Complications

Mark A. Peppercorn

Beth Israel Hospital, Harvard Medical School, Boston, Massachusetts

Disease processes affecting many organ systems are associated with both ulcerative colitis and Crohn's disease. Many of these are directly associated with activity of the underlying inflammatory bowel disease (IBD), especially active colonic disease. Others are related to small bowel pathophysiology (1). Unlike the extraintestinal disorders related to IBD, both colon and small intestinal adenocarcinomas are complications of ulcerative colitis and Crohn's disease which occur in areas of involved bowel. This chapter reviews the treatment options available for these complications of IBD.

I. THROMBOEMBOLIC DISEASE

Ulcerative colitis and Crohn's disease may predispose to a hypercoagulable state manifested, most often, clinically by thrombophlebitis involving the lower extremities, with or without pulmonary embolism. Less frequent presentations of thromboembolic disease include arterial thrombosis which may involve the retina, glans penis, or large cranial vessels, and a form of vasculitis resembling periarteritis nodosum which may involve multiple organ systems (2). The hypercoagulable state in IBD is likely multifactorial since elevations of Factor V, fibrinogen, and platelets, as well as a reduction in the level of antithrombin 3 have been found.

Therapeutic intervention in thromboembolic disease can present an especially difficult dilemma. The initial therapy of choice is heparin, clearly fraught with hazards in the patient who is already actively bleeding from colitis. Massive colonic hemorrhage during anticoagulation will necessitate vena caval interruption, with or without colectomy. In the patient who tolerated heparin without increased colonic bleeding, the drug should be given as a continuous intravenous infusion with careful monitoring of the partial thromboplastic time. Coumadin can then be added and continued long-term.

In patients whose colitis activity disappears or decreases, the Coumadin can be stopped after a three- to six-month course. In the patient who has demonstrated hypercoaguability and has ongoing disease activity not severe enough for colectomy, indefinite anticoagulation has to be considered.

II. SKIN

A. Erythema Nodosum

The cutaneous manifestation most often associated with IBD is erythema nodosum characterized by raised erythematous, tender subcutaneous nodules most prominent along the extensor surfaces of the arms and legs (4). Although occasionally seen prior to an attack of ulcerative colitis or Crohn's disease (usually involving the colon as well), these lesions generally parallel the activity of the bowel disease and will respond to therapy directed at the colitis. On those occasions when the colitis is dormant or when there is no response to treatment with nonsteroid medications, a course of prednisone (e.g., 40 mg/day for one week with reduction by 10 mg/wk) usually leads to prompt resolution of the erythema nodosum.

B. Pyoderma Gangrenosum

A less common but potentially more serious problem is pyoderma gangrenosum which parallels disease activity in only about 50% of patients (5). These lesions which may appear initially at the site of trauma and have the appearance of a boil, result in progressive necrosis of the dermis with deep ulceration associated with purulent-appearing material which contains white cells but generally no bacteria. High-dose prednisone (e.g., 60 mg/day) directed at the colitis when active or at the skin lesions when the colitis is mild or inactive usually results in healing of the skin lesions. Other treatment modalities reported at times to be successful include intralesional steroids, sulfasalazine, immunosuppressives, clofazamine, and topical and systemic antibiotics for most cases in which bacterial superinfection appears to delay healing. Additional treatments include topical potassium permanganate and acetic acid soaks as well as hyperbaric oxygen (6). A recent report describes impressive improvement of a severe case of pyoderma gangrenosum with high-dose methylprednisone given as pulse therapy in association with dapsone (7). Moreover, topical application of disodium cromoglycate appears to be an effective and safe therapy (8-10). On rare occasions, persistent severe pyoderma gangrenosum will itself be an indication for proctocolectomy.

III. OCULAR LESIONS

Episcleritis, characterized by inflammation of the episcleral tissues and injection of the deep ciliary vessels, parallels IBD activity and is associated with discomfort. Uveitis (iritis) often follows a course independent of the bowel disease and can cause acutely blurred vision, photophobia, and pain. An acute attack may be followed by synechiae, lens deposits, and atrophy of the iris. Immediate therapy with topical steroids should be instituted and if the colitis is active, systemic steroids directed at both the IBD and eye manifestations should be considered (11).

IV. ORAL MANIFESTATIONS

The most common oral lesion associated with both ulcerative colitis and Crohn's disease is the aphthous ulcer, which is also characteristic of the early lesions of Crohn's disease throughout the gastrointestinal tract (1). These lesions may signal disease activity elsewhere, but at times may precede the onset of overt IBD by weeks or months.

Oral aphthous ulcers often will respond to local treatment with hydrocortisone in a paste vehicle containing pectin, gelatin, and carboxymethylcellulose (Orabase) or to a paste-containing sucralfate. When the oral aphtha are seen in conjunction with active enteric disease, they will usually disappear when the bowel disease becomes quiescent on medical therapy.

Crohn's disease can involve the mouth and oral pharynx in a variety of other ways including large ulcerations, fissures, and localized mass lesions (12). The most advanced lesions usually develop progressively and are associated with active enteric disease and require therapy with corticosteroids or immunosuppressive agents (13).

V. JOINTS

Several rheumatologic conditions occur in association with IBD. The most common, occurring in up to 25% of patients, is a form of peripheral arthritis which tends to parallel the activity of the bowel disease although at times may antedate it (14,15). It tends to be monarticular and migratory, affecting most commonly knees, ankles, elbows, and wrists followed by proximal interphalangeal joints, metacarpophalangeal joints, and metatarsophalangeal joints (15). Patients complain of the acute onset of joint pain with limitation of motion and have evidence of synovitis with effusion, erythema, and tenderness. The most effective therapy for the acute arthritic symptoms is usually that directed at the IBD itself. The peripheral arthritis tends to be especially responsive to corticosteroids (15). Intra-articular injections of steroids may be effective as well. Aspirin and other nonsteroidal anti-inflammatory agents are frequently used in conjunction with therapy directed at the IBD, but should be used with caution in view of evidence linking these drugs with exacerbations of the colitis or ileitis (16). Physical therapy is an important aspect of therapy often neglected. Active and passive range of motion exercises should be employed to prevent contractures.

Two forms of axial arthropathy, ankylosing spondylitis and sacroiliitis are seen in association with IBD. The low back pain of spondylitis is characteristically insidious in onset associated with morning stiffness, and improves with exercise. In contrast to the peripheral arthritis, symptoms of spondylitis tend to be unrelated to exacerbations and remissions of the IBD and the process follows a chronic progressive course (15).

Sacroiliitis is often asymptomatic and is diagnosed because of the radiographic changes observed on barium studies. It may be associated with spondylitis and when symptomatic in its own right, activity does not correlate with the activity of the IBD.

Treatment for these forms of axial arthropathy include heat, physical therapy to maintain posture and muscle strength, the use of a bedboard and a firm mattress, and nonsteroidal anti-inflammatory drugs. Treatment of the IBD, especially with corticosteroids may provide some symptomatic relief (6,15).

A fourth category of clinical rheumatologic problems seen in association with IBD include entities such as "metastatic" granulomas involving bone and joint, amyloidosis, psoas abscess leading to septic arthritis, osteomalacia secondary to malabsorption, and complications of steroid therapy including osteoporosis compression fractures and aseptic necrosis. These disorders are treated by therapy directed at the IBD, replacement of calcium and vitamin D, or withdrawal of the offending steroid agent.

VI. HEPATOBILIARY

Fatty infiltration, chronic active hepatitis primary biliary cirrhosis, and amyloidosis have all been described in association with IBD, especially in patients with colitis. The most frequently described disorder related to IBD and involving both the liver and biliary tree is primary sclerosing cholangitis (17). This entity, much more common in ulcerative colitis than Crohn's disease, occurs primarily in men and has an insidious onset with gradual progressive fatigue and pruritis followed by jaundice. Clinical evidence of cholangitis appears to be unusual and may indicate the presence of a complication such as gallstones or bile duct carcinoma. A cholestatic biochemical picture is a consistent finding.

Both intra- and extrahepatic bile ducts are involved with short annular strictures separated by intervening segments of normal or slightly dilated ducts producing a "beaded" appearance. The process leads to secondary changes in the liver with the eventual development of biliary cirrhosis.

There is no therapy of proven benefit for primary sclerosing cholangitis. Isolated cases have been reported to benefit from corticosteroids, immunosuppressives, and cholestyramine. A recent report describes two patients who responded to low-dose oral pulse methotrexate treatment (18). Based on data in primary biliary cirrhosis, a trial of penicillamine is in progress. Finally, in those patients who present with acute symptoms of cholangitis, appropriate parenteral antibiotics should be used before assuming a superimposed bacterial infection is not present.

The role of surgery in the treatment of primary sclerosing cholangitis has not been well established. It has been suggested that hepatobiliary drainage be reserved for the patient with severe pruritis and jaundice with a dominant extrahepatic stricture in whom balloon dilation by transhepatic or endoscopic routes has failed or is not possible.

Although an early report suggested that proctocolectomy could favorably influence the course of primary sclerosing cholangitis (19), subsequent experience suggests that the hepatobiliary disease has a course independent of the colitis and is not an indication for colectomy (17).

Finally, although often technically difficult because of bile duct scarring or prior surgery, liver transplantation has become a major consideration for patients with end-stage liver disease secondary to sclerosing cholangitis. The one-year survival of such patients with the advent of cyclosporin therapy is approaching 70%. Without such surgery patients are doomed to progressive liver failure.

As mentioned above, gallstones may complicate sclerosing cholangitis and lead to septic cholangitis. Gallstones also occur with increased frequency in patients with Crohn's ileitis where disease or resection of the terminal ileum results in diminished bile salt absorption and a decrease in the bile salt pool with an increase in the ratio of cholesterol to bile salts in bile rendering it lithogenic (1). Indications for cholecystectomy are similar for other patients with symptomatic gallstones but without Crohn's disease.

VII. RENAL

Enterovesical fistulas occur in a small number of patients with Crohn's disease (1). Pneumaturia, the one symptom which establishes the diagnosis, may be absent and only a history of recurrent bouts of cystitis provide a clue to the presence of this complication. The management of these fistulas is discussed in Chapter 14.

Obstructive hydronephrosis with flank pain and occasional urinary tract infection may result from extension of ileal disease into the surrounding mesentery and retroperitoneum with entrapment of the ureter (20) usually on the right side against the psoas muscle. Intravenous pyelography and CT scan reveal noncalculus hydroureter and hydronephrosis. An associated psoas abscess may result, as well, from further extension of the inflammation with fistulization. A similar process can involve the left ureter when either the sigmoid or descending colon is involved. This presentation demands resection of the involved intestine with ureterolysis.

Amyloidosis involving the kidneys is a rare complication. However, renal calculi are found in up to 10% of patients with IBD. Uric acid stones are especially common in patients with ileostomies due to chronic dehydration and low urine pH. Maintaining an adequate level of hydration and alkalinizing the urine by administration of bicarbonate may be all that is needed to prevent this complication.

In recent years, much interest has focused on the increased incidence of caclium oxalate stones in patients with IBD. These can present with with renal colic and oxalate deposition in the kidney may lead to renal impairment. Patients most prone to oxalate stones are those with intact colons who have steatorrhea usually secondary to extensive ileal disease and/or resection. In this setting, calcium is preferentially bound to fat in the gut lumen rendering oxalate more soluble and allowing it to be "hyperabsorbed" in the colon and to be excreted at high concentrations in the urine where calculi form. The increased colonic absorption also results from increased permeability of the colon probably related to calcium chelation by fat in the tight junctions (21).

Oxalate stone formation may be controlled in part by following a diet low in oxalate. High oxalate-containing foods include beets, rhubarb, spinach, cocoa, leeks, peanuts, raspberries, green beans, carrots, onion, grapes, squash, and chocolate. Tea and colas have a high oxalate content. A low-fat diet with medium chain triglyceride supplementation should be used to decrease steatorrhea. This will not only decrease the amount of fat available for calcium binding but also decrease diarrhea and hence fluid losses. Agents which bind to both oxalate and bile acids are also useful. Cholestyramine at a dose of 4 g three times a day can be effective, but should be avoided when fecal fat excretions exceed 20 g of fat per day since it will tend to worsen steatorrhea. Camelox, a combination of calcium carbonate, aluminum hydroxide, and magnesium hydroxide has been suggested as an especially effective agent to bind oxalate.

VIII. MALIGNANCY

Patients with ulcerative colitis involving the entire colon begin to be at risk for the development of colon cancer after 8 to 10 years of disease, regardless of the degree of colitis activity. Some have estimated a 20-fold increased risk after 20 years compared with age-matched controls. Macroscopically defined left-sided colitis produces an increased risk after 12-15 years, while disease limited to the rectum apparently does not place the patient at increased risk (22,23).

Although data for Crohn's disease patients are less extensive than for ulcerative colitis, there appears to be a four- to sixfold increased risk of colon cancer development for patients with Crohn's colitis. Patients with ileitis, especially those who have a bypassed segment, are also at increased risk for the development of small bowel adenocarcinoma (24,25).

Surveillance programs utilizing barium enema, rigid sigmoidoscopy, occult blood testing, and serum colonic embryonic antigen (CEA) determinations have not proved useful. On the other hand, prophylactic colectomy is not well accepted by the patient with relatively quiescent, albeit longstanding disease.

Recent attention has focused on colonic mucosal dysplasia as a marker for colon cancer. High-grade dysplasia consists of dysplastic cytologic changes in the colonic epithelium similar to preinvasive neoplastic changes in the epithelium of organs such as the cervix (26,27). In limited prospective studies involving colonoscopic surveillance of patients with longstanding extensive colitis, if high-grade dysplasia is noted, about one-quarter to one-half will have a carcinoma (28). In the future, flow cytometric DNA analysis may complement the search for dysplasia in early cancer detection (29).

On the basis of current available data, ulcerative colitis patients with pancolitis of 8-10 yearss duration should have colonoscopic surveillance with biopsies every 10 cm from inactive areas or areas of thickened mucosa or plaques. The procedure should be repeated at least every two years if no dysplasia is found. If the biopsies are read as indefinite or low-grade dysplasia, the colonoscopy should be repeated in three months after treatment of any active disease. If high-grade dysplasia is found and confirmed by a second pathologist, colectomy is suggested. A similar surveillance program is recommended for patients with Crohn's colitis of 10 years duration and for patients with left-sided ulcerative colitis for more than 12 years.

REFERENCES

1. Greenstein, A. J., H. D. Janowitz, D. B. Sachar, The extraintestinal complications of Crohn's disease and ulcerative colitis: A study of 700 patients, Medicine, 55:401-412 (1976).
2. Yassinger, S., R. Adelman, D. Cantor, Association of inflammatory bowel disease and large vascular lesions, Gastroenterology, 71:844-846 (1976).
3. Lam, A., I. Borda, M. Inwood, Coagulation studies in ulcerative colitis and Crohn's disease, Gastroenterology, 68:245-251 (1975).
4. Basler, R., Ulcerative colitis and the skin, Med. Clin. N. Am., 64:941-954 (1980).

5. Thornton, J. R., R. N. Teague, T. S. Low-Beer, Pyoderma gangrenosum and ulcerative colitis, Gut, 2:247–248 (1980).
6. Schorr-Lesnick, B., L. J. Brandt, Selected rheumatologic and dermatologic manifestations of inflammatory bowel disease, Am. J. Gastroenterol., 83: 216–223 (1988).
7. Galvin, E., M. Y. Flugelman, D. Rachmilewitz, Pyoderma gangrenosum complicating ulcerative colitis: Successful treatment with methylprednisolone therapy and dapsone, Am. J. Gastroenterol., 81:988–989 (1986).
8. DeCock, K. M., M. G. Thorne, The treatment of pyderma gangrenosum with sodium cromoglycate, Br. J. Dermatol., 102:231–233 (1980).
9. Saffouri, B., B. M. Horn, J. M. Mertesdorf, Treatment of pyoderma gangrenosum weith disodium cromoglycate, Dig. Dis. Sci., 29:183–185 (1984).
10. Cave, D. R., R. Burakoff, Pyoderma gangrenosum associated with ulcerative coliits: Treatment with disodium cromoglycate, Am. J. Gastroenterol., 82: 802–804 (1987).
11. Pitrello, E. A., M. McKinley, F. J. Taniole, Ocular manifestations of inflammatory bowel disease, Ann. Opthalmol., 14:356–360 (1982).
12. Basu, M. K., M. P. Asqui, R. A. Thompson, Oral manifestations of Crohn's disease, Gut, 16:249–254 (1975).
13. Schnitt, S. J., D. A. Antonioli, B. Jaffe, M. A. Peppercorn, Granulomatous Inflammation of minor salivary gland ducts: A new oral manifestation of Crohn's disease, Human Pathol., 18:405–407 (1987).
14. McEwen, C., C. Linug, J. B. Kirsner, Arthritis accompanying ulcerative colitis, Am. J. Med., 33:9230–9241 (1962).
15. Gravallese, E. M., F. G. Kantrowitz, Arthritic manifestations of inflammatory bowel disease, Am. J. Gastroenterol., 83:703–708 (1988).
16. Kaufman, H. J., H. C. Taubin, Nonsteroidal anti-inflammatory drugs activate quiescent inflammatory bowel disease, Ann. Intern. Med., 107:513–516 (1987).
17. LaRusso, N. F., R. H. Wiesner, J. Ludwig, R. L. MacCarty, Primary sclerosing cholangitis, N. Engl. J. Med., 310:899–903 (1984).
18. Kaplan, M. M., S. Arora, S. Pincus, Primary sclerosing cholangitis and low dose oral pulse methotrexate therapy, Ann. Intern. Med., 106:231–235 (1987).
19. Eade, M. N., W. J. Cooke, B. N. Brooke, Liver disease in ulcerative colitis: The long-term effect of colectomy, Ann. Intern. Med., 72:489–497 (1970).
20. Present, D. H., J. G. Rabinowitz, P. A. Banks, Obstructive hydronephrosis—a frequent but seldom recognized complication of granulomatous disease of the bowel, N. Engl. J. Med., 280:523–528 (1969).
21. Dobbins, J. W., Hyperoxaluria and nephrolithiasis in current therapy in gastroenterology and liver disease. (Bayless, T. M. ed.) Toronto, Philadelphia, B.C. Decker, Inc., pp. 175–179 (1986).
22. Greenstein, A. J., D. B. Sachar, H. Smith, Cancer in universal and left-sided ulcerative colitis: factors determining risk, Gastroenterology, 77:390–394 (1979).

23. Sachar, D. B., A. J. Greenstein, Cancer in ulcerative colitis: Good news and bad news, Ann. Intern. Med., 95:642–644 (1981).
24. Hamilton, S. R., Colorectal carcinoma in patients with Crohn's disease, Gastroenterology, 89:398–407 (1985).
25. Petras, R. E., S. H. Mir-Modjilessi, R. G. Farmer, Crohn's disease and intestinal carcinoma: a report of 11 cases with emphasis on associated epithelial dysplasia, Gastroenterology, 93:1307–1314 (1987).
26. Morson, B. C., L. S. C. Pang, Rectal biopsy as an aid to cancer control in ulcerative colitis, Gut, 8:413–434 (1967).
27. Lennard-Jones, J. E., B. C. Morson, J. K. Ritckie, Cancer in colitis: assessment of the individual risk by clinical and histological criteria, Gastroenterology, 73:1280–1289 (1977).
28. Nugent, F. W., R. C. Haggitt, P. A. Gilpin, Cancer in ulcerative colitis: results of a 13 year prospective biopsy surveillance program, Gastroenterology, 94:A327 (1988).
29. Hammargerg, C., C. Rubio, P. Slezak, Flow-cytometric DNA analysis as a means for early detection of malignancy in patients with chronic ulcerative colitis, Gut, 25:905-908 (1984).

11

Pregnancy and Nursing

Francis A. Farraye*

Beth Israel Hospital, Harvard Medical School, Boston, Massachusetts

Idiopathic inflammatory bowel disease (IBD) most commonly affects young adults. Issues dealing with management and potential risks of IBD during pregnancy are often raised by our patients.

Several recent studies have examined in detail the effects of IBD and its treatment on fertility and the outcome of pregnancy as well as the effects of pregnancy on the activity of the IBD (1-10). This chapter summarizes the information in these areas and stresses the medical management of IBD during pregnancy.

I. PREGNANCY AND IBD INTERACTIONS

A. Fertility in IBD

Although earlier literature suggested decreased fertility in women with ulcerative colitis, more recent studies have noted no impairment of fertility in these women. No effect of ulcerative colitis on male fertility has been seen. Unlike rectal surgery performed for cancer, total colectomy for ulcerative colitis in men has a low incidence of impotency. In Crohn's disease the data are more controversial with most studies suggesting impaired fertility in women with Crohn's

**Present affiliation*: Brigham and Women's Hospital, Beth Israel Hospital, Harvard Medical School, Boston, Massachusetts.

disease. Fielding and Cook (11) reported an infertility rate of 32%; patients with colonic disease had a higher incidence than those with small bowel disease (67% vs. 26%). More recently, Mayberry and Weterman reported the results of a multicenter review of women with Crohn's disease (12). They noted a 42% infertility rate in married women with Crohn's disease who practiced no method of birth control. The site of disease did not affect the incidence of infertility. These results are in contrast to results of Khosla and colleagues who noted an infertility rate of 12% in 112 married women with Crohn's disease which is similar to the general population (13).

As many as 86% of men who take sulfasalazine for the treatment of IBD have low sperm counts with impaired sperm motility as well as abnormal morphology (14,15). Men with inflammatory bowel disease not using sulfasalazine do not have these findings (16). These abnormalities which lead to infertility are reversible within 3 months of discontinuation of sulfasalazine (17,18). Recently it was demonstrated that switching from sulfasalazine to an oral 5-aminosalicylate (5-ASA) preparation leads to resolution of these abnormalities (19,20). Children born to fathers taking sulfasalazine do not have an increased risk of spontaneous abortion, prematurity, or congenital abnormalities.

B. Effect of Pregnancy on IBD

In general, pregnancy has no adverse effects on the activity of ulcerative colitis or Crohn's disease (21). Nielsen et al. studied 97 women with ulcerative colitis over 12 years and found that the risk of relapse was 34% during pregnancy and 32% in the same women when not pregnant (22). Willoughby and Truelove found similar results with 30% of women in remission at conception relapsing during pregnancy (23). If reactivation is to occur, it tends to do so in the first and second trimesters. These studies and others have noted that if the ulcerative colitis was active at the time of conception it will likely remain active and that fetal outcomes in these patients were worse when compared with patients with inactive disease. Overall, over half of the women with active disease at the time of conception had no change or increase in symptoms during pregnancy. The first attack of ulcerative colitis during pregnancy and the puerperium does not seem to be more severe than in the nonpregnant patient.

If Crohn's disease is in remission at the time of conception it will likely remain so. In the study by Khosla et al. from England, 44 of 52 (89%) women with Crohn's disease in remission at the time of conception remained in remission (13). Relapse, when it occurs usually does so in the first trimester. In women with active Crohn's disease at the time of conception only 7 of 20 (35%) attained a remission. Additionally, this group of women had a 35% rate of spontaneous abortions. Results from Denmark support these observations (24). Previous data suggested an increased risk of relapse in patients with Crohn's disease during the postpartum period, but these recent studies are not confirmatory.

C. Effect of IBD on Pregnancy

Disease activity appears to be the major determinant of fetal outcome in patients with IBD. In women with inactive ulcerative colitis or Crohn's disease, approximately 85% will have an uncomplicated pregnancy (2). This rate is similar to that in the general population. Patients with active disease at the time of conception have a higher rate of premature delivery and spontaneous abortion (13,22-24). Crohn's disease patients with active disease have the highest incidence of complications. The course of subsequent pregnancies is not related to the outcome or course of previous pregnancies.

The presence of IBD is not a contraindication to pregnancy. Ideally pregnancy should be delayed until the underlying IBD is inactive. Therapeutic abortion has not been shown to reverse the course of either ulcerative colitis or Crohn's disease.

II. DRUG THERAPY

The following sections will discuss the use of individual drugs during pregnancy and nursing. The use of total parenteral nutrition and pregnancy after ileostomy or ileal pouch-anal anastomosis also will be reviewed.

Drug use during pregnancy and nursing should be minimized and reserved for clear indications (25-27). However, as noted above, favorable maternal and fetal outcomes in pregnant women with inflammatory bowel disease are most dependent on the activity of the underlying disease. Measures to keep the bowel disease in remission or to control flares are more likely to lead to an uncomplicated pregnancy. The theoretical risks of certain drugs, therefore, should not obscure their ability to successfully treat the underlying bowel disease.

A. Corticosteroids

1. Use in Pregnancy

Prednisone can cross the placenta. However, in humans prednisone is rapidly converted to prednisolone and bound to serum proteins. Consequently, transplacental passage of prednisone is low with maternal serum concentrations 8-10 times greater than the fetus (28). Cortisol secretion rates in infants born to mothers receiving chronic prednisone treatment have been normal. Furthermore, fetal pituitary suppression is rarely seen in infants born to mothers taking corticosteroids.

In animals, prednisone use is associated with intrauterine growth retardation, cleft palates, and occasional other birth defects. Placental insufficiency is felt to be responsible for these effects. A number of past studies raised concerns about the use of steroids based on observations of intrauterine growth retardation and an increased rate of spontaneous abortions in pregnant women taking prednisone (29,30). It remains difficult, however, to dissociate the effect of the drug from the severity of the underlying systemic disorder which required steroid therapy.

Recent studies have supported the safety of steroids during pregnancy. A study of 264 infants did not suggest any fetal toxicity from the steroids (31). In a study of 56 pregnancies in 51 women with severe asthma requiring steroid therapy, there was a slightly higher incidence of premature and low-birthweight infants when compared with that expected in the general population. This appeared attributable in part to infants born to mothers who required emergency room visits or developed status asthmaticus (32). In a retrospective study, Mogadam and co-workers examined the fetal outcome, spontaneous abortion rate, and presence of birth defects in 186 pregnancies of women with IBD treated with steroids or steroids and sulfasalazine (33). No statistically significant complications could be attributed to drug therapy. Furthermore, low fetal weight was less common in these patients when compared with historical controls. In another study of 147 pregnancies, the frequency of fetal complications was higher in IBD patients requiring prednisone or sulfasalazine during pregnancy than in those IBD patients not treated (34). This was especially prominent in patients with underlying Crohn's disease. The authors felt that these results, however, were more likely related to disease activity rather than to drug treatment. Smaller studies from England and Denmark add further support to the safety of corticosteroid use in pregnancy when the underlying illness dictates their use (13,22-24). Close monitoring of serum glucose values is essential to detect hyperglycemia.

No studies on the safety of topical steroid therapy in pregnancy are available. However, in patients with markedly symptomatic ulcerative proctitis, steroid enemas should be considered as an alternative to systemic therapy.

2. Use in Nursing

Low levels of prednisone and its metabolite prednisolone can be found in breast milk. McKenzie et al. found a mean concentration of 0.14% (range 0.07-0.23) per liter of breast milk after a 5 mg oral dose of prednisone in 7 healthy women over a 48-hr period (35). In six women on variable doses of long-term prednisolone (10-80 mg/day), the milk concentration was 5-25% of the maternal serum concentration. At a daily dose of 80 mg of prednisolone the infant would ingest <0.1% of the dose corresponding to <10% of the endogenous cortisol production (36). At high doses of prednisone, these authors recommend avoiding breast feeding for 4 hr after the dose of prednisone.

It appears that breast feeding is safe, especially if low-dose prednisone is being used. The American Academy of Pediatrics feels that breast feeding is compatible with ongoing prednisone use (37).

B. Sulfasalazine

1. Use in Pregnancy

Although isolated case reports of birth defects in infants born to mothers taking sulfasalazine can be found in the literature (38-40), the bulk of data suggest that its use in pregnancy and during nursing is safe. A recent study reported that lymphocytes in IBD patients treated with sulfasalazine have a higher incidence of chromosomal abnormalities (sister chromatid exchange and micronucleus formation). Although of concern, the prognostic significance of these preliminary findings is not clear (41).

Sulfasalazine and its metabolite sulfapyridine are found in cord blood at concentrations between 50% to 100% of maternal blood (42,43). 5-ASA levels are negligible in cord blood. In Mogadam et al.'s review of 531 pregnancies in women with inflammatory disease (33), 186 patients were treated with either sulfasalazine or sulfasalazine and corticosteroids. The frequency of fetal complications was similar to patients with inflammatory bowel disease not requiring treatment. As in other studies, patients with active Crohn's disease had the highest rate of complications. In a study from England involving 147 women, treatment with sulfasalazine or sulfasalazine and corticosteroids in 54 pregnancies did not lead to an increased risk of birth defects or spontaneous abortion (23). Furthermore, a study from Denmark of 97 women having 173 pregnancies over a 12-year period found that treatment with sulfasalazine or sulfasalazine and corticosteroids in 68 pregnancies had no influence on the course or outcome of the pregnancy (22).

There are no data in humans as to the safety of topical or oral 5-ASA in pregnancy. In animal studies, using 5-8 times the maximum recommended dose in humans, no adverse fetal effects were detected. However, since serum levels after topical 5-ASA administration are similar to those seen in patients on sulfasalazine, it is likely that use of topical 5-ASA is as safe as sulfasalazine in pregnant women.

The available data support the continued use of sulfasalazine to maintain remission or its initiation to treat flares in the pregnant woman as in the patient who is not pregnant (44). Supplemental folic acid should be administered to such patients.

2. Use in Nursing

Although earlier reports in the literature suggested avoidance of sulfasalazine in women nearing parturition and advocated exchange transfusions prophylactically in infants born to mothers taking sulfasalazine (45), more recent studies have documented no risk of kernicterus. Studies of mammary transfer of sulfasalazine during nursing have shown that the concentration of sulfasalazine in milk varies from negligible amounts to approximately 30% of that found in maternal serum (42). Serum levels of 5-ASA in the mother are low, and consequently, 5-ASA levels in breast milk are not detectable. Although sulfapyridine levels in breast milk approach 40–60% (42,46,47) of the mother's serum level, sulfapyridine itself has minimal ability to displace bilirubin from albumin. Studies have documented that sulfasalazine-treated mothers and their infants have no significant changes in their albumin binding sites (48). Janerot and Into-Malmberg have calculated that a mother taking 2 g of sulfasalazine daily would expose her nursing infant to 3–4 mg/kg of sulfapyridine, which is considered negligible (46). There has been no well-documented case of kernicterus in the neonatal period attributable to sulfasalazine.

The American Association of Pediatrics places no restriction on the use of sulfasalazine during breast feeding (37).

C. Metronidazole

Although metronidazole causes malignancy in animals and is mutagenic in bacteria, it has not been shown to cause cancer in humans (49). Nevertheless the use of metronidazole in pregnancy and during nursing remains controversial. The drug crosses the placenta freely and can be found in amniotic fluid and in cord blood. Although the drug has been given to women throughout pregnancy without obvious adverse effect (50), its routine use cannot be recommended especially given the prolonged course often necessary in patients with Crohn's disease. Metronidazole is excreted into the breast milk (51) and found in infant serum at levels 20% that of the mother (52). Consequently, it should not be given to nursing mothers.

D. Immunosuppressives

Azathioprine and 6-mercaptopurine are being used more frequently in patients with inflammatory bowel disease unresponsive to conventional therapy. Both drugs cross the palcenta and can be found in cord blood (53). Several hundred normal pregnancies have been reported in patients with renal transplants and several in women with inflammatory bowel disease (54) on azathioprine and prednisone. However, intrauterine growth retardation and multiple fetal abnormalities have been seen in animals treated with azathioprine (55,56). Consequently, every effort must be made to taper the patient off immunosuppressives prior to conception. Although the risk to a particular patient is hard to define, if pregnancy occurs while on azathioprine or 6-mercaptopurine, termination of the pregnancy should be considered.

E. Antidiarrheal Agents

In animal studies, diphenoxylate with atropine (Lomotil) has been reported to cause impaired fertility and decreased maternal weight gain at 50 times the human dose (57). Teratogenic effects were not seen in these studies. In similar studies using loperamide (Imodium) no teratogenic effects were documented at 30 times the human dose (57). Although prospective human studies have not been performed, there are reports of malformations in humans after first trimester exposure to diphenoxylate with atropine (27). The use of these agents should be reserved for patients unresponsive to the addition of bulk agents or dietary manipulation. Although the American Academy of Pediatrics feels that the use of diphenoxylate with atropine is compatible with nursing (35), the drug is excreted into breast milk and adverse effects of the agent have been reported in neonates (27). No data are available for loperamide but use in nursing mothers is not recommended (27).

Cholestyramine has not been shown to have any adverse effects in animal studies (58) and the drug has been used in treatment of women with benign cholestasis of pregnancy (59). The lack of systemic absorption suggests that its use in pregnancy is safe. Vitamin supplementation should be given and prothrombin times monitored (25). As in nonpregnant patients, the drug should not be given simultaneously with other medications. No human data are available about breast feeding, but one would not anticipate problems in nursing mothers if vitamin supplementation is given. Kaopectate and bulk-forming agents (e.g., Metamucil) are safe in pregnancy (25).

III. TOTAL PARENTERAL NUTRITION (TPN)

In some clinical situations disease activity requires complete bowel rest (e.g., rectovaginal fistula, IBD flare unresponsive to conventional therapy, extensive small bowel strictures). TPN has safely been used in pregnant patients with many different disorders including Crohn's disease, pancreatitis, and radiation-induced strictures (60,61). In Crohn's patients, TPN has effectively supported fetal growth in both short-term situations as well as throughout pregnancy (62–64).

It remains controversial whether fat emulsion can be safely used in pregnancy as a source of calories and essential fatty acids. Although several successful pregnancies have been reported, some authors feel that use of lipid emulsions leads to prematurity secondary to placental insufficiency as a consequence of fat emboli.

IV. PREGNANCY WITH AN ILEOSTOMY OR ILEAL POUCH-ANAL ANASTOMOSIS

Many women with a Brooke ileostomy have successfully completed term pregnancies (65,66). Occasional problems with the ileostomy stoma can develop as the uterus enlarges, but these usually can be managed conservatively. The most serious complication, although infrequent, is small bowel obstruction which may require surgical correction (67). There is no contraindication to vaginal delivery in patients with a Brooke ileostomy. It seems prudent to recommend a one-year waiting period after creation of the stoma before becoming pregnant.

More recently, successful term pregnancies have been reported in women who have had an ileal pouch-anal anastomosis (68). In three of six patients reported from the Lahey clinic there was some transient deterioration of anorectal function in the third trimester which resolved after delivery (69). Both vaginal and Cesarian deliveries have been performed.

V. SUMMARY

Based on the data reviewed above and clinical observations made over the past 30 years several conclusions can be drawn (10).

1. The majority of pregnant women with inflammatory bowel disease will have a normal infant.
2. There does not appear to be any adverse effect of pregnancy on IBD nor inactive IBD on pregnancy.
3. Active disease at the time of conception or during pregnancy requiring drug treatment is associated with a higher rate of complication. Overall, patients with Crohn's disease do less well than those with ulcerative colitis.
4. Initiation of drug treatment in women with active disease with sulfasalazine and/or prednisone is safe in pregnancy and during nursing. Sulfasalazine may be continued if needed to maintain remission in ulcerative colitis. The lowest dose of sulfasalazine and/or prednisone necessary to control symptoms should be used.
5. Immunosuppressive agents and metronidazole should be avoided if possible during pregnancy and nursing.
6. Total parenteral nutrition can be used safely in pregnancy when alternative therapy fails.
7. Successful full-term pregnancy can be expected in the patient with ileostomy or ileal pouch-anal anastomosis.

REFERENCES

1. Vender, R. J., H. M. Spiro, Inflammatory bowel disease and pregnancy, J. Clin. Gastroenterol., 4:231–249 (1982).
2. Jarnerot, G., Fertility, sterility and pregnancy in chronic inflammatory bowel disease, Scand. J. Gastroenterol., 17:1–4 (1982).
3. Warsolf, S. L., Medical and surgical treatment of inflammatory bowel disease in pregnancy, Clin. Obstet. Gynecol., 26:822–831 (1983).
4. Sorokin, J. J., S. M. Levine, Pregnancy and inflammatory bowel disease: a review of the literature, Obstet. Gynecol., 62:247–252 (1983).

5. Fielding, J. F., Pregnancy and inflammatory bowel disease, Irish J. Med. Sci. 151:194-202 (1982).
6. Donaldson, R. M., Management of medical problems in pregnancy—inflammatory bowel disease, N. Engl. J. Med., 312:1616-1619 (1985).
7. Hanan, I. M., J. B. Kirsner, Inflammatory bowel disease in the pregnant woman, Clin. Perinatol., 12:669-682 (1985).
8. Gilat, T., Y. Buganover, Inflammatory bowel disease and reproduction. In: Bockus Gastroenterology, 4th edition. (J. E. Berk, ed.) Philadelphia, Saunders (1985).
9. Miller, J. P., Inflammatory bowel disease in pregnancy: a review, J. R. Soc. Med., 76:221-225 (1986).
10. Korelitz, B. I., Fertility and pregnancy in inflammatory bowel disease. In: Inflammatory Bowel Disease. (J. B. Kirsner, R. G. Shorter, eds.) Philadelphia, Lea & Febiger (1988).
11. Fielding, J. F., W. T. Cooke, Pregnancy and Crohn's disease, Br. Med. J., 2: 76-77 (1970).
12. Mayberry, J. F., I. T. Weterman, European survey of fertility and pregnancy in woman with Crohn's disease: a case control study by European collaborative group, Gut, 27:821-825 (1986).
13. Khosla, R., C. P. Willoughby, D. P. Jewell, Crohn's disease and pregnancy, Gut, 25:52-56 (1984).
14. Birnie, G. C., T. I. F. McLead, G. Watkinson, Incidence of sulfasalazine-induced male infertility, Gut, 22:452-455 (1981).
15. Toovey, S., E. Hudson, W. F. Hendry, A. J. Levi, Sulphasalazine and male infertility: Reversibility and possible mechanism, Gut, 22:445-451 (1981).
16. O'Morain, C., P. Smethurst, C. J. Dore, A. J. Levi, Reversible male infertility due to sulphasalazine: Studies in man and rat, Gut, 25:1078-1084 (1984).
17. Levi, A. J., A. M. Fisher, L. Hughes, W. F. Hendry, Male infertility due to sulfasalazine, Lancet, 2:276-278 (1979).
18. Toth, A., Reversible toxic effect of salicylazosulfapyridine on semen quality, Fertil. Steril., 31:538-540 (1979).
19. Cann, P. A., C. D. Holdsworth, Reversal of male infertility on changing treatment from sulfasalazine to 5-aminosalicylic acid, Lancet, 1:1119 (1984).
20. Shaffer, J. L., A. Kershaw, M. H. Berrisford, Sulfasalazine induced infertility reversed on transfer to 5-aminosalicylic acid, Lancet, 31:1240 (1984).
21. Mogadam, M., B. I. Korelitz, S. W. Ahmed, W. O. Dobbins, The course of inflammatory bowel disease during pregnancy and postpartum, Am, J. Gastroenterol., 75:265-269 (1981).
22. Nielsen, O. H., B. Andreasson, S. Bondesen, S. Jarnum, Pregnancy in ulcerative colitis, Scand. J. Gastroenterol., 18:735-742 (1983).
23. Willoughby, C. P., S. C. Truelove, Ulcerative colitis and pregnancy, Gut, 21:469-474 (1980).

24. Nielsen, O. H., B. Andreasson, S. Bondesen, Pregnancy in Crohn's disease, Scand. J. Gastroenterol., 19:724–732 (1984).
25. Berkowitz, R. L., In: Handbook for Prescribing Medications During Pregnancy. (D. R. Coustan, T. K. Mochizuki, eds.). Boston, Little Brown and Company (1986).
26. Briggs, G. G., R. K. Freeman, S. J. Yoffe, Drugs in Pregnancy and Lactation. Baltimore, Williams & Wilkins (1986).
27. Lewis, J. H., A. B. Weingold, The use of gastrointestinal drugs during pregnancy and lactation, Am. J. Gastroenterol., 80:912–923 (1985).
28. Beitins, I. Z., F. Bayard, I. G. Ances, A. Kowaiski, C. J. Migeon, The transplacental passage of prednisone and prednisolone in pregnancy near term, J. Pediatr., 81:936–945 (1982).
29. Warrell, D. W., R. Taylor, Outcome for the foetus of mothers receiving prednisolone during pregnancy, Lancet, 1:117–118 (1968).
30. Reinisch, J. M., N. G. Simon, W. G. Karow, R. Gandelman, Prenatal exposure to prednisone in humans and animals retards intrauterine growth, Science, 202:436–438 (1978).
31. Bongiovanni, A. M., A. J. McPadden, Steroids during pregnancy and possible fetal consequences, Fertil. Steril., 11:181–186 (1960).
32. Fitzsimmons, R., P. A. Greenberger, R. Patterson, Outcome of pregnancy in women requiring corticosteroids for severe asthma, J. Aller. Clin. Immunol., 78:349–353 (1988).
33. Mogadam, M., W. O. Dobbins, B. I. Korelitz, S. W. Ahmed, Pregnancy in inflammatory bowel disease: effect of sulfasalazine and corticosteroids on fetal outcome, Gastroenterology, 80:72–76 (1981).
34. Baiocco, R. J., B. I. Korelitz, The influence of inflammatory bowel disease and its treatment on pregnancy and fetal outcome, J. Clin. Gastroneterol., 6:211–216 (1984).
35. McKenzie, S. A., J. A. Selley, J. E. Agnew, Secretion of prednisolone into breast milk, Arch. Dis. Childhood., 50:894–896 (1975).
36. Ost, L., G. Wettrell, I. Bjorhom, A. Rane, Prednisolone excretion in human milk, J. Pediatr., 106:1008–1011 (1985).
37. Committee on drugs, American Academy of Pediatrics. The transfer of drugs and other chemicals into human breast milk, Pediatrics, 72:375–383 (1983).
38. Craxi, A., F. Pagliarello, Possible embryotoxicity of sulfasalazine, Arch. Intern. Med., 140:74 (1980).
39. Newman, N. M., J. F. Correy, Possible teratogenicity of sulphasalazine, Med. J. Aust., 1:528–529 (1983).
40. Hoo, J. J., T. A. Hadro, P. Von Behren, Possible teratogenicity of sulfasalazine (letter), N. Engl. J. Med., 318:1128 (1988).
41. MacKay, J. M., D. P. Fox, P. W. Brunt, G. M. Hawkins, J. E. Brown, Sulphasalazine causes chromosome changes in patients with inflammatory bowel disease, Gut, 27:A1271 (1986).
42. Azad Khan, A. Z., S. C. Truelove, Placental and mammary transfer of sulphasalazine, Br. Med. J., 2:1553 (1979).

43. Jarnerot, G., M. B. Into-Malmberg, E. Esbjorner, Placental transfer of sulphasalazine and sulfapyridine and some of its metabolites, Scand. J. Gastroenterol., 16:693-697 (1981).
44. Peppercorn, M. A., Sulfasalazine: pharmacology, clinical use, toxicity and related new drug development, Ann. Intern. Med., 101:377-386 (1984).
45. Hensleigh, P. A., R. E. Kauffman, Maternal absorption and placental transfer of sulfasalazine, Am. J. Obstet. Gynecol., 127:443-444 (1977).
46. Jarnerot, G., M. B. Into-Malmberg, Sulphasalazine treatment during breast feeding, Scand. J. Gastroenterol., 14:869-871 (1979).
47. Berlin, C. M., S. J. Yaffe, Disposition of salicylazosulfapyridine (Azulfidine) and metabolites in human breast milk, Dev. Pharmacol. Ther., 1:31-39 (1980).
48. Jarnerot, G., S. Anderson, E. Esbjorner, B. Sandstrom, Albumin reserve for binding of bilirubin in maternal and cord serum under treatment with sulphasalazine, Scand. J. Gastroenterol., 16:1049-1055 (1981).
49. Beard, C. M., K. L. Noller, W. M. O'Fallon, L. T. Kurland, M. B. Dockerty, Lack of evidence for cancer due to use of metronidazole, N. Engl. J. Med., 301:519-522 (1979).
50. Roe, F. J. C., Toxicologic evaluation of metronidazole with particular reference to carcinogenic, mutagenic and teratogenic potential, Surgery, 93:158-164 (1983).
51. Erickson, S. H., G. L. Oppenheim, G. H. Smith, Metronidazole in breast milk, Obstet. Gynecol., 57:48-50 (1981).
52. Heisterberg, L., P. E. Branebjerg, Blood and milk concentrations of metronidazole in mothers and infants, J. Perinat. Med., 11:114-120 (1983).
53. Saarikoski, S., M. Seppala, Immunosuppression during pregnancy: transmission of azathioprine and its metabolites from the mother to the fetus, Am. J. Obstet. Gynecol., 115:1100-1106 (1973).
54. Levy, N., I. Roisman, I. Teodor, Ulcerative colitis in pregnancy in Israel, Dis. Colon Rectum, 24:351-354 (1981).
55. Rosenkrantz, J. C., J. H. Githens, S. M. Cox, Azathioprine (Imuran) and pregnancy, Am. J. Obstet. Gynecol., 97:387 (1967).
56. Scott, J. R., Fetal growth retardation associated with maternal administration of immunosuppressive drugs, Am. J. Obstet. Gynecol., 128:668-676 (1976).
57. Physicians Desk Reference. 42nd edition. Oradell NJ, Medical Economics Company, (1988).
58. Innis, S. M., Effect of cholestyramine administration during pregnancy in the rat, Am. J. Obstet. Gynecol., 146:13-16 (1983).
59. Laatikainen, T., Effect of cholestyramine and phenobarbital on pruritis and serum bile acid levels in cholestasis of pregnancy, Am. J. Obstet. Gynecol., 132:501-6 (1978).
60. Hew, I. R., M. Deitel, Total parenteral nutrition in gynecology and obstetrics, Obstet. Gynecol., 55:464-468 (1980).

61. Rivera-Alsina, M. E., L. R. Saldana, C. A. Stringer, Fetal growth sustained by parenteral nutrition in pregnancy, Obstet. Gynecol., 64:138-141 (1984).
62. Main, A. N. H., A. Shenkins, W. P. Black, R. I. Russell, Intravenous feedings to sustain pregnancy in a patient with Crohn's disease, Br. Med. J., 283: 1221-1222 (1981).
63. Tresadern, J. C., G. F. Falconer, L. A. Turnberg, M. H. Irving, Successful completed pregnancy in a patient maintained on home parenteral nutrition, Br.Med. J., 286:602-603 (1983).
64. Nugent, F. W., M. Rajala, R. A. O'Shea, Total parental nutrition in pregnancy conception to delivery, J. Parent. Enteral. Nutr., 11:424-427 (1987).
65. Morowitz, D. A., J. B. Kirsner, J. B., Ileostomy in ulcerative colitis: a questionnaire study of 1803 patients, Am. J. Surg., 141:370-5 (1981).
66. Gopal, K. A., A. L. Amshel, I. L. Shonberg, Levinson, K. A., VonWert, M., VonWert, J., Ostomy and pregnancy, Dis. Colon Rectum, 28:912-916 (1985).
67. Hudson, C. N., Ileostomy in pregnancy, Proc. R. Soc. Med., 65:281-283 (1972).
68. Pezim, M. E., Successful child birth after restorative proctocolectomy with pelvic reservoir, Br. J. Surg., 71:292 (1984).
69. Metcalf, A., R. R. Dozois, R. W. Beart, Wolff, B. G. Pregnancy following ileal pouch-anal anastomosis, Dis. Colon Rectum, 28:859-861 (1985).

12
The Pediatric Patient

Richard J. Grand

Boston Floating Hospital, New England Medical Center, Tufts University School of Medicine, Boston, Massachusetts

Kathleen J. Motil

USDA/ARS Children's Nutrition Research Center, Baylor College of Medicine, Houston, Texas

In general, the management of pediatric patients with inflammatory bowel disease (IBD) is based on the same principles as in adults, however, certain features of the diseases in the young patient demand age-specific concepts of treatment and therapeutic approaches.

Guidelines for the management of inflammatory bowel disease in children are summarized in Table 1. The aims of treatment are to induce and maintain a remission of disease activity, to correct nutritional deficits, and to restore normal growth and sexual maturation. These goals may be accomplished by the use of individual or combined modalities including drug therapy, nutritional support, surgery, and psychological support.

I. DRUG THERAPY

A. Ulcerative Colitis

The treatment of ulcerative colitis in children is directed toward control of disease activity, prevention of relapses, and maintenance of long-term remission. Although some patients will have one episode of illness without frequent recurrences, most children have more active and extensive disease than adults (1). Regardless of the severity of the disease, ulcerative colitis can usually be controlled medically or cured surgically.

A mild attack of ulcerative colitis characterized by diarrhea, abdominal pain, minimal rectal bleeding, and weight loss usually responds to sulfasalazine (40–50

Table 1 Guidelines for the Management of Inflammatory Bowel Disease

Aims of treatment
Induction and maintenance of remission of disease activity
Correction of body nutrient deficits
Restoration of normal growth and sexual maturation
Modalities of treatment
Pharmacologic agents
Nutritional support
Surgery
Psychologic support

mg/kg/day, in three divided doses, maximum 3-4 g/day), and does not require administration of systemic corticosteroids (Table 2). When disease is confined to the rectum, particularly in the presence of tenesmus, topical 5-aminosalicylate or corticosteroid preparations may be effective. Hydrocortisone foam is retained more easily than a liquid enema; however, the topical treatments penetrate unpredictably and may extend only as far as the sigmoid colon. Young children frequently fail to retain therapeutic enemas, and this may limit the efficacy of these forms of treatment.

In moderate attacks, bloody diarrhea, more than six times per day and occurring at night, colicky abdominal pain, and tenesmus are common symptoms. In addition, fever, malaise, anorexia, weight loss, leukocytosis, and mild anemia may be present. Children in this clinical category should be admitted to the hospital. Prednisone or prednisolone is effective when given as a single dose, orally or parenterally (1-2 mg/kg/day, maximum 3 mg/kg/day), or in divided doses. Using this regimen, clinical improvement should occur within 2 weeks. The dose should then be reduced by 5 mg decrements weekly or every two weeks. As an alternative, a 24-hr intravenous infusion of ACTH (1.6-2.0 U/kg) may be more efficacious than steroids in controlling an attack of ulcerative colitis when given for a first episode or when the patient has not received corticosteroid therapy recently (2).

Anticholinergics, opioids, and their analogues should be avoided because they may precipitate the development of a toxic megacolon (3). In addition, dehydration, serum electrolyte disorders, anemia, and hypoalbuminemia should be corrected. Hemoglobin and serum albumin levels should be maintained above 9 g/dl and 2.5 g/dl, respectively. Magnesium deficiency may complicate diarrheal disorders, particularly colitis (4). However, total body magnesium status is not always reflected by hypomagnesemia; hence, the diagnosis rests upon the excretion of less than 40% of a test dose of parenteral magnesium in 24 hr (5). Overall nutritional status should be maintained by total parenteral nutrition during a severe attack.

As in adults, sulfasalazine has both a prophylactic and therapeutic effect in ulcerative colitis (6). Therefore, once an improvement from corticosteroids is evident, sulfasalazine therapy should be initiated in an effort to maintain remission when corticosteroids are reduced. Children at risk for glucose-6-phosphate dehydrogenase deficiency should be screened prior to therapy. Complete blood counts should be obtained routinely in children on long-term sulfasalazine to detect potential side effects, and folic acid (1 mg daily) should be prescribed concurrently to avoid folate malabsorption.

Although corticosteroids are effective in the induction of remission in 75% of patients, the role of these drugs in prophylaxis is limited. Immunosuppressives, for example, azathioprine (2 mg/kg/day) or 6-mercaptopurine (1.5 mg/kg/day), may have a corticosteroid-sparing effect in chronic active ulcerative colitis (7). However, a child who requires long-term corticosteroids in doses high enough to produce significant side effects or to require an immunosuppressive, may benefit more from colectomy. Recent studies failed to detect a beneficial prophylactic or therapeutic effect of disodium cromoglycate in ulcerative colitis. There is no evidence that nutritional therapy, such as elemental diets or total parenteral nutrition induces a remission or shows greater beneft than that obtained from corticosteroids. However, the maintenance of good nutritional status is imperative in all patients with active disease.

Fulminant ulcerative colitis in children is a medical emergency (Table 3). The major features of a fulminant attack include grossly bloody diarrhea, fever, tachycardia, anemia, leukocytosis, hypoalbuminemia, and electrolyte disturbances (8). Most such children require blood transfusions and albumin infusions. Correction of fluid and electrolyte disturbances is necessary in all patients. Parenteral corticosteroids (methylprednisolone 3 mg/kg/day, maximum 90 mg daily) or ACTH (2.0 U/kg/day continuous IV) should be administered, as well as broad-spectrum antibiotics (synthetic penicillins, gentamicin, and clindamycin). Although parenteral nutrition does not induce remission with greater frequency

Table 2 Treatment of Ulcerative Colitis Mild to Moderate Attack

Rest at home
Low-residue, high-protein and energy diet, ± lactose-free
Multivitamins with minerals, elemental iron (6 mg/kg/day in three divided doses), folate (1 mg daily)
Loperamide (0.1–0.2 mg/kg/day, in three divided doses, maximum 6–8 mg daily) as needed
Sulfasalazine (40–50 mg/kg/day, in three divided doses, maximum 3–4 g daily)
Prednisone (1–2 mg/kg/day, as a single or two divided doses, maximum 40–60 mg daily)
Hydrocortisone, topical (1-2 rectal suppositories or foam treatments, twice daily)

Table 3 Treatment of Ulcerative Colitis—Fulminant Attack

Acute phase
- Hospitalize
- NPO
- Correct dehydration, electrolyte (K, Mg) losses, anemia, hypoalbuminemia
- Abdominal x-rays (upright, supine), avoid barium enema
- Intravenous corticosteroids (methylprednisolone 2 mg/kg/day, in two divided doses, maximum 3 mg/kg/day; ACTH 2 U/kg by continuous 24-hr infusion)
- Intravenous broad-spectrum antibiotics (semisynthetic penicillins, gentamicin, clindamycin)
- Total parenteral nutrition

Recovery phase
- Prednisone (1-2 mg/kg/day, as single or two divided doses, maximum 40-60 mg daily)
- Sulfasalazine (40-50 mg/kg/day, in three divided doses, maximum 3-4 g daily)
- Low-residue, high-protein and energy diet, ± lactose-free
- Multivitamins with minerals, elemental iron (6 mg/kg/day, in three divided doses), folate (1 mg/daily)

than corticosteroids alone, most children with fulminant disease are in a catabolic state and require nutritional therapy for this reason alone.

Careful clinical observation and hematologic and biochemical monitoring of the child with fulminant colitis must be emphasized. Toxic megacolon should be searched for by erect and supine abdominal radiographs, performed twice daily if necessary. Frequent changes of the child's position in bed and nasogastric suction may reduce the risk of toxic megacolon. Approximately one-third of children with fulminant colitis respond to medical treatment within 2 weeks; prolongation of medical therapy beyond this time is associated with a substantial increase in the incidence of complications (8). More than 50% of these children require surgery within 2 months because of failed medical treatment, massive bleeding, colonic perforation, or toxic megacolon. The majority of children responding to medical treatment require colectomy within 2 years (8).

The development of toxic megacolon in conjunction with fulminant colitis is indicated by marked abdominal distention and tenderness, paucity or absence of bowel sounds, and the persistence of dilated loops of gas-filled colon with or without areas of mucosal edema as seen on plain abdominal radiographs. The child appears ill, febrile, and has increasing tachycardia. Leukocytosis, electrolyte disturbances, and hypoalbuminemia usually are present. Gram-negative sepsis and massive hemorrhage may occur. Colonic perforation is indicated by increasing abdominal distention and tenderness, and confirmed by free intraperitoneal gas on a lateral decubitus radiograph. The clinical signs of this life-threatening complication may be masked by concomitant corticosteroid therapy. The initial management of toxic megacolon is the same as that for fulminant colitis; however, it is essential to avoid persistent medical management unless there is unequivocal and objective evidence of rapid improvement within 48 to 72 hr. Prolonged medical treatment is associated with a 30% mortality rate; in the presence of a perforation, even with surgical treatment, the mortality rate is 50%. Thus, early colectomy is indicated in the absence of rapid improvement following the institution of intensive medical treatment. Children who develop toxic megacolon require early colectomy; therefore, it is important to prepare the child and the family for this outcome early in the course of a fulminant attack.

B. Crohn's Disease

In contrast to ulcerative colitis, there is no evidence that any drug alters the long-term natural history of Crohn's disease. However, a variety of agents are useful in the management of various manifestations of the disease. Corticosteroids have been the mainstay of treatment in Crohn's disease. Remission may be achieved in about 70% of patients, but often is short-term. Approximately 70% of patients treated with corticosteroids will relapse within 12 months. Moreover, their use may be associated with an increased relapse rate following surgery. Although corticosteroids may interfere with normal growth, not infrequently the use of corticosteroids in the control of inflammation results in the reversal of growth arrest (9,10). The indications for corticosteroid therapy in children with Crohn's disease include symptomatic disease too extensive for surgery, systemic and extraintestinal complications, and postoperative recurrences of disease that preclude further surgery (Table 4).

For the induction of remission, prednisone is begun in high dosages (2 mg/kg/day), maximum 40-60 mg daily) and reduced within 2 to 3 weeks following symptomatic improvement and evidence of remission by laboratory testing.

Table 4 Indications for Corticosteroids in Crohn's Disease

Severe symptomatic disease unresponsive to usual supportive therapy
Diffuse small bowel disease too extensive for surgery
Malnutrition, malabsorption
Fever
Severe, recurrent pain
Extraintestinal disease (eye, skin, joints, hemolytic anemia)
Postoperative recurrence when further surgery is to be avoided

The dose is further reduced gradually by 5 mg decrements over 4-6 weeks, tapered first to alternate day dosage, then reduced and stopped if feasible. Some patients experience a recurrence of their symptoms when the dose is lower than 0.3 mg/kg per day. In these patients, alternate day corticosteroids may control their symptoms without affecting growth (9).

Immunosuppressives (azathioprine, 6-mercaptopurine) have a useful role in the maintenance of remission while corticosteroid dosing is reduced in children (7,10). However, the average time for improvement with immunosuppressive therapy may be as long as three months. In our personal experience with 30 young patients, azathioprine has been effective in facilitating a remission in 75% while allowing reduction of corticosteroid dosage (7). Treatment should be monitored with frequent blood counts, liver function tests and amylase determinations, and other surveillance as in adults. Withdrawal of immunosuppressive agents usually is initiated slowly after 12 to 24 months of a symptom-free remission, but may be maintained at lower doses for longer periods of time. Sulfasalazine (40-50 mg/kd/day, maximum 3-4 g/day) is useful in the management of symptomatic Crohn's colitis; however, in contrast to ulcerative colitis, this drug does not have a prophylactic effect in Crohn's disease. Some children experience nausea, vomiting, or bloody diarrhea after the initiation of treatment (11); such symptoms can be avoided by beginning with small doses that are increased gradually or by replacing sulfasalazine with another 5-aminosalicylate preparation. Oligospermia appears to be reversible, but is worrisome in children on long-term treatment.

Recently, metronidazole has been shown to be effective in the treatment of Crohn's disease, particularly in patients with colonic and perianal disease and fistulas (12). Metronidazole (15-20 mg/kg/day, maximum 1 g/day) currently is recommended in patients with colitis who fail to respond to sulfasalazine, those with significant perianal disease, and in patients with small bowel bacterial overgrowth.

In some patients, *Clostridium difficile* may be a pathogen associated with persistent diarrhea and rectal blood loss. Vancomycin (40 mg/kg/day, maximum 2 g/day) or metronidazole (15 mg/kg/day) should be administered to those patients with toxin-positive stools. In children in whom diarrhea follows extensive ileocolic resection or dysfunction, loperamide (0.1-0.2 mg/kg/day, maximum 6-8 mg/day) may provide symptomatic relief. The dose of loperamide should be titrated such that intestinal transit time is lengthened and the frequency of diarrhea is reduced. Diarrhea due to increased amounts of bile acids entering the colon following the partial resection of terminal ileum may respond to oral cholestyramine (0.25 g/kg/day in four divided doses, maximum 16 g/day). There is no evidence that dietary manipulation aids in the induction of remission in ulcerative colitis; however, foods high in residue that aggravate diarrhea should be avoided until disease activity is controlled.

II. NUTRITIONAL THERAPY

Indications for nutritional therapy include its use as primary or supportive therapy for active disease, to correct specific nutrient deficiencies, or to manage complications of inflammatory bowel disease (13-22, Table 5). With respect to disease activity, nutritional regimens have been advocated as primary modes of therapy in certain clinical settings: (1) Newly diagnosed inflammatory bowel disease; (2) chronic disease unresponsive to medical management; (3) short bowel syndrome; (4) acute obstruction; (5) closure of fistulas; (6) healing of ostomy sites; (7) as supportive therapy for disease that is too extensive and diffuse for surgical excision; or (8) in the preparation for surgical procedures related to disease activity. Nutritional supplementation also has a primary role in the treatment of the nutritional complications of inflammatory bowel disease, including malnutrition. In Crohn's disease, disease activity diminishes and nutritional status improves with nutritional therapy, as does body weight, erythrocyte sedimentation rate, and serum total protein, albumin, and transferrin levels. Moreover, with adequate nutritional support, it is often possible to reduce or

Table 5 Indications for Nutritional Therapy in Inflammatory Bowel Disease

Primary therapy for disease activity
Active acute inflammatory bowel disease
Chronic disease unresponsive to medical therapy
Closure of fistulas
Short bowel syndrome
Small bowel obstruction
Ostomy care
Supportive therapy for disease activity
Preoperative nutritional rehabilitation
Inoperable diffuse disease
Drug–nutrient interactions
Sulfasalazine (increases folate requirements)
Specific nutrient deficiencies
Anemia (microcytic, macrocytic)
Hypoproteinemia
Fat malabsorption
Lactose intolerance
Serum mineral deficiency (Fe, K, Ca, Mg)
Serum vitamin deficiency (folate, B_{12}, A, D)
Prolonged prothrombin time (vitamin K)
Depressed alkaline phosphatase (Zn)
Complications of inflammatory bowel disease
Malnutrition
Growth failure

discontinue entirely the dosage of corticosteroids administered, even in the corticosteroid-dependent patient (14-16). This feature is extremely important in children in order to minimize the potential side effects of these drugs.

The impact of malnutrition on growth failure in inflammatory bowel disease is emphasized by the findings of studies of nutritional repletion. Improved linear and ponderal growth rates are commonly observed in adolescents with Crohn's disease who receive continuous enteral feedings (>2.5 g/kg protein and >90 kcal/kg daily) via the nasogastric route, as well as those who are supplemented orally with daily protein and energy intakes of 13-26 g and 600-2100 kcal, respectively. These observations demonstrate that the gastrointestinal tract can be utilized in the nutritional rehabilitation of many children and adolescents with inflammatory bowel disease.

In our own clinics, a program of long-term nutritional supplementation is initiated for severely growth-retarded children with Crohn's disease (20,22,23). Adolescents who have sustained significant deficits in their lean body and visceral protein masses are supplemented with a commercially prepared liquid formula that provides up to 1500 ml nightly via a silastic nasogastric feeding tube or feeding gastrostomy. The addition of a nutritional supplement to the customary dietary intake provides the patients with a daily protein and energy intake of approximately 3.0 g/kg and 95 kcal/kg, respectively. In published studies, after three weeks of nutritional supplementation, body weight increased by 10%, nitrogen, calcium, magnesium, and phosphorus balances improved two- to fourfold, and total body potassium (^{40}K), a measure of lean body mass, increased significantly (22,23) (Table 6). The mechanisms responsible for this improvement in nutritional status include increased rates of amino acid incorporation into newly synthesized protein and reduced rates of amino acid oxidation. Basal metabolic rates also increase to accommodate the deposition of nutrients and the synthesis of new tissues. After 7 months of nutritional supplementation, the average height and weight velocities are five times greater than those observed prior to supplementation, and equal or exceed the growth velocities of normal adolescents (20). Thus, malnutrition and growth failure in inflammatory bowel disease are unrelated to intrinsic defects in the pathways of body protein and energy metabolism. In addition, although fecal nutrient losses in adolescents with Crohn's disease are greater than those in healthy children, nutritional supplementation does not augment fecal nutrient losses in these patients. Moreover, neither the presence of inflammation nor the use of corticosteroids interfere with the ability to rehabilitate these children nutritionally.

When abdominal symptoms, such as severe diarrhea, abscesses, or fistulas prevent enteral nutrition, intravenous nutritional therapy can produce a remission, provide nutritional rehabilitation, and reverse growth arrest (15,18,21). Adolescents who receive intravenous energy intakes of nearly 140% of their oral allowances for height age demonstrate an average weight gain of 5 kg after

Table 6 Effect of Nutritional Supplementation on Body Composition, Mineral and Protein Metabolism, and Growth in Adolescents with Inflammatory Bowel Disease

Measurement	Dietary Interval	
	Presupplement	Postsupplement
Body composition, weight (kg)	39	41
Nitrogen retention (mg/kg/d)	36	137
Total body potassium (g)	80	87
Calcium retention (mg/kg/d)	7	19
Magnesium retention (mg/kg/d)	0	4
Phosphorus retention (mg/kg/d)	18	34
Whole body protein and energy metabolism		
Amino acid incorporation (mg/kg/day)	269	447
Amino acid oxidation (mg/kg/day)	262	154
"Basal" oxygen consumption (ml/min/m^2)	156	206
Growth velocity		
Height (cm/6 mo)	0.6	3.0
Weight (cm/6 mo)	1.3	7.3

8 weeks of parenteral therapy. A significant proportion of the total body weight accrued is lean body mass as determined by total body potassium (^{40}K) content and urinary creatinine excretion. Moreover, after intravenous alimentation, the growth rate increases threefold compared with the pretreatment rate and equals that of healthy adolescents (21). These studies emphasize the importance of nutritional considerations in the management of malnutrition and growth failure in children with inflammatory bowel disease.

In the nutritional care of ill children and adolescents, the goals are: (1) to promote normal metabolic functions, (2) to replace nutrient losses associated with inflammatory processes, (3) to correct body deficits, and (4) to promote catch-up growth. To achieve these goals, appropriate assessment of nutritonal status should be performed in all children with inflammatory bowel disease, but should be reviewed at least every 6 months. The history should focus on previous growth measurements, the type, extent, and duration of inflammatory bowel disease, and the medications used by the patient. A three-day diet record provides an overall evaluation of dietary intake and identifies potential nutrient insufficiencies. Clinical anthropometry and Tanner staging are essential elements of the physical examination. Selected laboratory tests should be obtained when the nutritional or clinical status of the child warrants further diagnostic studies.

The methods available for the treatment of nutritional disorders in inflammatory bowel disease include enteral and parenteral routes (Table 7). The easiest way to provide nutritional supplementation is to increase oral dietary intakes. Although elimination diets may be advocated, there is no good evidence that the consumption or avoidance of specific foods alters the course of disease. Therefore, children are encouraged to eat a well-balanced diet of favorite foods. When specific foods exacerbate symptoms or when laboratory tests suggest specific abnormalities, the diet should be modified accordingly. Multivitamins with minerals should be administered routinely to replace potential deficits in the diet. Oral iron and folate supplements should be provided when laboratory findings are consistent with deficiency states. Parenteral administration of vitamin B_{12} may be necessary in children with extensive small bowel disease or ileal resection. The role of zinc supplementation remains controversial; however, low serum zinc levels in the presence of low serum alkaline phosphatase levels indicate zinc deficiency and this responds readily to zinc therapy.

If a child is unable to increase dietary protein and energy intakes with palatable snacks, oral supplementation with a commercially available liquid formula

Table 7 Nutritional Therapy of Inlammatory Bowel Disease

Well-balanced, high-protein and energy diet	
± Low residue	
± Lactose-free	
± Low fat, MCT or cholestyramine supplemented	
Enteral supplementation (140% to 150% of Recommended Daily Allowances for height age)	
Continuous or intermittent nasogastric tube feeding	
Feeding gastrostomy, continuous or intermittent	
Total parenteral nutrition (140% to 150% of Recommended Daily Allowances for height age)	
Peripheral	
Central	
Vitamins and minerals	
Supplemental multivitamins with minerals (daily)	
Therapeutic	
Folate	1 mg p.o. daily
Vitamin B_{12}	1000 μg every three months IM
Iron	6 mg (Fe^{+2})/kg/d PO
Ferrous sulfate (20% Fe)	
Ferrous gluconate (11.5% Fe)	
in three divided doses	
Iron dextran (Imferon)	Follow directions on package insert
Magnesium	200–400 mg Mg^{2+}/day IV
Zinc sulfate (22% Zn)	50–100 mg Zn^{2+}/day PO in three divided doses

should be attempted. Unfortunately, many children will experience early satiety when consuming these formulas and will not increase their total nutrient intake substantially. Under these circumstances, nutritional supplementation can be accomplished by intragastric feedings or parenteral nutrition.

Continuous intragastric infusions effectively improve the nutritional status, growth rates, and clinical well-being of children with inflammatory bowel disease. A silicone nasogastric tube of small diameter is passed into the stomach each evening for continuous, overnight, slow-drip or pumped feedings, then removed upon awakening to prevent interference with the child's school attendance and social activities. If the child does not tolerate the nasogastric regimen, a gastrostomy may be performed and utilized in the same manner. The major complication associated with intragastric feeding is reversible diarrhea secondary to rapidly administered nutritional supplements. The amount of formula administered via the intragastric tube will vary, depending upon the nutritional requirements and the tolerance level of the child (13).

In children who have active inflammatory disease and are unable to tolerate sufficient amounts of enteral alimentation, parenteral alimentation may provide substantial benefits. Peripheral solutions of 12% glucose, 2% amino acids, 10% lipids, vitamins, and minerals may be an acceptable form of short-term therapy. Alternatively, central venous alimentation appropriately influences nutritional status, linear growth rates, lean body mass deposition, and postoperative recovery (13). Parenteral alimentation also may induce clinical remission without the use of sulfasalazine or corticosteroid therapy, although as a primary treatment modality, it has been less effective in patients with ulcerative colitis, intestinal obstruction, abdominal masses, or fistulas (13). Home parenteral alimentation currently is available for those children who require long-term nutritional support for active disease, short bowel syndrome, or growth failure (15).

III. SURGICAL THERAPY

A. Ulcerative Colitis

Indications for surgery in ulcerative colitis (24) include persistent disease unresponsive to medical management, significant corticosteroid-induced side effects, complications of the disease such as hemorrhage, perforation, toxic megacolon, or growth failure, and colonic dysplasia (Table 8). In emergencies, a subtotal colectomy with a Hartman pouch or a mucous fistula and terminal ileostomy is the procedure of choice; simultaneous removal of the rectum in these circumstances increases mortality and morbidity considerably. Although postoperative complications of the retained rectum are few, this site may have a persistent inflammatory process with mucopurulent discharge from the anus or mucous fistula. These symptoms may be treated effectively with topical corticosteroids,

Table 8 Indications for Colectomy in Ulcerative Colitis

Emergency
Uncontrollable massive bleeding
Perforation or imminent perforation (toxic dilation)
Acute fulminant colitis not responding within two weeks to intensive medical treatment
Toxic megacolon not responding within 48–72 hr of intensive medical treatment or deterioration following initiation of medical therapy
Elective
Continuous incapacitating disease despite one year of adequate medical treatment
Chronic intermittent course with recurrent severe attacks or long periods of disability
Retardation of growth and sexual maturation despite aggressive nutritional therapy
Duration of disease more than ten years and epithelial dysplasia of the colonic mucosa

or 5-aminosalicylate or sulfasalazine enemas; however, if symptoms persist longer than 6 to 12 months, further surgery is advisable. The extraintestinal manifestations of ulcerative colitis may continue until both colon and rectum are excised. Short-chain fatty acid enemas may provide control of diversion colitis.

Removal of the rectal disease may be achieved either by mucosectomy with ileal endorectal pull-through or followed later by the construction of a continent ileostomy. Ileoanal and ileorectal anastomosis are contraindicated in pediatric patients with ulcerative colitis. The precise timing for elective surgery should take into account the symptoms and complications of chronically active disease as well as important milestones in the child's educational and psychosocial development. The child and parents should be prepared psychologically before colectomy, based on advice from the appropriate physician, surgeon, psychiatrist, and stoma therapist experienced in the management of inflammatory bowel disease in children. A preoperative visit from the Ostomy Association Visiting Program or a successfully treated patient is also helpful. Current surgical procedures available include a proctocolectomy with either a terminal ileostomy or continent ileostomy (Kock pouch), or rectal mucosectomy and ileal endorectal pull-through (Table 9). Proctocolectomy with terminal ileostomy is a curative procedure and has been used with success despite the loss of the rectum and the placement of an ileostomy. Although the volume of ileal fluid lost decreases within weeks after surgery, the loss of sodium (100 to 130 mEg/L) and fluid (500 ml/day) predisposes the child to dehydration and renal calculi. Proteolytic enzymes within the ileostomy fluid may cause stomal ulcerations if local care is not scrupulous. Sucralfate may provide protection of the peristomal skin. With current surgical techniques, impotence in the male and dyspareunia in the female are very uncommon. Provided that appropriate preparation is made, the psychosocial adjustment of children and adolescents to a permanent stoma is very good (25).

Proctocolectomy with a continent ileostomy also is a curative operation. A conventional terminal ileostomy is replaced by a pouch of terminal small bowel with a nipple valve on the efferent loop, thereby rendering the stoma continent. The pouch is emptied three to four times a day by means of a catheter. The quality of life with this type of ileostomy is better than that with the standard type, but it is not recommended for young children (24).

Colectomy with mucosal proctectomy and ileal endorectal pull-through is a relatively new procedure, but it has been performed with extremely encouraging results in young patients (26-29). In this procedure, the colon and diseased rectal mucosa are removed, but the anorectal musculature is preserved. The terminal ileum is placed inside the retained muscular wall of the rectum and anastomosed to the anus. As a result, all diseased mucosa is resected while preserving anorectal continence. Satisfactory results are obtained in 70% to 90% of patients. Nearly all patients are able to distinguish between flatus and fluid, have good anal sphincter tone, and experience voluntary rectal control. Because the rectal musculature remains in situ, the risk of impotence in the male or bladder dysfunction virtually is eliminated. The frequency of bowel movements diminishes gradually during the first year to approximately five or six times per day and once or twice at night. Although postoperative complications are infrequent, the procedure is surgically demanding. Moreover, questions regarding the risk of late development of cancer in unresected islands of rectal mucosa remain unanswered.

B. Crohn's Disease

Surgical treatment of Crohn's disease in children is less well defined than for ulcerative colitis and should be reserved for acute and chronic complications of the disease. Indications for surgery include intestinal perforation, obstruction or bleeding, abscesses, and fistulas (Table 10). Whether or not nutritional therapy will alter the natural history of Crohn's disease or lessen the frequency of

Table 9 Operations for Ulcerative Colitis

Proctocolectomy with standard ileostomy
Protocolectomy with continent ileostomy (Kock procedure)
Proctocolectomy with rectal mucosectomy and ileal endorectal pull-through

Table 10 Indications for Surgery in Crohn's Disease

Perforation
Obstruction
Massive bleeding
Abscess
Fistula
Growth failure (limited response to nutritional therapy)

surgical intervention currently is unclear. Presently, nutritional therapy is indicated before surgery, particularly in debilitated malnourished patients who require long-term, continuous corticosteroid therapy.

Before the advent of nutritional therapy, Crohn's ileocolitis often presented special problems in management with a high incidence of local complications such as development of fistulas and abscesses. The incidence of reoperation in this group currently is low, although in one-third of children followed for an average of 17 years, disease extended proximally into the ileum within a few weeks to as long as 11 years (30).

In intractable colonic disease, a total proctocolectomy is the operation of choice, except in rare patients with total sparing of the rectum, in whom an ileorectal anastomosis may be possible. Perianal disease is sometimes severe enough to require proctectomy, but may be managed conservatively. Drainage of abscesses sometimes is required (12,31).

In children with small bowel disease, the recurrence rate following local resection is less than in patients with ileocolitis. Thus, children with small bowel disease alone have a reoperation rate of 3% at one year and 23% at ten years compared with 10% and 65%, respectively, when small bowel and colon both are involved (32,33).

The response of growth arrest to surgical resection in Crohn's disease is variable. In some instances, a significant increase in growth velocities following surgery was observed, while in other reports, the response was less optimal (10,33) At present, a conservative approach is indicated when growth failure is the sole indication for surgery, particularly when nutritional therapy also is likely to be effective in the reversing growth arrest. Growth following surgery is most likely to occur in the prepubertal child with a retarded bone age in whom all macroscopically abnormal bowel can be resected and when a sustained, disease-free period follows surgery.

IV. PSYCHOSOCIAL SUPPORT

Inflammatory bowel disease in childhood inflicts on the child and family many years of chronic ill health and multiple visits to the hospital. For this reason, a team approach should be adopted, with physician, psychiatrist or psychologist, social worker, nutritionist, and nurse coordinator pooling their resources to support the child and the family. While there is not good evidence that psychologic factors are etiologically important, symptoms often are worse at times of stress. However, at present, psychological intervention has not altered the long-term course of inflammatory bowel disease.

Marked changes in mood, behavior, outlook, and personality occur during adolescence. A newfound sexual awareness coupled with a need to rebel against authority implies that all children in this age group require special care. This observation is particularly true of children with inflammatory bowel disease where chronic illness and, perhaps, a stoma or growth failure hinder close identification with the peer group. New problems arise, such as poor drug compliance or erratic outpatient attendance. Parents also require support in relinquishing the responsibility for the care of a sick child to the patient, particularly when the child shows little interest in self-care. Community self-help groups in conjunction with local or regional chapters of the National Foundation for Ileitis and Colitis (444 Park Avenue South, New York, New York 10016) provide a support structure for families of children with inflammatory bowel disease. The Foundation also is a major resource for adult patients. The timing of transfer of care from the pediatric to adult gastroenterologistis is best avoided until the problems of adolescence have subsided and the concerns of the child and his or her parents have been considered.

V. PROGNOSIS

Although 10% of patients with ulcerative colitis with onset in childhood or adolescence will experience only one episode, the remainder will have further symptoms. Approximately 20% will have intermittent symptoms, 50% will have chronic but not incapacitating disease, and 20% will have chronically active, incapacitating disease (34). Fully a third of patients require a colectomy, but this procedure is curative provided the rectal mucosa is removed; subsequent life expectancy is normal (34,35). In disease confined to the recutm or distal colon, 10% of patients experience progression to pancolitis, 75% resolve, and in 15%, symptoms continue intermittently.

The risk of carcinoma in patients with colitis probably has been overestimated (35,36). Recent arguments favor examination of the colon by sigmoidoscopy and biopsy every 6 to 12 months and by colonoscopy every 2 years in place of colectomy for patients with pancolitis of greater than 10 years' duration. The presence of persistent severe dysplasia should be regarded as precancerous and proctocolectomy should be advised. At present, the question of the efficacy of routine long-term surveillance versus prophylactic colectomy is unanswered.

The prognosis in Crohn's disease is difficult to determine due to the different treatment regimens employed, particularly with respect to the frequency of surgical intervention, and the extent to which corticosteroids have been used. Furthermore, the effect of nutritional therapy on long-term prognosis also is unknown. In general, the long-term prognosis of Crohn's disease in childhood is fairly good; most children experience good health and lead productive lives, although morbidity during childhood and adolescence may be high (37). Despite increased morbidity, mortality is low; 2.4% of a large series of patients died (38), and after 5 and 20 years of disease, the actuarial probability of survival was 98% and 89%, respectively, of that expected.

The onset of Crohn's disease before the age of 15 years also has been associated with a significantly shorter adult height than the normal population. However, a more concerted attempt toward achieving and maintaining a good nutritional status during the course of the disease may prevent this complication in the future.

Although the incidence of colorectal carcinoma in patients presenting with Crohn's disease below the age of 21 years is greater than that in a control population, the exact risk requires further clarification. Currently, the risk of developing colonic cancer does not justify prophylactic colectomy, although in the future a larger number of patients surviving without colectomy as a result of successful medical therapy may result in a revision of this view (39).

REFERENCES

1. Ament, M. E., Inflammatory disease of the colon: Ulcerative colitis and Crohn's colitis, J. Pediatr., 86:322–334 (1975).
2. Meyers, S., D. B. Sachar, J. D. Goldberg, H. D. Janowitz, Corticotropin versus hydrocortisone in the intravenous treatment of ulcerative colitis. A prospective, randomized double-blind clinical trial, Gastroenterology, 85: 351–357 (1983).
3. Binder, S. C., J. F. Patterson, D. J. Glotzer, Toxic megacolon in ulcerative colitis, Gastroenterology, 66:909–915 (1974).
4. Grand, R. J., A. H. Colodny, Increased requirement for magnesium therapy during parenteral therapy for granulomatous colitis, J. Pediatr., 81:788–790 (1972).
5. Harris, I., A. W. Wilkinson, Magnesium depletion in children, Lancet, 2:735–736 (1971).
6. Dissanayake, A. S., S. C. Truelove, A controlled therapeutic trial of long-term maintenance therapy for ulcerative colitis, Gut, 14(12):923–926 (1973).
7. Verhave, M., H. Winter, R. J. Grand, Efficacy and safety of azathioprine in children with IBD, Gastroenterology, 92(5):1682 (1987).
8. Werlin, S. L., R. J. Grand, Severe colitis in children and adolescents: Diagnosis, course and treatment, Gastroenterology, 73:828–832 (1977).
9. Whittington, P. F., H. V. Barnes, T. M. Bayless, Medical management of Crohn's disease in adolescence, Gastroenterology, 72:1338–1344 (1977).

10. Gryboski, J. D., H. D. Spiro, Prognosis in children with Crohn's disease, Gastroenterology, 74:807-817 (1978).
11. Werlin, S. L., R. J. Grand, Bloody diarrhea—a new complication of sulfasalazine, J. Pediatr., 92:450-451 (1978).
12. Markowitz, J., F. Daum, H. Aiges, E. Kahn, M. Silverberg, S. Fisher, Perianal disease in children and adolescents with Crohn's disease, Gastroenterology, 86:829-833 (1984).
13. Motil, K. J., R. J. Grand, Nutritional management of inflammatory bowel disease, Pediatr. Clin. North Am., 32:447-469 (1985).
14. Morin, C. L. et al., Continuous elemental enteral alimentation in the treatment of children and adolescents with Crohn's disease, J. Parent. Ent. Nutr., 6:194-199 (1982).
15. Strobel, C. T., J. Byrne, M. E. Ament, Home parenteral nutriton in children with Crohn's disease: An effective management alternative, Gastroenterology, 77:272-279 (1979).
16. Navarro, J. et al. Prolonged constant rate elemental enteral nutrition in Crohn's disease, J. Pediatr. Gastroenterol. Nutr., 1:541-546 (1982).
17. Kirschner, B. S., J. R. Klich, S. S. Kalman, M. V. DeFavaro, I. H. Rosenberg, Reversal of growth retardation in Crohn's disease with therapy emphasizing oral nutritional restitution, Gastroenterology, 80:10-15 (1981).
18. Layden, T., J. Rosenberg, B. Nemchausky, C. Elson, I. Rosenberg, Reversal of growth arrest in adolescents with Crohn's disease after parenteral alimentation, Gastroenterology, 70:1017-1021 (1976).
19. Morin, C. L., M. Roulet, C. C. Roy, A. Weber, Continuous elemental enteral alimentation in children with Crohn's disease and growth failure, Gastroenterology, 79:1205-1210 (1980).
20. Motil, K. J., R. J. Grand, C. J. Maletskos, V. R. Young, The effect of disease, drug, and diet on whole body protein metabolism in adolescents with Crohn's disease and growth failure, J. Pediatr., 101:345-351 (1982).
21. Kelts, D. G., R. J. Grand, G. Shen, J. B. Watkins, S. L. Werlin, C. Boehme, Nutritional basis of growth failure in children and adolescents with Crohn's disease, Gastroenterology, 76:720-727 (1979).
22. Motil, K. J., R. J. Grand, D. E. Matthews, D. M. Bier, C. J. Maletskos, V. R. Young, Whole body leucine metabolism in adolescents with Crohn's disease and growth failure during nutritional supplementation, Gastroenterology, 82:1359-1368 (1982).
23. Motil, K. J., S. I. Altchuler, R. J. Grand, Mineral balance during nutritional supplementation in adolescents with Crohn's disease and growth failure, J. Pediatr., 107:473-479 (1985).
24. Telander, R. L., S. L. Smith, H. M. Marciner, W. M. O'Fallon, J. A. Van Heerden, J. Perrault, Surgical treatment of ulcerative colitis in children, Surgery, 90:787-794 (1981).
25. Hyams, J. S., R. J. Grand, A. H. Colodny, S. R. Schuster, A. Eraklis, Course and prognosis after colectomy and ileostomy for inflammatory bowel disease in childhood and adolescence, J. Pediatr. Surg., 17:400-405 (1982).

26. Martin, L. W., C. LeCoultre, W. K. Schubert, Total colectomy and mucosal proctecomy with preservation of continence in ulcerative colitis, Ann. Surg., 186:477–480 (1977).
27. Fonkalsrud, E. W., M. E. Ament, W. J. Byrne, Clinical experience with total colectomy and endorectal mucosal resection for inflammatory bowel disease, Gastroenterology, 77:156–160 (1979).
28. Telander, R. L., J. Perrault, Colectomy with rectal mucosectomy and ileo-anal anastomosis in young patients, Arch. Surg., 116:623–629 (1981).
29. Perrault, J., R. L. Telander, A. R. Zinsmeister, B. Kaufman, The endorectal pull-through procedure in children and young adults: A follow-up study, J. Pediatr. Gastroenterol. Nutr., 7:89–94 (1988).
30. Korelitz, B. I., D. Gribetz, F. B. Kopel, Granulomatous colitis in children: A study of 25 cases and comparison with ulcerative colitis, Pediatrics, 42: 446–457 (1968).
31. Biller, J. A., R. J. Grand, B. H. Harris, Abdominal abscesses in adolescents with Crohn's disease, J. Pediatr. Surg., 22:873–876 (1987).
32. Castille, R. G., R. L. Telander, D. R. Cooney, D. M. Ilstrup, J. Perrault, J. Van Heerden, G. B. Stickler, Crohn's disease in children: Assessment of the progression of disease, growth, and prognosis, J. Pediatr. Surg., 15: 462–469 (1980).
33. Homer, D. R., R. J. Grand, A. H. Colodny, Growth, course and prognosis after surgery for Crohn's disease in children and adolescents, Pediatrics, 59:717–725 (1977).
34. Michener, W. M., R. G. Farmer, E. A. Mortimer, Long-term prognosis of ulcerative colitis with onset in childhood or adolescence, J. Clin. Gastroenterol., 1:301–307 (1979).
35. Devroede, G. J., W. F. Taylor, On calculating cancer risk and survival of ulcerative colitis patients with the life table method, Gastroenterology, 71:505–509 (1976).
36. Lennard-Jones, J. E., B. C. Morson, J. K. Ritchie, D. C. Shove, C. B. Williams, Cancer in colitis: An assessment of the individual risk by clinical and histological criteria, Gastroenterology, 73:1280–1289 (1977).
37. Farmer, R. G., Factors in the long-term prognosis of patients with inflammatory bowel disease, Am. J. Gastroenterol., 75:97–103 (1981).
38. Farmer, R. G., W. M. Michener, Prognosis of Crohn's disease with onset in childhood or adolescence, Dig. Dis. Sci., 24:752–757 (1979).
39. Butt, J. H., J. E. Lennard-Jones, J. K. Ritchie, A practical approach to the risk of cancer in inflammatory bowel disease, Med. Clin. North Am., 64: 1203–1220 (1980).

13

Psychosocial Issues

Karen A. Kurlander and Mary F. O'Brien

Charlesbridge Counseling and Resource Center for People with Chronic Gastro-intestinal Illnesses, Watertown, Massachusetts

Views of the psychological needs and treatment of inflammatory bowel disease (IBD) patients have evolved in the shadow of controversy and confusion concerning the possible role of emotional factors in the etiology of these illnesses. The literature reveals two conflicting views. According to one view, the psychic distress of these patients reflects underlying psychopathology, which in some manner contributes to the physical condition (1-32). A large body of research, retrospective in nature, and for the most part, reflecting either anecdotal or poorly controlled data, was published in this country in support of this position over a 40-year period extending into the early 1970s. From the second, and more recently developed, perspective, the origins of these illnesses are believed to be physiological, and emotional disturbance associated with the IBD is then, by implication, seen as a secondary response to chronic and debilitating illness (33-48).

Clearly, the two positions have profoundly different implications for mental health treatment. The first suggests working within a psychopathological model, treating the defective personality as a way of impacting the illness. The other, accepting the illness as a "given," encourages practitioners to help people with the full range of complex, interactive problems which these illnesses impose on patients, regardless of their prior level of emotional stability.

The view of psychopathology as being a major causal or contributory factor in these illnesses has proved surprisingly enduring (49,50), and has largely suppressed development of this second form of treatment, even though a number of well-controlled studies conducted over the past two decades largely discount a greater frequency of psychopathology in these patients than in either normal control groups or groups with chronic nongastrointestinal illnesses (34-36,40,41, 43,44,46,48). The result is that very little has been written to help professionals understand the dilemma of the IBD patient (51-53). Furthermore, we failed to find a single description of psychological treatment which dealt with the distress of this population as normal and secondary to the illness.

This review attempts to close both gaps, to help professionals better understand the reactive processes likely to arise in IBD patients, regardless of their pre-existing level of mental health, and then to suggest a treatment approach congruent with the realities which they face. In the interest of clarity we have separated our discussion of the processes into three sections: the emotional, the social, and the cognitive. First, however, we will briefly describe the powerful physical experience which launches these processes.

I. THE PHYSICAL EXPERIENCE OF THE IBD PATIENT

Although IBD is not the only illness that imposes a heavy burden of misery and distress on the victims, it is particularly treacherous in both its symptoms and its prognosis (54-56). We have seen patients who have a history of as many as 16-20 bowel movements on a good day and who continue to lead productive lives. Many are incontinent to a degree that they are forced to live with a conceptual map of geographical space structured around the availability of public toilets.

Even with less severe cases, there may be urgency that reaches the level of panic, along with smells and sounds that are so socially repugnant and unacceptable that patients often live in great dread of having to use a bathroom in any space but their own. On top of these problems, people with IBD can expect to be so fatigued that engaging in the normal routine of living is more than they can even think about. They can expect to be anorexic and nauseated, and in pain. They may bleed. They may not sleep for the indescribable sensations afflicting a body that has major systemic inflammatory process going on within it. At times, often indefinitely, they will be on medications that are not only dangerous, but disfiguring, possibly even crippling. And this only touches the ordinary effects of the illness. The extraordinary are another level of disorder, pain, and misery. More than 100 systemic complications involving virtually every organ system in the body have been identified in IBD. As Kirsner has pointed out in a major article, this is a "constellation of biomedical problems unmatched in any other human illness" (54).

Over time, patients will learn to fear what all too often comes to pass, that the illness will flare up and ruin the sacred as well as the ordinary experiences of their lives—dating, sexual encounters, marriages, pregnancies, and job promotions. IBD will loom as a dark shadow over their lives, vicious, unpredictable, and all too often ending in psychic trauma. The degree to which people are able to adjust and adapt to the predicament in which they find themselves will depend not only on their own coping resources but on the support and assistance which professional caregivers will be able to mobilize and provide (53). This will require a fine-tuned understanding on the part of these professionals of the psychosocial aspects of these diseases

II. THE EMOTIONAL CRISIS OF IBD

The nature of some illnesses—cancer, cerebral palsy, muscular dystrophy—will secure a person's right to intense emotion in the minds of others. In fact, much great drama is based on how people cope with such conditions. This is not true of IBD. It is difficult indeed to image any great drama based on bowels and diarrhea. Instead, famillarity with some of the milder symptoms, coupled with the repugnant feelings that most people feel toward them will make it hard for others to relate to the depths of despair involved in living with a chronic debilitating intestinal illness.

The difficulty others have in empathizing with the IBD sufferer is compounded by the enduring tendency of professionals and nonprofessionals alike to view these illnesses as emotionally caused. The writings of the Austrian psychiatrist Elizabeth Kubler-Ross have encouraged people to view what might have been regarded as pathological emotions and behavior in dying people as legitimate adaptation to loss and grief (57). Seeing a process rather than emotional pathology, people have been moved to participate in the world of the dying patient and to interact with them in a supportive manner. Unfortunately, this has not tended to be the case with IBD patients. Instead, as the literature reveals, their distress has been largely misunderstood or discounted as psychopathology.

What sort of process might be triggered by illness of this type and magnitude? A long line of researchers have written extensively about loss and depression in these patients. In fact, in a classic study completed in the 1940s, noted psychoanalyst Erich Lindemann identified a syndrome based on grief and loss in people with IBD (17). This is certainly not surprising considering that IBD has the potential to threaten and disrupt virtually every aspect of a person's present and future. What is surprising is that so many researchers interpreted these emotions to be signs of pathology, rather than realistic reactions to the illness itself.

In what sense might IBD provoke an experience of grief and depression? The chronicity of the illness, the spoiled self-image, the associated loss of energy, and the diminished capacity to live fully will hold IBD patients uncomfortably close to the awareness of bodily deterioration, permanent debilitation, and death. This awareness is painfully heightened by the fact that when the illness flares the patient is removed from all the great and small pleasures and comforts of everyday life. Dinner with the family, plans with a friend, an evening's entertainment—all of this is denied for an indeterminate period of time by the ravages of the illness. Even the pleasure of eating, which is the last to leave for most of us, is now gone. For those who live with consistent unremitting symptoms, these losses may be permanent.

Unfortunately, certain factors will tend to get in the way of an IBD patient successfully resolving the grieving process. One is that IBD patients often do not feel a sense of legitimacy for the powerful emotions they are likely to experience. As Cooley describes in his concept of "the looking-glass self" (58), we tend to see ourselves as reflected in the eyes of others. If, in the height of their distress, people see themselves being judged negatively, they may begin investing psychic energy toward hiding and repressing, rather than in expressing and coping. Their capacity to experience their feelings may, over time, become compromised, making successful adaptation impossible. Furthermore, the course of the illness, as it waxes and wanes, will encourage the part of people that wants to deny. It is only the unremittingness of a loss that forces the psyche to finally surrender and let go.

Thus, what one may see in the IBD patient is a varying emotional course in which they will be in denial of illness and deterioration until the condition worsens and throws them back into an intense and often silent state of grief and depression. It is not surprising that Engel and the psychoanalysts saw so many fearful, anxious patients, unable to express their emotions because they had been given no mechanism for either understanding or expressing them, nor permission to do so without being thought crazy.

In addition to being portrayed in the early literature as depressed, IBD patients were also seen as angry (3,30,55,59,60), anxious (2,32,33,61,62), and dependent (3,8,12,30,62,63). These emotions were interpreted as further indications of the underlying psychopathology believed to be in some central way involved with the disease process. Rather than as pathological, such emotions can be seen as realistic reactions to severe threat and deprivation. Both these conditions rob their victims not only of control over their bodies, but also over their lives. In adolescents and young adults, IBD threatens the capacity of these young people to complete their identities, to establish independence, to build relationships, to establish families, and to become self-sufficient (52,56). We have found in our clinical experience that these are areas of grave concern, provoking many realistic fears in IBD patients.

For all of the effects of these diseases on young adults, it is obvious that from a dynamic developmental point of view the impact has to be potentially much more serious for children. The younger they are, the more powerful the consequences are likely to be. Children with IBD are sicker than adults, their symptoms are harder to manage, and their prognosis is poorer. Their identities are also less formed and their psyches less capable of defending themselves against trauma than their adult counterparts. Consequently, their physical and psychic pain is bound to be greater.

As Bluebond-Langner has documented, professionals may seriously underestimate the potential for young children to understand and react to illness (64). In an anthropological study of children dying of leukemia, this researcher reported that children as young as 3 years of age were aware of their prognoses, but held this knowledge a secret from the adults around them. Instead, the children created a world of their own to deal with their emotional distress and to insure that their caretakers, in grief or helplessness, did not abandon them.

While the world of the IBD child touches more peripherally on issues of death, it is full of its own demons. Pain, bleeding, surgery, impaired growth, bodily disfigurement, and highly intrusive medical procedures must often be incorporated into the developing psyches of these children. Like the leukemic chldren, they are forced to live in dread of the drugs failing them. Nowhere in the literature, however, has the magnitude of their struggle been fully recognized. Instead, like their adult counterparts, they have been caught in the etiological controversy, being described either as crazy or normal, with the character and intensity of legitimate distress lost in the argument.

We believe, from our experience with IBD children and adults who were diagnosed as children, that professionals need to assume the same sort of pressures in this group as in the leukemic children. Otherwise, seeing no permission in the eyes of their caretakers and loved ones, the IBD children may, like their adult counterparts, become involved in hiding or suppressing their feelings and their fears, rather than risk losing the support of those they so desperately need. Both children and adults with IBD will need people who can accept and encourage them to express the intensity of their distress without judgement as a first step toward a resolution based neither in denial or helplessness.

III. FITTING AND MISFITTING INTO THE SOCIAL ARENA

Patients with IBD will have to contend not only with physical and emotional pain but with serious problems in the social arena—problems which often have no satisfactory resolution. This is because the illness will significantly compromise their ability to fit into the social fabric of life (55,65). The uncertainty of the illness, often compounded by the side effects of medications and surgeries, leaves them vulnerable to frequent changes in physical well-being which make their participation in social events problematic. Plagued by bowel difficulties and fatigue, they often cannot guarantee when they will be present, and when they are absent they cannot say for how long it will be.

This inability to be certain of their availability to others is a problem for many chronically ill patients, but particularly so with IBD since incapacitation from the illness is often a sudden occurrence. When this occurs repeatedly there is a limit to how understanding others will be. "People in my family say, 'But I spoke with her just this afternoon and she was okay'," one woman told us as she tried to convey her distress over the disruptions her absences from family functions had caused.

Added to this, the social difficulty of the IBD patients is vastly complicated by the potential for these illnesses to be seen in a stigmatized light. According to the sociologist Goffman, a stigma is an undesirable difference which will lead others to preceive the bearer of the stigma as being inferior or having defects that go beyond and may even be unrelated to the original difference (66). He describes it as a matter of "spoiled identity," a case of a single difference influencing more broadly the way a person is seen.

The physical nature of IBD lends itself to stigmatization. The symptoms of the disease are widely held to be socially unacceptable and appropriate objects of social ridicule and expressions of disgust. Thus, patients find themselves unable to control in public behavior which they themselves may have previously found repellent and the basis of invalidating others.

The following experience of a colostomy patient, as recounted by Goffman (66), reflects the potential for social embarrassment and self-rejection with which the IBD patient must live: "When I smelled an odor on the bus or subway before the colostomy I used to feel very annoyed. I'd think that the people were awful, that they didn't take a bath or that they should have gone to the bathroom before traveling. I used to think that they might have odors from what they ate. I used to be terribly annoyed; to me it seemed that they were filthy, dirty. Of course, at the least opportunity I used to change my seat and if I couldn't it used to go against my grain. So naturally, I believe that the young people feel the same way about me if I smell" (p. 34).

The issue here is not whether the colostomy smells but rather the fear of rejection and embarrassment that all IBD patients live with, since they are all vulnerable to similarly unpleasant symptoms. Interestingly enough, this is especially so in hospital rooms, where much of the research concerning the emotionality of these patients was conducted. Hospital rooms represent close quarters from which there is little escape when symptoms get out of control. When the loss of control coincides with mealtimes or visiting hours, roommates, visitors, and staff members alike become affected by the symptoms. The medically sophisticated and compassionate observer may struggle to hide repugnance; others may not be so kind.

The stigmatization associated with the symptoms of IBD is compounded by the surprisingly prevalent view of the public that these are not true physical conditions (65). Many people who know nothing else about these illnesses—about the pain, the bleeding, the threat of cancer, the destruction of tissue, the wide variety of extraintestinal symptoms—"know" that they are psychosomatic

(65). While the sophistication of the public understanding of this concept will vary, for many it implies that people with IBD are not really physically ill but rather mentally ill. As an example of this, a professional woman with IBD whom we see was taken aback by a co-worker's advice to her upon hearing she had been out sick with a very serious Crohn's attack. He informed her that she would "really be much better off to just go home and throw dishes at the wall."

Being judged as emotionally disturbed creates additional social pressures for the IBD patient. For example, although it is not acceptable to reject someone physically ill, unfortunately these norms do not apply to the mentally ill. And while a physically ill person will be accorded the rights and privileges of the sick, this is often not true for those seen as psychologically ill. There is always suspicion of a voluntary component or at the very least a lapse of will involved in their difficulties.

According to Goffman, when one has a stigmatized condition that is potentially concealable, like IBD, the central issue becomes that of managing information about the defect. "To display or not to display, to tell or not to tell, to let on or not to let on, to lie or not to lie, and in each case to whom, how, when and where" (p. 42). For IBD patients these are not very easy questions to answer because either decision–to reveal or not to reveal–places them in a potentially treacherous social situation.

While revealing the illness exposes them to embarrassment and suspicions of mental illness, choosing to conceal the condition vastly compounds tensions provoked by the uncertainty of social availability. People are then left without a valid reason for failing to meet family, social, and work responsibilities, and therefore, become vulnerable over time to being socially ostracized.

It might be assumed that such fears are unrealistic and outgrowths of the social anxieties of the patient, but nothing could be further from the truth. We have listened to people anguish as they come under excruciating social pressure from co-workers who have come to suspect them of being work shirkers. We have watched as old friendships come to an end because people tire of plans being broken without a seemingly legitimate excuse.

Unfortunately, the social dilemma of the IBD patient is essentially one without resolution. To conceal the illness in an effort to keep one's identity as a person unsullied by negative associations with the illness means to expose oneself to the wrath of others for frequent social lapses without a viable excuse (ironically, to follow this course over time may lead one to be seen as having emotional problems anyway). On the other hand, to reveal the stigma is to risk being seen as a discredited human being by others. Furthermore, revealing does not guarantee people the right to the legitimate privileges that they will need as people with a chronic illness, the implication of which we will discuss in the next section.

Finally, there is the drama of IBD as played out within the family. For many IBD patients—like other stigmatized people—the family will become a sanctuary (66). It may be the only place where people will witness first-hand the ravages and suffering of the illness. Because of this, the family is much less likely to question the validity of the physical component of the illness. Within its boundaries the IBD patient is likely to be accorded appropriate privileges (66), and treated like a legitimately ill person. The problem is that this is an illness that will not go away. Over time, the family may become overwhelmed by the burden, a situation which may result in anger and resentment directed toward the sick member.

An alternative scenario which we have observed on more than one occasion is for the stigmatization process to extend into the family. In such situations, the credibility of the sick member may begin to be questioned in much the same way it is in the outside world. The person comes to be increasingly seen as mentally rather than physically ill. One can only imagine the pain involved in losing legitimacy within one's own family during the times of greatest physical and emotional need. The problem may be greatly aggravated if the shame of the stigmatization bleeds by association onto the family itself. The less healthy a family is, the more they may need to reject the IBD patient in an attempt to free themselves of suspicion. The patient's increasingly agitated efforts to find help and to force the family to acknowledge genuine illness may only end up confirming the diagnosis of mental instability. Trapped in dilemmas which have no really good solutions, it is not surprising when some patients begin to fulfill the negative picture of them as presented by the early researchers.

IV. ACHIEVING AN UNDERSTANDING OF IBD IS DIFFICULT AND CRUCIAL FOR PATIENTS

Another critical aspect of adjustment for IBD patients will be in the cognitive area, the arena of ideas and beliefs. A diagnosis of IBD will initiate a struggle within these patients to develop a belief system that will incorporate both the illness and also their role as sick people (67). Once derived, these ways of understanding will have great power in guiding both their experience and their behavior.

The belief system of those with IBD is likely to be highly idiosyncratic for a number of reasons. According to the literature and in our clinical experience, patients often have relatively little information about their illness, and even less about how to live with it (51,67-71). In addition, they cannot establish first-hand physical information because the actual area of disease cannot be viewed. Furthermore, all of this will be compounded by confusion over what it means to have an illness that is chronic, as opposed to acute (67).

In this vacuum, IBD patients will develop ways of seeing themselves and their illnesses that will be composed of varying degrees of information, misinformation, wishful thinking, and personal experience (67). This highly personal perspective will be, in all likelihood, the guiding force in determining how people will interact with the medical care system—whether and when they use it, whether or not they comply with the advice of the physician, and whether and how they take care of themselves.

Kelly's autobiographical description (67) of how he came to understand the chronicity of his illness illustrates several critical features of how such a belief system is derived. It further depicts the difficulty in developing a system that will facilitate wise rather than destructive behavior in relation to the illness. For him, the concept of chronicity evolved through a series of hypotheses that changed over a period of five years as a result of his experience of the illness. Over time he progressed from his initial hypothesis that the illness was nothing more serious than an ordinary stomach ache to a phase during which he considered himself to be well when he felt well and ill when he felt ill. With recurrent bouts he came to believe that he was "not yet cured but on the way to recovery." This was followed by the belief that he had an illness that was difficult to get better from. Only after five years did Kelly finally understand that this was an illness from which he would never fully recover and to which he would have to accommodate for life.

The core difficulty for Kelly, as it is for other IBD patients, was in constructing a functional belief system that allowed for the possibility of feeling well while still having an illness. Instead, when he felt sick he thought of himself as sick. When he felt well, he thought of himself as totally well. This is a significant problem, since a different set of rights and responsibilities are associated with wellness than with illness.

A central difference between wellness and illness in our culture is the relative weight we are expected to give to taking care of ourselves on the one hand, and to meeting our responsibilities on the other. When we are well the priorities are clear; we are expected to find time to take care of ourselves within the context of meeting our responsibilities. When we are sick, the order of our priorities is shifted, and it is considered permissable to put taking care of ourselves above meeting our responsibilities. The price for release from responsibility is that it is implicitly assumed that we will not participate fully in other aspects of life. As children we quickly learn that if we are too sick to go to school we are too sick to go out and play even if we feel well enough to do so.

The problem for IBD patients is that much of the time they do not clearly fit into either category. As an example of how this process works to the detriment of people with IBD, a patient of ours complained of a long-standing pattern in which just as he thought he was getting better he would get sick again.

In discussing this with him the pattern became obvious. When he became very ill, he would stay home from work and rest and sleep almost all of the time, as his body required. When he began to feel better, and placed himself in the well category, he would work overtime to make up to his colleagues for all the extra work they had needed to do while he was ill. Soon, the course of his recovery would again reverse itself. This young man would go abruptly from seeing himself as ill, and being able to appropriately use the privileges associated with that state, to seeing himself as well and therefore required to assume the full responsibilities that went along with that condition. Clearly his decision was based on the category in which he placed himself, rather than on cues from his body which would almost certainly have gradually inclined him back to work. What is sad about this is the likelihood that if he had chosen to listen to his body those at work would have, over time, become impatient and suspicious in the face of the ambiguity of his symptoms when not acutely ill. There is no category in the culture that defines an appropriate role for a chronically ill person whose illness has a varying course.

As a result, IBD sufferers are forced to choose between two equally undesirable alternatives, neither of which captures their situation. They may see themselves as well, a choice which robs them of the right to the much-needed privileges of the sick, or they may see themselves as sick—a choice which puts them to varying degrees in the invalid category, unable to participate fully in life (67,72). We believe that neither choice will serve them. Rather than choosing between these two options, what they need to acknowledge and have accepted by those around them is the fact that even when they are not obviously sick they still carry the illness submerged within them and that futhermore, in their own best interests, they must often claim the privileges of illness.

In our experience, given the options, most people will choose to believe themselves well. Unfortunately, there are a number of distortions involved in maintaining the concept that one is well when one has a chronic illness. The first is one of accommodation. In this process the abnormal comes to seem normal as it becomes more familiar and habitual. After years of having pain and diarrhea, only a marked change will be perceived as problematic. This encourages people to see themselves as well and to dismiss the need to do anything about their condition. The other is denial. In our practice we see many IBD patients who, in the absence of strong physical cues to the contrary, will simply "forget" about the existence of the disease. This form of distortion is seen in a typical remark which patients make to us: "When I am well I can do anything, and it doesn't bother me." The implication here is that "Since I am no longer sick, I can eat anything I want, work as unrelentingly as I choose, stay up 'til all hours as often as I fell like, and it never bothers my systemic illness."

Kelly came to believe that denial of the illness can be functional because it allows IBD patients to avoid a certain amount of depression and encourages them to stay fully engaged in life, as opposed to slipping into some version of invalidism (67). But this logic holds only if the singular alternative to being well is being sick. And the price of denial is not small, since from this position taking care of oneself will remain relatively low on one's priority list. Furthermore, there may be a tendency to avoid medical care, because any visit to the physician may yield information that will threaten their belief that they are well.

Those whose illness is unremitting are likely to develop a different, but equally distorted vision of the illness as being totally intractable, regardless of what they do. The tendency for this group is to fall into the state of helplessness and hopelessness which a number of early researchers reported finding in their patients (5,17,73). From this stance they proceed to make other kinds of self-destructive decisions. A common example involves people who eat foods that they know will make them feel worse. When asked why they do this, they often reply, "I'm going to be sick all the time anyway, so what difference does it make?" The assumption is that they can do nothing to help themselves, even though information from their bodies is clearly telling them otherwise.

The examples we have given are outcomes of the inadequate cognitive structure within which most patients will struggle to understand and contain their illness. Many, if not most, patients will need help in sorting through and understanding the issues involved. In addition, the pathways and issues involved are not obvious to either patient or observer. Psychological help which relates to patients totally through issues around emotionality is very likely to leave them ill-prepared for the realities they face. They will need help to develop a cognitive structure that is a good fit with the realities of chronic illness.

V. TREATMENT ISSUES

The last four sections discussed the impact of IBD at several levels: the physical, the emotional, the social, and the cognitive. The question remains: What kind of psychological help will meet the specific needs of these patients?

As noted, all of the studies of psychological treatment which we found in our search focused primarily on psychopathology in these patients. Furthermore, nearly all of this research was conducted on ulcerative colitis, although this is confounded by the fact that ulcerative colitis and Crohn's disease of the colon were not formally distinguished from each other until the 1960s and are still at times difficult to separate diagnostically (74). This confound is not of major interest here, however, since the literature and our own clinical experience both indicate that the diseases are largely similar from the psychological aspect (75,76).

Within this body of literature the studies tend to fall into two broad categories. The first group is comprised of studies in which various methods of outpatient psychotherapy from classical psychoanalysis to supportive therapy were used. Included are a number of case studies in which researchers reported positive physiological results after treatment of patients with IBD (77-83). Results of these studies are clouded, however, by the inherent methodological weakness of case research, complicated by the tendency of these illnesses to run a highly variable course.

A number of larger studies both support and contradict these finding. Grace and Wolff (62), Karush et al. (84), Langford (85), and Paulley (86), all reported psychological improvement in patients treated with psychotherapy, although none of these researchers used controls. Grace et al. (87), using superficial psychotherapy with emphasis on stress reduction, indicated finding similar results in a study using matched controls. Psychotherapy did not result in physical improvement for the patients of Crohn and Yarnis (88), or any long-term physical improvement for patients who received short-term hospital psychotherapy and then were followed-up by Weinstock (89). Weinstock later, however, compiled reports from psychoanalysts of 28 patients who benefitted from long-term psychoanalysis (90). Other researchers, in a major study at Columbia Presbyterian Hospital in the 1960s (14,84,91,92), noted that psychotherapy appeared to reduce social and personal disability caused by IBD, but that psychological improvement was not correlated with physiological benefit.

A second major approach to working with IBD involved the creation of therapeutic environments for patients hospitalized because of their illness. This body of studies developed out of the so-called "analytic approach" used by the Massachusetts General Hospital team in the 1940s under the leadership of Lindemann. The MGH team based their intervention on the theory that the grief and depression which numerous researchers had reported finding in ulcerative colitis patients were rooted in object loss, that is, the real or imagined loss of a significant person in the patient's life. Within the context of a highly supportive therapeutic environment, they specifically encouraged transference of the emotions and the dependency previously assigned to that person to the physician in hopes of resolving the conflict.

Other researchers reported using similar strategies, sometimes from somewhat different theoretical bases. Groen and Bastiaans (93), Groen and Birnbaum (94), Marder (95), and Nichols et al. (96), all suggested using therapeutic hospital environments in the belief that fostering regression in IBD patients would help them to a more mature reorganization of the personality. Only the last two teams reported any actual data or follow-up, indicating that approximately 50% of the patients in both studies remained well for periods ranging from 1 to 9 years. Freyberger (97), with a German team of researchers, concentrated on building a close relationship between the doctor and hospitalized patients, as well as an environment in which staff members were particularly sensitive to the needs and wishes of these patients. Nichols et al. (96) refer to the creation of these sorts of therapeutic environments as one of the sheet anchors of the approach to medical management, even in the era of steroid therapy.

What can be concluded about the role of psychological treatment in the care of IBD patients on the basis of these studies? Although more extensive follow-up is in order, overall they suggest that some form of such treatment may be a meaningful component of care for people with IBD. Furthermore, certain common elements emerge in these interventions which support a possible framework for delivering such help to people.

First, whether physicians, psychoanalysts, or other mental health experts were in contact with the patients, the professionals seem to have been secure in their own belief that they could help and were able to convey that attitude to the patient, to the relatives, and to other members of their team. Karush and colleagues report that interest, empathy, and optimism on the part of the therapists were more predictive of success even than the type of therapy, the skill of the interpretations, or the amount of experience of the therapist (84).

Second, all successful interventions provided extensive emotional support for their clients in whatever form that took. Whether is was provided by a single person as in intensive psychoanalysis or by a team as in the hospital studies, in all cases patients were enveloped in an environment in which it was both normal and acceptable to express even the deepest feelings. A third common element in successful treatment approaches is that when teams were involved in the treatment, the whole team was in synchrony with the plan. Sometimes even extended families, employers, and fellow employees were invited into the circle of people committed to creating a peaceful environment for these clients. Finally, many of these studies stress the beneficial effects of supporting clients in making positive environmental changes in their lives.

But why were these elements of use to the IBD patients? Was it because they alleviated the underlying psychopathology of these patients which had caused the illness to begin with? Or was it for some other reason? Another and simpler explanation would be that not only IBD patients, but patients with other illnesses might do better physically as well as psychologically in environments that offer intensive support for their total well-being. The four elements described above, positive attitude on the part of the practitioner, an environment in which expression of distress is permitted, synchrony among practitioners from various fields working with a patient, and finally support in making positive environmental changes, might be thought of as minimum requirements for programs designed to meet the psychological needs of any chronically ill population.

VI. CREATING A BROADER APPROACH

In our work with IBD patients we have chosen to incorporate these elements into a normative as opposed to a psychopathological approach. By normative we mean that we do not see these people as necessarily suffering from psychopathology by virtue of their diagnosis. Instead, we see them as emotionally healthy until proven otherwise, although often subject to a difficult adjustment process. From our perspective there are a number of advantages to operating from such a position. First, and most importantly, it encourages practitioners to develop a systematic way of addressing the reactive distress that IBD will inevitably cause, while at the same time it permits them to help people with the life-style issues involved in making an optimal adaptation to their illness. In addition, such an approach also avoids alienating the patients, who consider that they have a physical illness and will strongly resist being labeled mentally ill. Furthermore, it allows the therapist to be in synchrony with the issues uppermost in the minds of patients.

Based on the conclusions of numerous investigators, certain tasks have been defined in the literature as vital to such an adaptation process. As summarized by Cohen and Lazarus (98), patients must reduce harmful environmental conditions, tolerate or adjust to negative events and realities, maintain a positive self-image, maintain emotional equilibrium, and continue satisfying relationships with others. To these social and emotional goals we would add the need to construct a conceptual model through which they can interact with their illness in some manner not based on either denial or hopelessness, in other words, a model that will directly address the issue which is uppermost in their minds: "How am I going to live with a body that has gone functionally awry in a very nasty and threatening way and over which I no longer seem to have any control?" The distress and the confusion implied in this question is so pervasive for most IBD patients that to isolate emotional concerns and treat them in a vacuum will not meet their needs.

A central aspect of the approach we use involves helping people to regain some measure of control over their lives. For us this means encouraging them to understand that they are not totally helpless before the onslaught of the illness, that there are nonmedical interventions they themselves can engage in to support the efforts of their physicians. We encourage them, therefore, to raise their vision of their systemic illness to the systemic level and to understand that when you have a chronic illness of unknown cause for which there is no known cure, it makes sense to take excellent care of yourself in hopes of impacting the illness.

For this purpose we identify six interacting physical and emotional areas as needing consideration: stress management, activity level, nutrition, emotional well-being, relationships, and lastly, purpose and meaning. In each area the goal is the same. It is helping people to program balance into their lives at all levels to assist their bodies in regaining the lost homeostasis and to restore psychological well-being. Many IBD patients live markedly unbalanced lives as they strive to replace satisfactions lost to their illness with other satisfactions.

Within this approach, the responsibility for defining what is to be addressed is shared by the professional and the client. We do not label IBD patients as having emotional problems that need to be dealt with simply because they have IBD.

Rather, we work with them to identify what the work is that needs to be done in each area. This may involve learning stress management techniques, getting more sleep, working on relationships, broadening and improving their nutritional intake, taking time off from work, getting a new job, or dropping a class or two in an academic program. It may mean entering into dynamic psychotherapy aimed at uncovering and resolving longstanding issues from the past that create unneeded stress in the present. Or it may involve searching for meaning and purpose not only in their lives as a whole but also in the experience of having IBD. The research on grief has shown the importance of being able to attach meaning to traumatic events (99). People seem to do better if they can, as the folk wisdom goes, make "lemonade out of the lemon" fate has handed them.

We believe that the approach we have described has a number of important psychological implications which separate it from earlier approaches based on models of psychopathology. First, people begin to regain some sense of control over their lives. They move into an autonomous mode, as opposed to a heteronomous one in which they simply sink into the role of being managed by experts (100).

In addition, such an approach restores a more functional role to people by encouraging them to acknowledge the chronicity of their illness. It gives them permission to claim their rights as a sick person ("I am not well; therefore, I have a right to resist impossible demands on my strength and to take special care of myself"). But at the same time, since it is based upon people taking some responsibility for their own health, it keeps them from claiming the inappropriate liberties of the chronically ill that go along with denying the illness or becoming trapped in a hopeless position. Furthermore, from the viewpoint of the practitioner, it allows for avoiding the undesirable trap of telling patients they need something that is not congruent with their perceptions.

Will this kind of psychological support impact the physical condition? Only time and research will tell for certain. Certainly, the obverse of this statement, that poor psychological conditions will have a negative impact, has been borne out in the studies (101,102).

What are the limitations of this approach? One is that most people look for immediate short-term feedback. With our systemic approach we are asking them to compare results over much longer periods of time and to measure systemic outcomes. Instead of counting their bowel movements day by day, now they ask themselves such questions as "Am I a happier, more functional person than I was six months ago?" "Do I have more energy than I did six months ago?"

Another difficulty is that this approach will arouse resistance in some people. It means taking care of oneself at a high level. Some people are not interested in taking on this sort of responsibility; some are not able to. Others have not yet acknowledged the threat of the illness and may be in what has been defined as a defensive retreat stage of adaptation to crisis (103). Even for those who are interested and motivated, making changes in aspects of life-style, as anyone who has ever tried to diet or exercise knows, can be difficult and trying, and people will need much support. Although the literature has very little to say about support groups for IBD patients, we have found that when members are reasonably congenial and well-matched around degree of illness, they can be very helpful in this regard. Groups offer a setting in which IBD patients can engage in a mutual learning and discussion process centered on what it means to have a chronic illness of this magnitude. They provide a forum for exploring life-style issues, as well as the factors in peoples' past and present lives that inhibit change.

Even within the normalizing view we take of these patients, it is obvious that not all IBD patients will fall within a normal mental health range. Considering people with these illnesses as a whole, one can expect to find the same wide ranges of psychopathology that one would find in any group. Both the literature, as well as our own clinical experience, indicate that when IBD strikes someone already afflicted with severe psychopathology, the whole is more than the sum of the parts. Karush et al. reported that in schizophrenic patients, for example, the occurrence of IBD flare-ups greatly exacerbated the schizophrenic symptomatology (102). Furthermore, the medical prognosis for schizophrenics tended to be poor, despite the fact that diagnostic categories in general seemed unrelated to medical outcomes (101,102). In our experience, for patients who have extremely weak senses of self, the additional stress of having a body that is out of control creates a level of disequilibrium in the psyche that is difficulty to stabilize. For most patients, though, the literature and our own experience strongly indicate that this will not be the case.

We do occasionally see people who are anxious and depressed enough to be candidates for medication (104-106). For most people, however, individual and/or group support will be the main approach. If one views distress in a normative light it becomes obvious that the goal is not to suppress the troubling emotions, but rather to help patients work through their feelings to resolution.

A final caution is in order. Mental health professionals need to be aware at all times that these are major illnesses with potentially very serious consequences and that the first line of treatment will always be that of the medical specialists. Beyond that fact, if they are willing to withhold judgement and to meet the patient on his or her own terms we believe they can make a significant contribution to the overall treatment plan.

REFERENCES

1. Alexander, F., Psychosomatic Medicine. New York, W.W. Norton & Co., pp. 116-131 (1950).
2. Bockus, H. L., Present status of chronic regional or cicatrizing enteritis, JAMA, 127:449-456 (1945).

3. Cohn, E. M., I. I. Lederman, E. Shore, Regional enteritis and its relation to emotional disorders, Am. J. Gastroenterol., 54:378–387 (1970).
4. Crohn, B. B., Psychosomatic factors in ulcerative colitis in children, NY State J. Med., 63:1456–1457 (1963).
5. Engel, G. L., Studies of ulcerative colitis, III, The nature of the psychologic processes, Am. J. Med., 19:231–256 (1955).
6. Fava, G. A., L. Pavan, Large bowel disorder, I, Illness configuration and life events, Psychother. Psychosom., 27:93–99 (1976–77).
7. Finch, S. M., J. H. Hess, Ulcerative colitis in children, Am. J. Psych., 118: 819–826 (1962).
8. Ford, C. V., G. A. Glober, P. Castelnuovo-Tedesco, A psychiatric study of patients with regional enteritis, JAMA, 208:311–315 (1969).
9. Freyberger, H., The doctor/patient relationship in ulcerative colitis, Psychother. Psychosom., 18:80–89 (1970).
10. Fullerton, D. T., E. J. Kollar, A. B. Caldwell, A clinical study of ulcerative colitis, JAMA, 181:463–471 (1962).
11. Grace, W. J., Life stress and regional enteritis, Gastroenterology, 23:542–553 (1953).
12. Groen, J., J. M. Van Der Valk, Psychosomatic aspects of ulcerative colitis, Gastroenterologia 86:591–608 (1956).
13. Hislop, I. G., Onset setting in inflammatory bowel disease, Med. J. Aust. 1: 981–984 (1974).
14. Karush, A., G. E. Daniels, C. Flood, J. F. O'Connor, A review of the psychosomatic literature on chronic ulcerative colitis. In: Psychotherapy in Chronic Ulcerative Colitis. Philadelphia, W.B. Saunders, Chap. 3 (1977).
15. Krasner, L., Personality differences between patients classified as psychosomatic and nonpsychosomatic, J. Abnor. Psychol., 48:190–198 (1953).
16. Leidtke, R., H. Freyberger, S. Zepf, Personality features of patients with ulcerative colitis, Psychother. Psychosom., 28:187–192 (1977).
17. Lindemann, E., Psychiatric problems in conservative treatment of ulcerative colitis, Arch. Neur. Psychiatr., 53:322–324 (1945).
18. McDermott, J. F. Jr., S. M. Finch, Ulcerative colitis in children. Reassessment of a dilemma, J. Am. Acad. Child Psychiatr., 6:512–525 (1967).
19. McMahon, A. W., J. F. Patterson, Personality differences between inflammatory bowel disease patients and their healthy siblings, Psychosom. Med., 35:91–103 (1973).
20. Murray, C. D., Psychogenic factors in the etiology of ulcerative colitis and bloody diarrhea, Am. J. Med. Sci., 180:239–248 (1930).
21. O'Connor, J. F., Psychological considerations in ulcerative colitis, NY State J. Med., 68:1055–1065 (1968).
22. Paulley, J. W., Ulcerative colitis. A study of 173 cases, Gastroenterology, 16:566–576 (1950).
23. Paulley, J. W., The emotional factors in ulcerative colitis, Gastroenterologia, 86:709–712 (1956).
24. Prugh, D. G., The influence of emotional factors on the clinical course of ulcerative colitis in children, Gastroenterology, 18:339–354 (1951).

25. Reinhart, J. B., R. A. Succop, Regional enteritis in pediatric patients, Psychiatric aspects, J. Am. Acad. Child. Psychiatr., 7:252-281 (1968).
26. Rigatelli, M., A global psychosomatic study of 16 consecutive patients with ulcerative colitis, Psychother. Psychosom., 35:22-33 (1981).
27. Rosenbaum, M., Ulcerative colitis, Psychosomatics, 24-515-529 (1983).
28. Sheffield, B. F., M. W. Carney, Crohn's disease: a psychosomatic illness?, Br. J. Psychiatr., 128:446-450 (1976).
29. Sperling, M., Ulcerative colitis in children. Current views and therapies, J. Am Acad. Child. Psychiatr., 8:336-352 (1969).
30. Stewart, W. A., Psychosomatic aspects of regional ileitis, NY State J. Med., 49:2820-2824 (1949).
31. Schwartz, R. A., I. K. Schwartz, Psychiatric disorders associated with Crohn's disease, Int. J. Psychiatr. Med., 12:67-73 (1982).
32. Whybrow, P. C., F. J. Kane, M. A. Lipton, Regional ileitis and psychiatric disorder, Psychosom. Med., 30:209-221 (1968).
33. Crocket, R. W., Psychiatric findings in Crohn's disease, Lancet, 1:946-949 (1952).
34. Esler, M. D., K. J. Goulston, Levels of anxiety in colonic disorders, N. Engl. J. Med., 288:16-20 (1973).
35. Feldman, F., D. Cantor, S. Soll, W. Bachrach, Psychiatric study of a series of 34 consecutive patients with ulcerative colitis, Br. Med. J., 3:14-17 (1967).
36. Feldman, F., D. Cantor, S. Soll, W. Bachrach, Psychiatric study of a consecutive series of 19 patients with regional ileitis, Br. Med. J., 4:711-714 (1967).
37. Goligher, J. C., F. T. de Dombal, J. Mc.K. Wattis, G. Watkinson, Ulcerative Colitis. Baltimore, William & Wilkins Co. (1968).
38. Hamilton, J. R., G. A. Bruce, M. Abdourhaman, D. G. Gall, Inflammatory bowel disease in children and adolescents, Adv. Pediatr., 26:311-341 (1979).
39. Helzer, J. E., S. Chammas, C. C. Norland, W. A. Stillings, D. H. Alpers, A study of the association between Crohn's disease and psychiatric illness, Gastroenterology, 86:324-330 (1984).
40. Helzer, J. E. W. A., Stillings, S. Chammas, C. C. Norland, D. H. Alpers, A controlled study of the association between ulcerative colitis and psychiatric diagnosis, Dig. Dis. Sci., 27:513-518 (1982).
41. Hendriksen, C., V. Binder, Social prognosis in patients with ulcerative colitis, Br. Med. J., 281:581-583 (1980).
42. Kraft, I. A., C. Ardali, A psychiatric study of children with diagnosis of regional ileitis, South. J. Med., 57:799-802 (1964).
43. Mendeloff, A. I., M. Monk, C. I. Siegel, A. Lilienfeld, Illness experience and life stresses in patients with irritable colon and with ulcerative colitis, N. Engl. J. Med., 282(1):14-17 (1970).
44. Monk, M., A. L. Mendeloff, C. I. Siegel, A. Lilienfeld, An epidemiological study of ulcerative colitis and regional enteritis among adults in Baltimore-III, J. Chronic Dis., 22(8):565-578 (1970).

45. Sloan, N. P., J. A. Nargen, R. B. Gage, Life histories of patients with chronic ulcerative colitis. A review of 2000 cases, Gastroenterology, 54 (Suppl):819–822 (1968).
46. Steinhausen, H-C., Comparative studies of ulcerative colitis and Crohn's disease in children and adolescents, J. Child. Psych. Psychiatr., 25:33–42 (1982).
47. Steinhausen, H-C., Life events in relation to psychopathology among severely and chronically ill children and adolescents, Child. Psychiatr. Human Dev., 13:249–258 (1983).
48. West, K. L., MMPI correlates of ulcerative colitis. J. Clin. Psychol., 26:214–219 (1970).
49. Eaton, M. T. Jr., M. H. Peterson, J. A. Davis, Psychiatry. Medical Outline Series, 4th ed. New York, Medical Examination Publishing Co., p. 186 (1981).
50. Kaplan, H. I., B. J. Sadock, Clinical Psychiatry from Synopsis of Psychiatry. Baltimore, Williams & Wilkins, p. 265 (1988).
51. Gazzard, B. G., H. L. Price, G. W. Libby, A. M. Dawson, The social toll of Crohn's disease, Br. Med. J., 2(6145):1117–1119 (1978).
52. Latimer, P. R., Crohn's disease: A review of the psychological and social outcome, Psychol. Med., 8:649–656 (1978).
53. Olbrisch, M. E., S. W. Ziegler, Psychological adjustment and patient information in inflammatory bowel disease: Development of two assessment instruments, J. Chronic Dis., 35:649–658 (1982).
54. Kirsner, J. B., Inflammatory bowel disease. Considerations of etiology and pathogenesis, Am. J. Gastroenterol., 69(3 Pt 1):253–271 (1978).
55. Simmons, M. A., Using the nursing process in treating inflammatory bowel disease, Nurs. Clin. North Am., 19(1):11–25 (1984).
56. Sparacino, L. L., Psychosocial considerations for the adolescent and young adult with inflammatory bowel disease, Nurs. Clin. North Am., 19(1):41–49 (1984).
57. Kubler-Ross, E., On Death and Dying. New York, Macmillan (1969).
58. Cooley, C. H., Human nature and the Social Order. New York, Schocken Books (1964).
59. Levitan, H. L., Infantile factors in two cases of ulcerative colitis, Int. J. Psychiatr. 1. Med., 8:185–190 (1977–78).
60. Goldberg, D., A psychiatric study of patients with diseases of the small intestine, Gut, 11:459–465 (1970).
61. Riemer, M. D., Case reports. Ileitis-underlying aggressive conflicts, NY State J. Med., 60:552–557 (1960).
62. Grace, W. J., H. G. Wolff, Treatment of ulcerative colitis, JAMA, 146:981–987 (1951).
63. Edmiston, F. G., R. C. Williams, A study of object relations in a case of ulcerative colitis, Comp. Psychiatry, 4(2):96–104 (1963).
64. Bluebond-Langner, M., The Private Worlds of Dying Children. Princeton, NJ, Princeton University Press (1978).
65. Myer, S. A., Overview of inflammatory bowel disease, Nurs. Clin. North Am., 19(1):3–9 (1984).

66. Goffman, E., Stigma, Notes on the Management of Spoiled Identity. Englewood Cliffs, NJ, Prentice-Hall (1963).
67. Kelly, M. P., The subjective experience of chronic disease: Some implications for the management of ulcerative colitis, J. Chronic. Dis., 39:653–666 (1986).
68. Mayberry, J. F., J. S. Morris, B. Calcraft, J. Rhodes, Information assessment by patients of a booklet on Crohn's disease, Publ. Hlth. Lon., 99: 239–242 (1985).
69. Rees, J. E. P., J. F. Mayberry, B. Calcraft, What the patient wants to know about Crohn's disease, J. Clin. Gastroenterol., 5:221–222 (1983).
70. Scholmerich, J., P. Sedlack, P. Hoppe-Seyler, W. Gerok, The information needs and fears of patients with inflammatory bowel disease, Hepatogastroenterology, 34:162–165 (1967).
71. Smart, H., J. Mayberry, B. Calcraft, J. S. Morris, J. Rhodes, Effect of information booklet on patients' anxiety levels and consultation rates in Crohn's disease, Pub. Health, 100:164–165 (1986).
72. Parsons, T., The Social System. New York, Free Press, p. 285 (1951).
73. Sperling, M., Psychoanalytic study of ulcerative colitis in children, Psychoanalyt. Q., 15:302–329 (1946).
74. Lockhart-Mummery, H. E., B. C. Morson, Crohn's disease of the large intestine, Gut, 5:493–509 (1964).
75. Steinhausen, H-C., H. Kies, Comparative studies of ulcerative colitis and Crohn's disease in children and adolescents, J. Child. Psych. Psychiatr., 25:33–42 (1982).
76. McKegney, F. P., R. O. Gordon, S. M. Levine, A psychosomatic comparison of patients with ulcerative colitis and Crohn's disease, Psychosom. Med., 32:153–166 (1970).
77. Bressler, B., Ulcerative colitis as an anniversary symptom. Emergency psychotherapy with remission of symptoms, Psych. Rev., 43(3):381–387 (1956).
78. Chambers, W. N., M. Rosenbaum, Ulcerative colitis. Psychosomatic Conference of the Cincinnati General Hospital, Psychosom. Med., 15(5):523–532 (1953).
79. Clark, L. D., Psychotherapy of ulcerative colitis. Dis. Nerv. Syst., 17(5): 149–154 (1956).
80. Daniels, G. E., Treatment of a case of ulcerative colitis associated with hysterical depression, Psychosom. Med., 2:276–285 (1940).
81. Joseph, E. D., Some psychiatric observations of ulcerative colitis with report of a case, J. Nerv. Ment. Dis., 51–57 (1958).
82. Klein, H. S., Notes on a case of ulcerative colitis, Int. J. Psychoanal., 46: 342–351 (1965).
83. Straker, M., Ulcerative colitis: Recovery of a patient with brief psychiatric treatment, Can. Med. Assoc. J., 82:1224–1227 (1960).
84. Karush, A., G. E. Daniels, J. F. O'Connor, L. O. Stern, The response to psychotherapy in chronic ulcerative colitis. II. Factors arising from the therapeutic situation, Psychosom. Med., 31:201–226 (1969).

85. Langford, W. S., The psychological aspects of ulcerative colitis, Clin. Proc. Child. Hosp., 20(4):89-97 (1964).
86. Paulley, J. W., Crohn's disease. Treatment by corticosteroids, antibiotics and psychotherapy, Psychother. Psychosom., 19:111-117 (1971).
87. Grace, W. J., R. H. Pinsky, H. G. Wolff, The treatment of ulcerative colitis II., Gastroenterology, 26:462-468 (1954).
88. Crohn, B. B., H. Yarnis, Present trends in treatment of ulcerative colitis, NY Med. J., 51:2129 (1951).
89. Weinstock, H. I., Hospital psychotherapy in severe ulcerative colitis, Arch. Gen. Psychiatr., 4:509-512 (1961).
90. Weinstock, H. I., Successful treatment of ulcerative colitis by psychoanalysis: A survey of 28 cases, with follow-up, J. Psychosom. Res., 6:243-249 (1962).
91. O'Connor, J. F., G. Daniels, C. Flood, A. Karush, L. Moses, L. Stern, An evaluation of the effectiveness of psychotherapy in the treatment of ulcerative colitis, Ann. Intern. Med., 60(4):587-602 (1964).
92. O'Connor, J. F., Ulcerative colitis: Emotional problems and their management, Med. Times, 11:106-113 (1966).
93. Groen, J., J. Bastiaans, Psychotherapy of ulcerative colitis, Gastroenterology, 18:344-352 (1951).
94. Groen, J. J., D. Birnbaum, Conservative (supportive) treatment of severe ulcerative colitis. Methods and results, Isr. J. Med. Sci., 4:130-139 (1968).
95. Marder, L., Symposium: Psychiatric aspects of ulcerative colitis, South. Med. J., 91:1281-1284 (1967).
96. Nichols, C. R., J. B. Nowlin, M. D. Bogdonoff, Some psychologic considerations in the medical management of ulcerative colitis, South. Med. J., 60:1285-1288 (1967).
97. Freyberger, H., H. W. Kunsebeck, W. Lempa, W. Wellman, H. J. Avenarius, Psychotherapeutic interventions in alexithymic patients, Psychother. Psychosom., 44:72-81 (1985).
98. Cohen, F., R. S. Lazarus, Coping with the Stresses of Illness, Health Psychology. San Francisco, Jossey-Bass, pp. 217-254 (1979).
99. Glick, I. O., R. S. Weiss, C. M. Parkes, The First Year of Bereavement. New York, Wiley-Interscience (1974).
100. Illich, I., Medical Nemesis: The Expropriation of Health. London, Calder and Boyars, (1975).
101. Karush, A., G. E. Daniels, J. F. O'Connor, L. O. Stern, The response of psychotherapy in chronic ulcerative colitis. 1. Pretreatment factors, Psychosom. Med., 30(3):255-276 (1968).
102. O'Connor, J. F., G. Daniels, A. Karush, C. Flood, L. O. Stern, Prognostic implications of psychiatric diagnosis in ulcerative colitis, Psychosom. Med. 28:375-381 (1966).
103. Fink, S. L., Crisis and motivation: A theoretical model, Arch. Phys. Med. Rehab., 48:592-597 (1967).
104. Chaplan, A., S. K. Vanov, GI illness. Treatment of the anxiety component, Psychosomatics, 18(4):49-54 (1977).

105. Furtado, J. D., Lorazepam in gastrointestinal disorders with anxiety overlay, Psychosomatics, 17:32–34 (1976).
106. Stokes, D. K. Lorazepam in anxiety associated with chronic enteritis and ulcerative colitis, J. Clin. Psychiatr., 39:53–57 (1978).

14 Case Studies

Mark A. Peppercorn The previous chapters presented in-depth reviews of individual therapeutic modalities or general topics in the management of patients with inflammatory bowel disease (IBD).

This chapter deals with many of the specific clinical presentations of IBD patients encountered by the practicing physician. The cases are drawn from actual clinical practice and the management of each case is discussed by two of our authors.

CASE 1. DISTAL ULCERATIVE COLITIS

A 26-year-old woman presents with a one-month history of rectal bleeding, tenesmus, and the passage of mucus associated with two to three soft stools per day. Her exam and lab tests including stool cultures are unremarkable. Flexible sigmoidoscopy to 60 cm reveals diffuse erythema, petechiae, loss of vascular markings, exudate and touch friability in the distal 28 cm, with normal mucosa above that area. Biopsies show a diffuse colitis with no granulomas.

Stephen B. Hanauer Although the presentation of distal ulcerative colitis remains one of the most common clinical scenarios of IBD, the optimal treatment remains undefined and usually depends on a combination of physician and patient preferences. Since most of my patients prefer oral versus rectal therapy, I usually offer sulfasalazine to individuals with mild distal disease. I begin with a 2 g daily dose and advance to 4 g daily if there is no initial response and the drug is tolerated.

If the patient does not respond quickly to the oral therapy or is very uncomfortable, then a course of hydrocortisone enemas usually produces a clinical response which, in most cases, should be maintained with oral sulfasalazine. Patients with a mild first attack may sometimes be treated with a course of steroid enemas without maintenance therapy as long as they are observed and cautioned against the risk of relapse.

5-Aminosalicylate (5-ASA) enemas also are a highly effective therapy for distal ulcerative colitis and can be administered for an acute flare after which patients may be weaned, treated expectantly for relapse, switched to an oral agent, or given 5-ASA enemas on a maintenance schedule (e.g., every other night, every third night, or nightly for one week per month). At the moment, the cost of the 5-ASA enemas and apparent need for maintenance enema therapy are problematic in prescribing these as first-line treatments.

Gerald Friedman I believe the treatment of choice for new onset distal ulcerative colitis is the use of nightly rectal instillations of 100 mg of hydrocortisone in 60 cc of diluent for 14 nights. Most patients in this category (e.g., first onset of disease, no prior history, and negative stools for ova and parasites and culture) will respond in a salutory manner with dramatic reduction of symptoms and endoscopic reversal of disease within two weeks. This being the initial episode, I could not add sulfasalazine at this time to prevent recurrences, but would rather observe the patient's future course. If this therapy did not prove effective, then I would consider the alternatives mentioned by Dr. Hanauer.

CASE 2. REFRACTORY DISTAL COLITIS

A 23-year-old man developed rectal bleeding and constipation four years earlier. Sigmoidoscopy revealed ulcerative proctitis involving the distal 8 cm of rectum. He was treated successfully with a course of hydrocortisone enemas which was repeated two years later when he had recurrent symptoms. Three months ago he again developed rectal bleeding now associated with three loose stools per day. When another course of steroid enemas failed to resolve his symptoms, he underwent flexible sigmoidoscopy to 60 cm which showed active colitis up to 20 cm. The steroid enemas were stopped and for the past two months he has been taking sulfasalazine at a dose of 3 g per day, but bleeding and diarrhea persist.

Gerald Friedman This patient has a typical history of proctitis progressing to proctosigmoiditis with recurrent episodes over a four-year period. Typically, such patients have an initial favorable response to absorbable steroid enemas, but later become refractory or relatively refractory to such therapy. Additionally, a

3-g dose of sulfasalazine has failed to prevent recurrent episodes of colitis. This patient is a candidate for the use of rectally instilled 5-ASA enemas administered nightly for a minimum period of three weeks. A significant percentage of patients in this category will respond both clinically and endoscopically to such treatment. The onset of action is not as rapid as seen with steroid enemas. To sustain the beneficial effect, it is often necessary to continue rectal instillations at night, reducing the frequency of administration to every other night or every third night. At this time it would be prudent to increase the oral dose of sulfasalazine to 4 g daily. If the beneficial effects of the combined therapy is sustained, further reduction of the rectally administered suspension is indicated.

Stephen B. Hanauer I agree that most patients with refractory distal colitis will respond to local therapy with 5-ASA enemas or suppositories, despite prior resistance to sulfasalazine and topical or oral steroids. As noted, the response may take up to 6–12 weeks, so an initial failure to completely resolve should not lead to early termination of the new therapy. Maintenance therapy with 5-ASA enemas (or possibly oral 5-ASA or sulfasalazine) will be necessary.

If the patient fails to improve with 5-ASA enemas, we have been able to recruit additional responses with the addition of topical steroids in conjunction with 5-ASA enemas (steroid enema or steroid foam every morning 5-ASA enema every evening). These patients typically require high doses of oral steroids to respond, in which case 5-ASA enemas may assist in steroid weaning.

Occasionally, an immunosuppressant will assist in steroid weaning. Less than 10% of our colectomies are for refractory distal disease. Finally, if the patients had ceased smoking cigarettes prior to the attack, a return to smoking may benefit the colitis. Prostaglandin enemas are being investigated for distal colitis and, in rare cases of "allergic proctitis," sodium cromoglycate enemas may be tried.

This is a frustrating group of patients to treat; many will have mild, nonprogressive symptoms which simmer along despite all attempts at therapy. Persistence with an optimistic attitude and alternating attempts to try new combinations will occasionally result in a remission. Many of these refractory ulcerative colitis patients will turn out to have Crohn's disease, so a trial of metronidazole may be of benefit.

CASE 3. MODERATE ACTIVE ULCERATIVE COLITIS

A 39-year-old man had noted intermittent rectal bleeding attributed to hemorrhoids for five years. Three weeks ago following an upper respiratory infection he began having diarrhea with four to six loose stools per day. Subsequently, rectal bleeding, abdominal cramps, and a painful swollen right ankle developed. His exam is normal except for mild left lower quadrant tenderness. Lab tests show a hematocrit of 38%, white blood cells 11,200, and stool cultures were negative. Flexible sigmoidoscopy reveals active colitis to 60 cm, with extension at least several centimeters beyond the reach of the scope.

Samuel Meyers My initial therapy of this patient includes a combination of oral and rectal medication. Even though I am not sure of the anatomic extent of the colitis, clearly there is involvement of the left colon. Topical enema therapy provides high doses of medication to the effected mucosa of the distal colon. This could be additive to the oral medication, with less potential for additional side effects. I introduce sulfasalazine at a dose of 500 mg/day. This is increased 500 mg each day to a dose of 6 g daily, in three or four divided doses. If the patient develops side effects at this high dose, I will determine the highest tolerable level. Two grams daily is the minimal therapeutic dose. Enema therapy consists of 5-ASA at the commercially available dose of 4 g daily, given at bedtime. An alternative is a 100 mg hydrocortisone enema. During this combined oral and enema therapy I monitor renal function periodically. The potential for renal side effects of the 5-ASA has been suggested by animal studies.

I allow 6 to 8 weeks for this combination to be effective. The temptation to use antibiotics for the upper respiratory infection is resisted. This will not be useful for this invariably self-limited viral infection and could induce further diarrhea or even an antibiotic colitis. The arthritis is treated symptomatically and will resolve when the colitis activity subsides.

If the patient deteriorates or fails to respond, I consider stopping the enemas and adding oral corticosteroids. I use prednisone at a dose of 45 mg to 60 mg daily for 10 to 14 days. Once a response occurs I lower the dose 5 mg every 7 to 10 days. If the colitis flares up during the withdrawal period, it may become necessary to raise the dose to attain control. Then I attempt withdrawal again. If the patient cannot be weaned to a dose of less than 10 mg daily within one year, I seriously consider a surgical approach. Once the condition stabilizes, it becomes important to determine the extent of disease. I would be more definite in my surgical recommendation if the patient has extensive disease, although even with left-sided disease, I would be reluctant to continue long-term, high-dose prednisone therapy. I would consider an immunosuppressive medication to aid in the withdrawal of the prednisone, but I do not enthusiastically support this approach in view of the limited data attesting to its efficacy and the potential for serious toxicity. This is especially true, since ulcerative colitis is a surgically curable disease.

If I am successful, a clinical remission will be achieved medically. Then the prednisone can be stopped. I will continue the sulfasalazine as indefinite maintenance therapy at a dose of 2 g/day.

Mark A. Peppercorn The patient is moderately ill but needs to be brought under control realtively quickly before he becomes sicker. My approach is similar to that of Dr. Meyers. I would use sulfasalazine getting the patient up to 3 or 4 g/day within one week and look for improvement within two to three weeks. Occasionally doses of 5 or 6 g/day are useful but usually not well tolerated. The addition of 5-ASA enemas or hydrocortisone enemas may be useful if they can be retained. I would try to avoid nonsteroidal anti-inflammatory agents for his arthritis because of their potential to aggravate the colitis. If he did not respond to the sulfasalazine or was intolerant and I had no access to an oral aminosalicylate, I would begin prednisone at 40-60 mg/day, depending on the severity of his condition, continue the initial dose for two weeks, and then, assuming he is better, begin to taper by 5 mg/week. I would continue the sulfasalazine while starting the steroid, and if he went into remission keep him on a maintenance dose of 2 g/day once he was off the prednisone, warning him about possible effects on fertility in case he wants to have children.

CASE 4. SEVERE ULCERATIVE COLITIS

A 59-year-old woman had a six-year history of left-sided colitis with intermittent episodes of bloody diarrhea and cramps treated with sulfasalazine and brief courses of prednisone. Shortly after a trip to the Dominican Republic while on maintenance sulfasalazine, she developed severe diarrhea with 12 to 15 stools per day, cramps, bleeding, fever to 102°F, and anorexia. On exam she appeared ill, with BP 90/60, P 130, T 102.6°F pr; bowel sounds were hypoactive and she had tenderness with mild guarding in the left midabdomen. Her WBC is 21,000 with 15% bands, Hct 34.6%, BUN 32 mg%, and serum K 2.9 mEq/l. A plain film of the abdomen shows thumbprinting of the left colon and some loss of haustration of the transverse colon which measures 6 cm. Three stools for parasites and bacterial pathogens are negative. Rigid sigmoidoscopy to 12 cm shows a friable mucosa with exudate.

Francis A. Farraye This woman has severe ulcerative colitis with many features seen in patients with toxic megacolon. Dilation of any segment of the colon greater than 6 cm in this clinical setting constitutes the diagnosis of toxic megacolon. Regardless of the colon diameter, this patient is clearly "toxic" with dehydration, fever, abdominal pain, ileus, leukocytosis, and electrolyte abnormalities and requires aggressive treatment.

The patient requires immediate hospitalization. Surgical consultation should be obtained and the patient made NPO. Deyhydration and electrolyte abnormalities should be corrected. Narcotic analgesics and antidiarrheal agents must be avoided. The trip to the West Indies raises the possibility of a superimposed bacterial or parasitic infection not detected by the routine culture techniques. I would exclude the presence of *C.difficile* by toxin testing and obtain serum for amebic hemagglutin assay. Blood cultures must be obtained. I would discontinue the sulfasalazine and initiate therapy with parenteral corticosteroids. Several different preparations can be used and include methylprednisolone (48-60 mg), or hydrocortisone (200–300 mg). I prefer methylprednisolone as a constant infusion because it is less salt-retaining than hydrocortisone. Others feel that ACTH is useful, especially in patients not previously on steroids (80-110 units/day). Given the clinical severity of her illness broad-spectrum antibiotics should be started concomitantly and would include an aminoglycoside and metronidazole. Depending on the extent of the colonic dilatation, a rectal tube and a nasogastric or long intestinal tube may be needed for decompression.

If there is evidence of significant protein malnutrition, a central line for total parenteral nutrition will be necessary, but need not be placed acutely. Peripheral parenteral nutrition should be instituted upon admission after correction of electrolyte abnormalities and dehydration.

The gastrointestinal surgeon should be involved in the patient's care from admission. Close serial observations are essential with daily or twice daily plain film assessment for perforation or progressive dilation of the colon. I would have the patient roll from supine to prone position in an effort to decompress the dilated colon. Surgery should be seriously considered if there is no improvement within 72 hours. Short of perforation, the actual timing of surgery will be dependent on the clinical response to this aggressive medical regimen, the duration of the ulcerative colitis and the patient's wishes. Persistent fever in a patient who seems to be improving should be evaluated by a CT scan of the abdomen.

If the patient improves, I would empirically continue the IV antibiotics for 5 to 7 days unless cultures are positive. The patient can usually be changed to oral steroids (prednisone 40-60 mg/day) after two weeks of parenteral therapy. Feedings are begun with clear liquids followed by a BRAT diet (bananas, rice, applesauce, toast) and finally a low residue diet. Sulfasalazine can be restarted at the time of discharge.

Samuel Meyers As described above, this woman presents with an acute exacerbation of her chronic ulcerative colitis and requires hospitalization. The clinical picture and the plain film of the abdomen suggests disease extension beyond the known left-sided involvement. She is toxic and has megacolon seen on the abdominal x-ray. My approach to her care is quite similar to that outlined by Dr. Farraye. Elimination of all oral intake as well as intravenous fluid repletion and correction of the electrolyte imbalances are a necessary first step. Blood transfusions and plasma are given as needed. I also use broad-spectrum antibiotics for presumed sepsis. The combination chosen includes an aminoglycoside and coverage for anaerobes as well as enterococci. This is to be adjusted once results of blood cultures are available. I prefer a long intestinal tube to help decompress the bowel and prevent further gas accumulation. A rectal tube and rotation of the patient from the supine to the prone position every 15 minutes while awake is recommended. This will help to expel the colonic gas and reduce the risk to perforation. Sulfasalazine is discontinued and a corticoid agent given. Unlike Dr. Farraye, I prefer ACTH in this patient who has not received corticosteroids. It is given as a continuous intravenous infusion of 120 units daily. Stool examination for parasites and bacterial pathogens will continue in view of the onset during vacation in a tropical area.

A surgeon is asked to examine the patient and become involved in the care on a regular basis. This is requested upon hospital admission. Clinical examination and abdominal x-ray are required at least twice daily. If she deteriorates, prompt surgery before perforation occurs may be lifesaving. If she fails to respond, I too will suggest surgery after about 72 hours. If there is some improvement, the therapy is continued for 10 days. If she is well enough, the intestinal tube is removed and oral intake slowly introduced.

Once the ACTH therapy is completed, oral prednisone is started at a dose of 60 mg daily in divided doses. If she remains stable after several days of observation she is discharged from the hospital. If clinical remission was achieved during the ACTH therapy, I would be optimistic, at least in the short term. However, if remission does not occur, I prepare her for the probability of surgery. This will be necessary in at least half of such patients within one year.

After 10 to 14 days, I start to lower the prednisone dose 5 mg every 7 to 10 days. Sulfasalazine is introduced as the prednisone is reduced to about 25 mg daily. The initial dose is 500 mg per day. This is increased 500 mg each day to a dose of 6 g daily, in three or four divided doses. If the patient develops side effects at this dose, as noted above, I will determine the highest tolerable level. The minimal therapeutic dose is 2 g daily.

If the colitis flares up during the withdrawal period, it may become necessary to raise the prednisone dose to attain control. Then I attempt withdrawal again. If the patient cannot be weaned to a dose of less than 10 mg daily within one year, I seriously reconsider a surgical approach. During the treatment period, once the condition stabilizes, it becomes important to determine the disease extent as in Case 3. I would be more definite in my surgical recommendation if the patient has extensive disease, although again even with left-sided disease, I would be reluctant to continue long-term, high-dose prednisone therapy. My concerns regarding immunosuppressives have been stated above.

If a clinical remission has been achieved, then the prednisone can be stopped. As before, I will continue the sulfasalazine as indefinite maintenance therapy, at a dose of 2 g/day.

CASE 5. CROHN'S COLITIS

A 42-year-old woman began noting supraumbilical burning pain, nonbloody loose stools, and canker sores. Five weeks later she saw her internist who obtained stool cultures which were negative and a barium enema read as normal. A trial of loperamide was not effective. Her exam is unremarkable except for guaiac-positive stools. Labs included Hct 33.2%, WBC 14,800 with 14% bands, albumin 3.1 g%. A colonoscopy shows normal mucosa in the distal 50 cm with focal ulcerations and edematous folds from 50 cm to the hepatic flexure. A small bowel x-ray is unremarkable.

Lawrence J. Brandt This woman appears to have a segmental colitis. The differential diagnosis of such a process in this age group includes Crohn's disease, infectious colitis, colitis of systemic diseases, drug-induced colitis, and rarely ischemic colitis—usually due to vasculitis (periarteritis, SLE or HBsAg) or oral contraceptives. A history of drug use, especially antibiotic and oral contraceptives, would be relevant. However, the presence of canker sores, perhaps reflecting an extraintestinal manifestation of IBD, would be unusual with medication-induced colitis. A history of travel also would be important as infectious colitis can present in this fashion. I also would take a careful social history including the patient's sexual contacts because now we are seeing infectious colitis as the initial presentation of AIDS. The patient has a mild anemia, a leukocytosis with an increase in band forms, and an albumin which is in the low range, showing that the process is both chronic and acute. It is important to biopsy the normal as well as the abnormal appearing areas. Blood cultures as well as a culture of the stool is crucial, and it might be important to culture the biopsy material for viruses such as cytomegalovirus and also herpes virus. If the patient was not on medications and had no systemic diseases such as lupus or periarteritis nodosa and no sexual contacts which might predispose to infection with human immunodeficiency virus or hepatitis B virus, and if the stool cultures and tissue cultures were negative, I would begin the patient on parenteral hyperalimentation, and parenteral broad-spectrum antibiotics. I would not use steroids because the patient does not appear to be toxic, although I am concerned about he leukocytosis and increase in bands. If the patient did not respond within a week to ten days or if she developed fever or abdominal signs, I would add intravenous ACTH to the regimen.

Mark A. Peppercorn This patient is moderately ill as reflected by her symptoms, serum albumin, and extent of disease. Once the likely diagnosis had been limited by the above studies to Crohn's colitis, I would begin her on sulfasalazine and gradually increase the dose over one week to 3 or 4 g/day depending on her response. From the case description, she does not seem ill enough to warrant initial parenteral therapy in hospital as preferred by Dr. Brandt. I would hope for improvement within one or two weeks, but as long as she was holding her own would not give up on it for three or four weeks. If she did improve, I would lower the dose to 2 g/day and in three months recolonoscope her. If signs of active disease were absent, I would taper and stop the sulfasalazine since it does not appear to have a prophylactic benefit. If she was not improving in that time or if she could not tolerate sulfasalazine, I would next use metronidazole at a dose of 250 mg p.o. three times a day. If she responded, I would continue this dose and followup as I would with sulfasalazine. Should she not have a full response within 2 to 3 weeks, or should her condition worsen, I would add prednisone at a dose of 40–60 mg/day. If she showed signs of toxicity, I would admit her to the hospital and place her on broad-spectrum antibiotics and parenteral steroids. Assuming she responded to prednisone, I would continue the initial dose for 2 weeks and then try to taper her off it by 5 mg/week. I would go to 6-mercaptopurine only if the above measures failed.

CASE 6. CROHN'S ILEITIS

A 36-year-old woman presents with several hours of crampy abdominal pain and vomiting. She gave a 10-year history of recurrent diarrhea and abdominal pain thought to be related to stress. In the prior month she has had a recurrence of diarrhea with four to five loose stools per day, severe cramps, and periods of postprandial nausea. She had a history of rash on sulfa drugs. A plain film of the abdomen shows dilated small bowel loops and air–fluid levels. She quickly improved with nasogastric suction and intravenous fluids. A small bowel x-ray is abnormal with a narrowed ulcerated distal 15 cm of ileum. A colonoscopy is unremarkable.

Samuel Meyers This patient has a history of Crohn's disease manifested by recurrent diarrhea and abdominal pain. She now presents with an exacerbation complicated by intestinal obstruction. The initial therapy with intestinal decompression and intravenous fluids was successful. The next priority is to replace any vitamin and nutrient deficiencies. Peripheral or central alimentation is not usually necessary until the patient has been without oral intake for about 10 days; it may be prudent however if she had a serious nutritional deficiency upon entering the hospital. I would also add antibiotics to her therapy aimed at any potential suppurative component that may be contributing to the obstruction. I use cefoxitin, or in sicker patients, a combination of drugs. This should include an aminoglycoside and agents that would be effective against anaerobes and enterococci. The antibiotic choice is reconsidered once the results of blood cultures are available.

I wait several days to evaluate the effect of the antibiotic and supportive therapy. If these are inadequate, then a parenteral corticoid agent is added. In any event, if she had been on one of these agents before hospitalization, it must continue. I use hydrocortisone, at a dose of 300 mg daily or its equivalent, given as a continuous intravenous infusion. If she has not recently been on corticosteroids, I use a continuous infusion of ACTH, 120 units daily as in Case 4.

If either the antibiotic or the corticoid therapies were effective, I continue them for 10–14 days. During this time the nasogastric suction is discontinued and oral feedings slowly introduced. At the completion of this treatment period, if ACTH was used it is stopped and oral prednisone, 40-60 mg is given in divided doses. This is then reduced by 5 mg every 7 to 14 days, hopefully being able to drop it as soon as possible. This attempts to avoid the often serious steroid side effects. I reduce the prednisone so that once a 15 mg/day dose is given, it is administered as a single morning dose.

During the initial treatment period I begin to consider the choice of maintenance therapy. An oral antibiotic could be continued in cycles of three weeks on and one week off until a drug-free remission is achieved. An alternative is to rotate drugs in 3- or 4-week cycles. These maneuvers are in an attempt to prevent the emergence of microbial resistance. I use ampicillin, cephalexin, or tetracycline in this manner. Trimethoprimsulfamethoxazole is not an acceptable choice since she is allergic to sulfa drugs. Once oral medications are possible, another alternative is the use of sulfasalazine in therapeutic and later maintenance doses. Since this is not possible due to her sulfa allergy, one of the newer oral 5-ASA drugs can be substituted. Presently these are not approved for routine use in the United States. However, they may be obtained from pharmaceutical companies on a case by case basis. Pentasa, Claversal, or Asacol may all be useful, since they release medication in the small bowel. I favor the latter two which deliver their medication more distally.

I expect improvement with medical therapy, at least initially. Only a minority of patients with Crohn's disease will require emergency surgery because of obstruction. However, if the improvement is not dramatic and continued, I strongly favor surgical removal of all diseased bowel. My leaning toward surgical therapy is also true in the maintenance phase. If there were to be a prompt recurrence of active disease, surgery would provide rapid relief. It is my experience that most patients with chronic Crohn's disease who have an episode of severe obstruction will require surgery. Therefore, I do not prolong ineffective medical therapy. This only results in a poor quality of life for the patient and the high likelihood of serious side effects from the drugs. In this patient with localized disease, I would not favor the use of immunosuppressive drugs over the effective results of surgical resection. The issue of postoperative recurrence must be carefully explained to the patient. However, this does not delay my choice of surgical therapy for this patient.

Mark A. Peppercorn This woman with stenosing Crohn's ileitis, probably of long-standing duration, appears to have recovered quickly from an episode of partial small bowel obstruction. If her obstructive symptoms truly resolved so quickly, then I would not initiate the parenteral antibiotic and steroid therapy outlined by Dr. Meyer. Although her current diarrhea might be controlled with loperamide or diphenoxylate, she would clearly benefit from an agent directed at the inflammatory process given her episode of obstruction and symptoms prior to and after the acute episode.

I have had no success with metronidazole in this setting but have seen some patients respond to sulfasalazine. Because of her history of sulfa-related rash, one of the new oral slow-release 5-ASA preparations would be an especially good consideration here.

If I could not obtain such an agent, I would place her on a low residue diet and begin a course of sulfasalazine desensitization taking her up slowly to a dose of 3 to 4 g/day over 4 to 6 weeks. If she could not tolerate the sulfasalazine or if cramps and diarrhea continued, I would begin prednisone at 40 mg/day, continue it for two weeks and then begin to taper her off at a dose of 5 mg/week. If she continued to be symptomatic and had evidence of an active inflammatory disease (e.g., an elevated sedimentation rate), I would offer her a course of 6-mercaptopurine before sending her for surgical resection.

CASE 7. RECURRENT CROHN'S DISEASE AFTER RESECTION FOR ILEOCOLITIS

A 43-year-old man had previously diagnosed Crohn's disease involving the distal ileum, cecum, and ascending colon. He had required two prior resections, four years apart, involving 60 cm of ileum and his right colon with an ileotransverse colostomy because of repeated episodes of bowel obstruction despite therapy with sulfasalazine and prednisone. Following his second resection, he did well except for watery diarrhea controlled with cholestyramine. Two years later he presents with three weeks of crampy abdominal pain, occasional vomiting, low-grade fever and a 10-lb weight loss. An x-ray reveals recurrent disease at the neoterminal ileum extending midway through the transverse colon.

Francis A. Farraye This patient has mild to moderately severe recurrent Crohn's disease manifested by abdominal pain, low-grade fever, and weight loss. He has had progressive disease requiring two resections despite treatment with sulfasalazine and prednisone.

Given this history I am not optimistic that another course of sulfasalazine will be effective but a several week trial using 4-5 g/day if tolerated remains an option. Instead I would treat this patient with metronidazole at a dosage up to 20 mg/kg as my first choice. The patient would be instructed to follow a low residue diet. Lactose intolerance should be excluded as well. If symptoms persist, especially fever, pain, or development of a mass, I would obtain a CT scan to exclude an abscess. If an abscess is identified, additional antibiotics would be indicated and he will likely need further surgical intervention. If symptoms persist on metronidazole and suppurative complications are excluded, prednisone at a dose of 40–60 mg would be indicated. In addition, I believe that this patient, given his progressive disease, is an ideal candidate for immunosuppressive therapy and would add 6-mercaptopurine (6-MP) to the corticosteroids. A prolonged course of therapy should be expected. It remains to be seen if the new oral 5-ASA agents will have a role in the routine management of Crohn's disease of this nature.

Burton I. Korelitz By current criteria this patient might have fared better if he had a trial of 6-MP therapy prior to his first resection. If his small bowel obstruction had been due more to inflammatory disease than fibrosis, it very well might have worked. In any case, 6-MP has been shown to have prophylactic value and I would have introduced it right after his second resection. I begin it at a dose of 50 mg/day increasing the dose to 100 mg/day in stepwise fashion if there is no adverse effect on the white cell count but no obvious efficacy after 3 to 4 weeks. Unquestionably it should be used now in this fashion although a course of steroids might be required "to buy time" for the 6-MP to be effective.

CASE 8. CROHN'S COLITIS WITH PERINEAL DISEASE

A 65-year-old man with a 6-year history of Crohn's colitis treated with intermittent courses of prednisone and sulfasalazine presents with a perirectal abscess and two draining sinus tracts as well as an exacerbation of diarrhea and abdominal cramps. Flexible sigmoidoscopy shows focal ulcers, edematous folds and pseudopolyps from 20 to 60 cm.

Lawrence J. Brandt This patient exhibits simultaneous manifestations of Crohn's perineal and intestinal disease. While prednisone might be useful in treating the intestinal aspect of the disease, it will typically not help the perineal manifestations. Primary therapy for a painful and fluctuant perirectal abscess is incision and drainage. Of course, at the time of the surgical drainage, material should be obtained for cultures after which metronidazole, a good antianaerobic agent, may be begun. Both the perineal and intestinal components of this exacerbation may be successfully treated with metronidazole, although the diarrhea and abdominal cramps may respond more quickly then the perirectal abscess and sinus tracts. In terms of predicting response to treatment it is likely that both the intestinal phase and the perineal manifestations will improve albeit several months may be required for perineal healing.

Gerald Friedman This patient with Crohn's colitis as noted by Dr. Brandt may require surgical drainage of the perirectal abscess in combination with medical therapy designed to reduce the activity of the disease and close the sinus tracts. Two acceptable medical therapies are available for this purpose, namely metronidizole as discussed above and 6-mercaptopurine (6-MP).

I, too, have utilized metronidizole, in a dosage of 20 mg/kg per day effectively to close draining sinuses and fistulas in Crohn's colitis and ileocolitis. In some patients, the onset of action may be one to two weeks with diminution of erythema, tenderness, and edema, but it may take from 6 to 8 weeks or more for closure of fistulas to occur. Alcohol should be interdicted and the patient should be followed carefully with CBCs and frequent clinical evaluations. Side effects of anorexia, nausea, emesis, metallic taste, and darkening of urine may occur. Peripheral neuropathy is the most significant side effect usually noted after several months of therapy. Discontinuation of therapy usually results in reversal of neuropathic symptoms.

As an alternative, 6-MP may be considered, particularly if the patient is refractory to metronidizole. Employing a dose of 1.5 mg/kg per day, effective closure of fistulas may ensue. Careful attention should be given to CBCs and the patient's clinical progress. The onset of action with this agent is usually longer than that seen with metronidazole (commonly 2 to 3 months).

With both of the above agents, maintenance therapy at a reduced dosage may be required.

CASE 9. CROHN'S ILEITIS WITH LOCALIZED PERITONITIS

An 18-year-old man had experienced 6 months of frequent loose stools associated with crampy right lower quadrant pain and a 12-lb weight loss. Evaluation revealed nonstenosing ileitis in the distal 2 feet of ileum. A sigmoidoscopy and barium enema were unremarkable. He had a prompt response to sulfasalazine and over the next two years remained on the drug with only occasional mild flares of disease activity responsive to increased doses of sulfasalazine. Three days prior to admission, he began to experience severe suprapubic and right lower quadrant cramps and a sense of urinary urgency and frequency without dysuria. On the morning of admission he had an abrupt worsening of pain now localized to the right lower quadrant and had a shaking chill and felt warm. On admission he had a BP of 130/80, pulse 120, temperature 102.6°F pr. His chest was clear but his abdomen revealed a 3 x 4 cm mass in the right lower quadrant associated with cough and percussion tenderness. Lab tests revealed a WBC of 18,000 with 23% bands, a Hct of 46%, serum ablumin of 3.2 g%, and urine analysis showed 5–10 WBCs/HPF (high power field) 0–5 RBCs/HPF and no bacteria.

Mark A. Peppercorn This patient has almost certainly suffered a complication of his ileitis with a microperforation leading to sepsis and a localized mass with peritoneal signs. The bladder symptoms may relate to inflamed bowel adjacent to the bladder rather than a frank ileovesical fistula as is suggested by the lack of bacteria in the sediment. Broad-spectrum antibiotics should be instituted at once after blood cultures are drawn. I would use intravenous ampicillin, gentamicin and either p.o. or intravenous metronidazole. A cephalosporin could be substituted for ampicillin in the penicillin-allergic patient. Because of the high fever and WBC and tender mass, the possibility of a frank abscess exists. I would therefore obtain a CT scan early in the course. If an abscess is obvious, I would push for early surgery after several days of antibiotics and bowel rest and hope that the abscess cavity and involved segment of bowel could be dealt with at the same time with a primary anastomosis.

If the CT scan was more suggestive of a phlegmon with matted edematous bowel loops, then a prolonged course of antibiotics with careful observation is reasonable. I would not institute steroids since they can mask findings and possibly promote infection. If the signs of peritonitis resolve, oral alimentation can begin and a small bowel x-ray obtained. Were a large fistulous tract noted, I would be reluctant in the future to use steroids but would try to again control symptoms with sulfasalazine and consider 6-MP before proceeding with surgery.

Burton I. Korelitz The patient has developed a worsening of this ileitis with mass, either due to peri-ileitis or even an abscess. Furthermore, he most likely now has an ileovesical fistula. The fever suggests sepsis, therefore, I too would start therapy with triple antibiotics. As soon as signs of sepsis were controlled, however, unlike Dr. Peppercorn, I would initiate therapy with intravenous steroids since the source of the entire clinical picture is still the ileitis. If I suspected still a true abscess, I would get a CT scan for monitoring and decision for using a skinny needle to drain an abscess, but I would continue with the basic program already established and anticipate remission without resection. Consideration would then arise as to chronic-phase therapy which would be influenced in part by the presence or absence of an actual ileovesical fistula.

CASE 10. CROHN'S ILEOCOLITIS WITH ENTEROVESICAL FISTULA

A 34-year-old man with a 7-year history of ileocolitis requiring intermittent courses of sulfasalazine and/or metronidazole was treated within 6 months for two *E. coli* urinary tract infections characterized by dysruia and urgency. He now presents with a repeat episode of dysuria and has noted the passage of gas for the first time while urinating. Urine culture again shows *E. coli*. An IVP is unremarkable. Barium enema shows extensive colitis involving the ascending and transverse colon with reflux into a stenotic ileum. During the study, barium is noted in the bladder although no fistulous tract is demonstrated. He currently has three loose stools per day with mild cramps.

Burton I. Korelitz The patient has an ileovescial fistula. Rarely does ascending infection and pyelonephritis occur as a complication. There should be no resection performed with this fistula alone as an indication. Clearly the patient now has Crohn's disease activity. If either of the two drugs mentioned above had been successful in the past, I would now reintroduce either or both, but I would also initiate treatment with 6-MP which stands the best chance of closing the fistula as well as favorably influencing the primary bowel disease. If this did not work, I would start prednisone at 60 mg daily, reduce the inflammation, and outline a program for steroid reduction. This would extend the period of opportunity for the 6-MP to be effective.

I would not resort to surgery for this indication unless the quality of life was poor as a result of combinations of the fistula, primary bowel symptoms, or drug therapy. I would favor surgery if the patient also had recurrent small bowel obstruction, failure of the other chronic phase drugs (sulfasalazine and metronidazole), and lack of desire to try 6-MP.

Lawrence T. Brandt This patient with Crohn's ileocolitis has now developed an enterovesical fistula. Rarely, if a suspected enterovesical fistula cannot be proven, a urachovesical fistula should be suspected. It is somewhat unusual that the cultures show just a single organism, namely *E. coli*. More typical is that multiple and various aerobic and anaerobic organisms would be identified at different times. The origin of the fistula is most likely the ileum, despite the fact that no fistula is noted on either IVP or barium enema. As Dr. Korelitz notes, patients with enterovesical fistulas usually tolerate the fistula well with only intermittent pneumaturia and cystitis; these fistulas are clinically silent most of the time. Most patients with enterovesical fistulas ultimately require surgery, albeit more often for the underlying bowel disease than for the fistula. The decision whether to operate depends in large part on the activity of the bowel disease and frequency of urinary infections, not the fear of developing renal insufficiency. Urinary infection is treated satisfactorily with conventional antibiotics, while both metronidazole and 6-MP may occasionally affect closure of the fistula. However, there is not a great deal of experience using metronidazole or 6-MP to treat these patients. Nonetheless, I personally would attempt a course of broad-spectrum antibiotics, followed by metronidazole, followed by 6-MP before resorting to surgical management. Many months may be required on these medications before the fistula heals and so failure to respond should not be considered before 3 to 6 months.

CASE 11. GASTRODUODENAL CROHN'S DISEASE

A 35-year-old man with a 5-year history of ileitis controlled with sulfasalazine presents with 6 months of epigastric pain, easy satiety, and vomiting. An upper GI and small bowel x-ray showed a narrowed antrum, thickened duodenal folds with ulceration and stricturing involving the second portion of the duodenum, as well as nonstenosing distal ileitis. Endoscopy reveals focal ulcers and edematous folds in the antrum and postbulbar duodenum. Biopsies show nonspecific inflammation.

Stephen B. Hanauer Many patients with symptomatic gastroduodenal Crohn's disease may respond to a low-fat, low-residue diet with acid reduction via an H_2-receptor antagonist and between-meal antacids. Some patients also will respond to sucralfate, although the drug may produce gastric bezoars if gastric emptying is significantly impaired.

If these measures fail, then a course of steroids should be attempted with concurrent acid suppression with or without sucralfate to avoid steroid-induced gastropathy. Failure to respond to steroids with persistent gastric outlet obstruction would be an indication for a gastroenterostomy, although in our hands this often results in a recurrence of Crohn's disease at the gastroenterostomy site with eventual stenosis. In the very refractory patient, bowel rest, total parenteral nutrition, and an immunosuppressive may be tried, although I am unaware of any controlled trials regarding the use of 6-MP for gastroduodenal Crohn's disease.

At times, the duodenum is involved secondarily to colonic or ileocolonic Crohn's disease. If this is the case, then a resection of the primary site will suffice.

The surreptitious use of nonsteroidals should be sought and these drugs discontinued. A local application of 5-ASA delivered to the stomach or duodenum via oral Pentasa, nonprotected 5-ASA, or even a "cocktail" of a 5-ASA enema may have a theoretical use as would a nonsystemic corticosteroid (tixocortol enema).

Burton I. Korelitz Most likely, Crohn's disease of the duodenum and antrum will not respond to sulfasalazine or metronidazole. It will improve on steroids, but the improvement will be transient and symptoms will recur as the dose is reduced or the drug terminated. In my experience, bypass surgery for this manifestation of Crohn's disease is often a disaster and recurrence results in miserable symptoms. On the other hand, our success rate for Crohn's disease of the duodenum with 6-MP so far has been 100%. 6-MP has the added advantage of favorably affecting the nonstenotic distal ileitis.

CASE 12. CROHN'S ILEITIS: DIARRHEA FOLLOWING RESECTION

A 42-year-old woman has recently undergone her second ileal resection for stenosing ileitis leading to recurrent small bowel obstruction. She has now had a total of 50 cm of ileum resected. She is seen 4 weeks after surgery complaining of four to six loose, watery stools per day not associated with pain or weight loss. Her examination and laboratory tests, including CBC, sedimentation rate, and albumin, are normal.

Mark A. Peppercorn Although this woman may have a very early recurrence postoperatively, it is much more likely that she is symptomatic from bile salt diarrhea following the further ileal resection. Although the diarrhea may respond to loperamide, diphenoxylate, or aluminum hydroxide, I have found cholestyramine to be the most effective therapy for this condition. It should be started at 4 g/day (1 packet or scoop in juice or water) and increased or decreased depending on the response. Given the amount of ileum resected, there may also be an element of steatorrhea contributing to the diarrhea. If a 72-hr fecal fat collection showed greater than 7 g/24 hr, then a low-fat diet with the addition of medium-chain triglyceride oil should be considered. If she had significant steatorrhea (e.g., >20 g of fat/day), then cholestyramine might make her worse. If she has steatorrhea, a low-oxalate diet should be advised to help prevent oxalate kidney stones. Finally, she is likely to have vitamin B_{12} malabsorption. This can be established with certainty with a Schilling test or it can be assumed and she can be started on monthly B_{12} shots (100 μg). A colonoscopy or small bowel x-ray looking for recurrence need not be done unless the diarrhea does not respond to the above measures.

Francis Farraye This woman has water diarrhea 4 weeks after her second small bowel resection for Crohn's disease. Given her recent surgery, I would first exclude *Clostridium difficile* infection. A careful review of her present medicatins is indicated to exclude drug-induced diarrhea. A lactose-free diet may also be helpful.

Recurrent Crohn's disease would be unlikely in the immedaite postoperative period. The pathophysiological consequences of an ileal resection can explain this patient's diarrhea. As Dr. Peppercorn notes, it is likely that she has bile salt-induced diarrhea. A terminal ileal resection (less than 100 cm) leads to malabsorption of bile salts with spillage into the colon, where they can stimulate colonic secretion. I agree on the use of cholestyramine (Questran) at a dose of 4–12 g/day, which acts to bind the bile salts in the proximal small bowel and decrease their effects on the colonic mucosa. I begin with 4 g given at breakfast. This is when the majority of bile salts are released into the intestinal tract in patients with a gallbladder. The dose can be increased and given in divided fashion if needed. Fat-soluble vitamin malabsorption and altered calcium metabolism may develop on long-term treatment. As an adjunct or alternative to cholestyramine, nonspecific antimotility agents such as loperamide are useful.

I have found that a combination of an antimotility agent and low dose of cholestyramine yields the best results.

Index

About the Editor

MARK A. PEPPERCORN is Senior Staff Physician, Division of Gastroenterology, Beth Israel Hospital, and Associate Professor, Department of Medicine, Harvard Medical School, Boston, Massachusetts. He also serves as a Consultant in Gastroenterology for New England Sinai Hospital, Stoughton, Massachusetts, and Huntington General Hospital, Jamaica Plain, Massachusetts. Dr. Peppercorn is actively involved in clinical research on new therapies for inflammatory bowel disease and publishes and lectures extensively on the subject. He is past-president of the Inflammatory Bowel Disease Forum, and a member of the American Gastroenterological Association (AGA), AGA Clinical Teaching Project Committee, National Foundation for Ileitis and Colitis, Phi Beta Kappa, and Alpha Omega Alpha, among other prestigious societies. Dr. Peppercorn received the A.B. degree (1964) from Harvard College and M.D. degree (1968) from Harvard Medical School, Boston, Massachusetts.